this book belongs to:

twelve moons

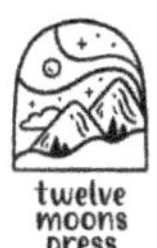

twelve
moons
press

twelve moons

A Lifelong Calendar Companion for Generations of Girls and Women: Making Space, Tuning In, and Protecting Your Sacred Health and Well-Being

by Jenny R. Austin

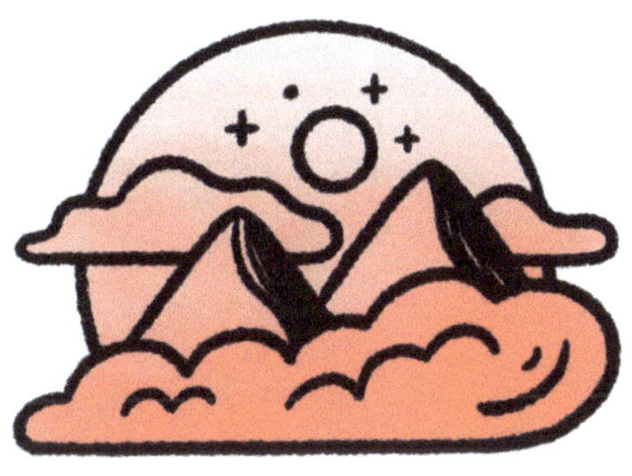

twelve moons press

Twelve Moons Press, LLC
P.O. Box 27469
Austin, Texas 78755 USA
www.twelvemoonspress.com

Names: Austin, Jenny R., and Twelve Moons Press, LLC., authors.
Title: Twelve Moons: a lifelong calendar companion for generations of girls and women: making space, tuning in, and protecting your sacred health and well-being / Jenny R. Austin

Trade Paperback ISBN: 978-3-9525958-0-0
First Edition, November 2023

For the magnificent girls beginning their female lifeline, to the
wise women who have seen and done astounding things in their time.
And for all the gutsy women and individuals navigating their lives in between.

You are seen, honored, and cherished.

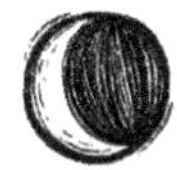

CONTENTS

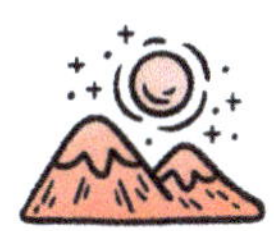

INTRODUCTION 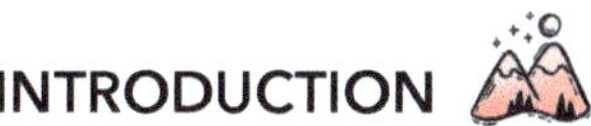

Twelve Moons is a lifelong personal calendar for growing girls and women of all ages, for chronicling our period cycles, changes in our bodies, as well as shifts in our head and heart spaces. The seeds of *Twelve Moons* first took form as a safe and empowering space with my daughter in mind, a private and sacred companion to accompany her throughout every stage of her life.

Our bodies are always giving us signals and messages, both powerful and subtle. They communicate themselves to us using the language of symptoms, as well as our intuition. Making ourselves truly at home in our ever-evolving bodies is essential to tuning in to and prioritizing our most important needs. Being able to quickly access our observations over the course of menstruation, as well as in our menopausal and postmenopausal years, provides a treasure trove of invaluable insights for a journey of health over the course of a lifetime. Listening to the cues, instincts, and synchronicities of our bodies is an act of grace and protection that can also serve as a silent advocate when medical care or other types of support are needed.

The momentous and seemingly everyday changes in our bodies — whether due to natural processes, medical interventions, or various kinds of trauma or imbalance — are so often forgotten and rarely documented. So, too, are our moments of peace and equilibrium. Astonishingly, most of us do not have intimate knowledge of our own bodies and the messages they are conveying to us.

Twelve Moons is a companion to accompany you throughout your life. You can bring it along with you to your healthcare appointments to provide helpful information, or chat about it with your family members and friends over a cup of tea. *Twelve Moons* is a testimonial to our most sacred rhythms, elevating their significance in our lives.

The Origins of *Twelve Moons*

I created *Twelve Moons* because I want girls and women[1] of all ages to have a way to record and celebrate the experience of our bodies over the course of a lifetime. Like every woman I know, I have been asked about my menstruation patterns by gynecologists and other physicians and practitioners countless times, and yet I have had no consistent record of my body's cycles, even though I have experienced significant changes throughout my life. Now in remission after completing breast cancer treatments, I have been emerging from a cocoon of protection and recovery, and focusing on true self-care for the first time in my life.

The journey I've been on, concentrating on my health and well-being, in addition to being the mother of a school-age daughter, has led me to deeply reflect on what women and girls need in order to feel whole, healthy, and valued in this world. But we shouldn't need a health crisis to sound the alarm before we notice our needs and give ourselves the well-deserved gift of reflection and nourishment. After all, our bodies are the magnificent vessels that carry each of us on our respective journeys.

The idea that each of us should have our own historical record of our bodies' changes just made perfect sense to me. I became overwhelmed with the desire to bring this idea to life and create a space for each of us, at all ages, to chart our lives, and for us to feel safe within the pages of our own book and story.

For All Ages — Where to Begin

Twelve Moons was specifically created to include girls and women of every generation. The book is intended for girls who are beginning their rite of passage into womanhood, for those of us who have had our menstrual cycles for a handful of years or decades, as well as

---

[1] *Twelve Moons* is for everyone who menstruates and experiences menopause, identifies with the female experience, or would simply like to use the book to record their body's rhythms, changes, and messages. While I use the terms *girl, woman, womanhood, female, and feminine* in the book, *Twelve Moons* embraces all humans and aims to provide a safe space for our optimal emotional, mental, and physical health and well-being.

women who want to meaningfully record their bodies' cadences and changes well into postmenopause and later in life.

This book was designed to be entirely customizable for you, based upon when you want to begin recording your cycle, changes, observations, and feelings. This can start now, or you can backdate your cycle by months, years, or even decades if you already have records of your monthly observations. This is your own personal archive, meant to be easily folded into your life. You can dedicate only a few minutes each month to record a change or thought, or you can create a mindful ritual that you put more time, intention, and heart into.

Girls can begin to use *Twelve Moons* as soon as they feel ready. It is powerful for girls to take note of the budding changes in their bodies and emotions, even when those begin a couple of years before their period starts. Understanding puberty as a gradual transition can help to make the onset of menstruation a lot less overwhelming, and soften the experience for girls who are undergoing deeply felt mental and emotional shifts that are not necessarily obvious from the outside.

Women and adolescents whose menses have already begun can reach into the past to record their period from the beginning, or as early as can be recalled. For those whose menses began a long time ago, being able to backdate our monthly changes can be highly beneficial. The process of recording our rhythms helps us to notice or identify a discernible menstrual pattern, puzzling changes, or need for healthcare support. The same is true for women experiencing perimenopause, the menopause transition, and postmenopause. Recording our body's cycles as far back as possible enables us to identify patterns and sweeping changes, and place our journey of health and well-being into context for the present and the future.

Women who are already in postmenopause need support in carefully observing changes in their bodies to safeguard their health. This is particularly important, as research shows that women develop disease at a higher rate than men. Healthy changes that we make in all stages of life — prioritizing our nutrition, exercise, sleep, and well-being — will have a positive impact on our overall health profile throughout our lifetime. Now more than ever before in human history, our life expectancy is increasing, and we have every reason to ensure that our health span — living in good physical, cognitive, and emotional health — is strong and vital for the duration of our life span.

The length of the calendar spans sixty-five years, so the journey of your body and its cycles can be chronicled throughout your lifetime and adapted to your needs.[2]

What *Twelve Moons* is Meant to Chronicle:

- your period cycle, ovulation, breast tenderness or changes, and various other observable body developments and changes;
- symptoms that occur in your everyday life, as well as during pregnancy, breastfeeding, pregnancy loss, the menopause transition, and postmenopause;
- signs of a discernible menstrual pattern for those with an irregular or unpredictable period;
- seasons of stress and vulnerability, health changes, traumas, and significant life transitions;
- life changes that affect our mind-body state and biorhythms, such as the loss of a loved one, long-held dreams that we've had to let go of, or other sources of considerable grief;
- side effects or reflections while taking medications;
- surprising symptoms or health concerns that may arise as we age and mature;
- times when we feel content, restored, renewed, or even invincible; and
- the quiet whisperings inside of us that we instinctively want to write down and reflect upon.

____

[2] The 65 calendar years can begin at the onset of puberty, when menstruation begins, or whenever feels best. If, for example, a girl gets her period at the age of 12, she can use the calendars until the age of 77 and carry on notating observations of her body and needs later in life in a supplementary journal. Additionally, a 30-year-old woman can begin using the book immediately, or date back her calendar to record her periods beginning at whatever age she began keeping records. The same is true for women experiencing the menopause transition in their 40s and 50s, or postmenopause in their 60s or 70s. They can backdate their monthly observations as far back in time as they'd like, and continue to record seminal body changes throughout their lives.

Even the smallest and most subtle observations matter. Whatever we are feeling and experiencing has tremendous value, and the clues provided by your calendar entries can prove to be vital to living a healthy and abundant life of self-advocacy. Chronicling our life cycles contributes to rest and contentment, and the reassurance that we are prioritizing something so deeply elemental and affirmative.

Paying Attention to Protect Our Health and Well-Being

In women's lives, we have our period for an average of thirty-eight years. Yet given global trends toward longevity, women can reasonably expect to live in the postmenopausal stages of our lives for as long as, or much longer than, we've had our period. We all want to thrive in wellness in every stage of our lives.

Our health at every age is tied to our nutrition, exercise, sleep, well-being, meaningful connection to the people in our lives, and the many other physical and emotional factors that comprise our complex human experience. And while our bodies alert us to take notice during our period or menopausal symptoms or health challenges, we may overlook what is happening in our bodies during the in-between times, when we may be symptom-free and bouncing back from those intense moments. Recording the common events in our cycles alongside the milestones serves to compile what can be powerful information that helps us stay more in tune with the needs of our physical, mental, and emotional health.

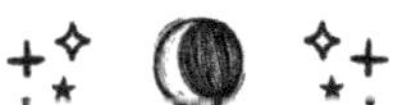

My hope is that *Twelve Moons* will become part of the powerful conversations that women and adolescents are having globally to shatter stereotypes and stigmas about menstruation and menopause, and to bring these amazing life cycle processes into the light. Women and girls are often confronted by false notions that we are tainted due to societal connotations or long-held cultural taboos about impurity during menstruation. In the same vein, recurring themes about menopausal women being undesirable or no longer relevant are still rampant. We know in our hearts and minds that the opposite is true. Fiercely.

Our intentions are our hearts' spotlight on what is of profound importance to us. We all want the girls in our lives to feel good about their bodies, develop the instincts to care about their health, and be their own advocates. Simply having this book is a step toward conveying this importance to ourselves and all girls and women in our lives. Using *Twelve Moons* is a commitment to our own precious lives — a love letter to past, present, and future versions of ourselves.

Twelve Moons was written and created from my very core. I want the book to feel like a soft, comforting nest to land in, a shield and a source of strength, a true friend holding tight to your hand, and a sanctuary for your heart and mind. *Twelve Moons* was handmade with love. I hope it feels like love.

Shine your heart brightly.

Jenny xo

P.S. My vision for *Twelve Moons* was to create the book together with my daughter, using her artwork within the sacred pages you are now creating for yourself. Her paintings are included in the front and back of the book, bookending its pages with her representations of the seasons of our lives and our connection to nature. A small drawing is also hidden in this book that was created by my young son.

PART 1: HOW TO USE *TWELVE MOONS* 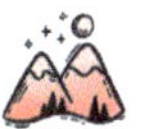

How to Organize the *Twelve Moons* Calendars

First, determine the month and year where you want to begin
recording your observations, whether it's this month, or a date in the
past (if you have kept records of your body's cycles). Next, be sure to
refer to an official calendar that represents the days and dates
correctly for that month and year, so the dates you enter into each
calendar month correspond with the day of the week.

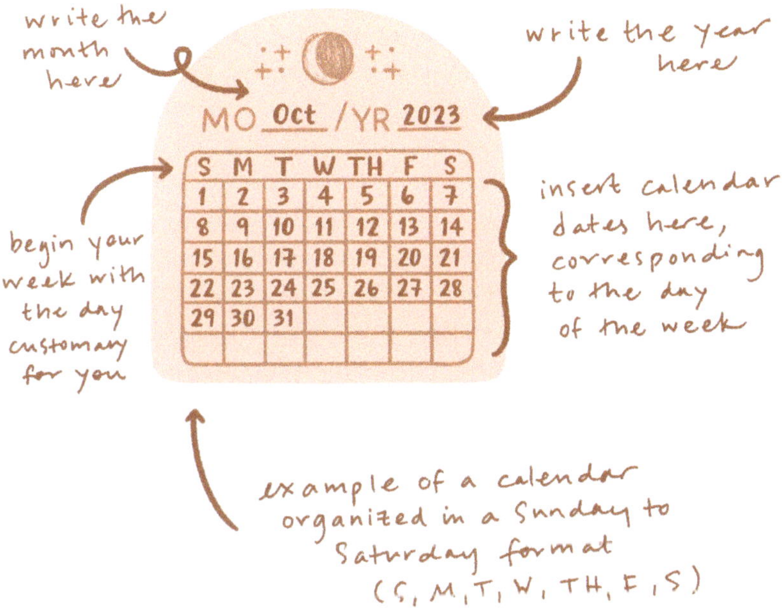

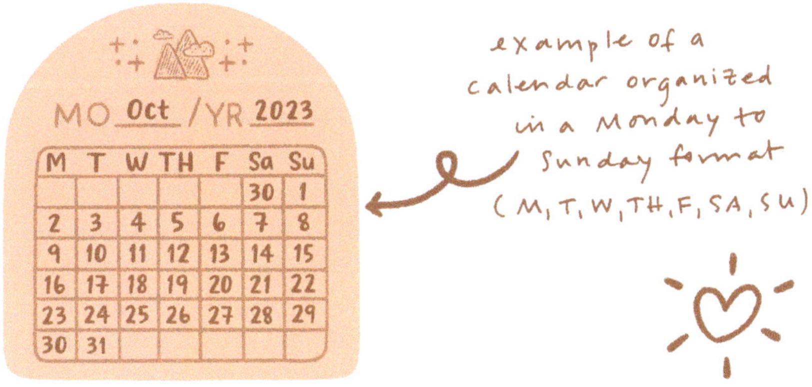

How to Make *Twelve Moons* Your Sacred Space and Lifelong Companion

Twelve Moons was designed to serve as a lifelong calendar companion with both beauty and function in mind. It includes a lifetime of monthly calendars that are customizable so that girls and women of all ages can tailor their book to their unique needs. This will enable you to create a storyline of your life that will empower you to observe, protect, and advocate for your physical and emotional needs.

Book Format

- Each page has three calendar months where you can circle or underline significant dates. Seeing your entries in a three-month format can help you notice seasonal changes and trends in your cycle, as well as notable observations that can help you achieve more balance.
- The calendar format is write-in and undated so you can begin charting where it makes the most sense for you.
- The days of the week are blank so you can start your week on Sunday, Monday, or whatever day best aligns with your routine or the standard in your country.
- The spaces accompanying each calendar month are unlined so that you can write notes and reflections, draw, doodle, create charts, lists, recall anecdotes, or whatever you can dream up. This book is yours, an invitation to make it your own.

Begin Where You Are Right Now, or Reflect on Your Past

- The pages are formatted so you can customize them to suit your exact needs and preferences.
- You can begin chronicling your menstrual, menopausal, and postmenopausal symptoms, and any other changes in your body from the moment you have the book.
- You can also start at the beginning of puberty or another significant time in your life to capture events that you may have previously recorded in calendars or notebooks.

Looking Ahead

- Sixty-five years of monthly calendars are included, so that events during your puberty, young and middle adulthood, menopause transition, and beyond have a place to be documented.[3] This means that the calendars in *Twelve Moons* can be used for 65 years from the start of puberty, the beginning of menstruation, or whenever you choose to begin, and carry on until well into postmenopause, capturing a lifetime of observations.
- This book is intended to hold space for reflecting on your life cycles — and, if you wish, sharing insights among the important people in your life — so that you can embrace the fullness of your journey.
- The book can include reflections from your parents or caregivers on their larger family medical history for healthcare purposes or for carrying on traditions.
- Supplementing *Twelve Moons* with other journals is also an excellent option.

Notes on the Calendar Format and Some Suggestions for Organizing Your Experiences

Because it is impossible to create a book that can accompany you throughout your life that is not massive, each calendar page is necessarily compact. You may want to create your own notation system, whereby you use color-coding or symbols for symptoms, changes, or feelings to accompany each month.

Similarly, in the notes area next to each calendar, you can use numbers or draw symbols or other images that have significant meaning to you and that will give you information at a glance when you need to have a more broad overview of seasons or years. You can create a map or legend in the book that helps you remember the significance for each color or symbol.

---

[3] The intent of the 65 calendar years is to capture the average 38 years of menstruation plus another 25+ years of notations covering both the menopause transition and the years well into postmenopause. You can supplement your calendar pages with a blank book or journal, such as the forthcoming *Twelve Moons Companion Journal,* or another special one you love.

My hope is that with this testament, we are able to give our bodies the attention they deserve, enabling us to better care for and listen to them. Putting pen to paper and seeing ourselves over months and years helps us to recognize trends, alert us to areas of concern, and realize what we really need. In turn, we'll get more comfortable creating boundaries, and shift our nurturing nature toward ourselves, not solely toward the people in our lives.

By being the historians of our lives and the bodies holding us strong everyday, we can navigate the complexities of our busy days with more intention and meaning. By committing your life to paper in this way, you can nurture yourself and live with more self-compassion.

PART 2: THE SEASONS OF OUR LIVES 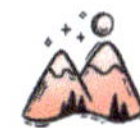

Each year, the rotating of the seasons signal internal changes in us and the traditions we treasure, giving us pause for reflection. We simultaneously look forward to the new season while already missing the joys of the one that has just passed. Many of us build rituals around marveling at the blossoming world around us, getting into nature and feeling the warmth of sunshine on our bare skin, cozying up with a cup of tea and a good book when the weather becomes chilly, lighting candles as the glittering night sky becomes dark, and spending time with family and friends over favorite dishes during our meaningful celebrations and holidays.

Just as each season expresses many different aspects of nature's beauty and the special rituals we create, we also experience seasons in our lives marked by our life cycles. In these seasons, or life cycles, we discover new and different aspects of ourselves. Our lifelong and layered experiences are the essence of our continual state of becoming, not just the aspirational best version of ourselves, but also our true self, for whom we ought to have love and compassion. Each new seasonal life stage encompasses all of the experience, knowledge, and wisdom we have gained that enables us to live more whole, intentional lives.

In the following sections, the four primary life stages of the female body after early and middle childhood are addressed, encompassing: the beginnings of puberty and menstruation; our young and middle adulthood; midlife, encompassing our menopause transition; and the postmenopausal stage of our later years:

Spring: Girlhood and Adolescence

Summer: Twenties and Thirties

Fall: Forties and Fifties

 Winter: Sixties and Beyond

These sections comprise our life stages, yet not everyone necessarily fits precisely into the above categories, as, for example, we may transition into menopause or postmenopause earlier or later than average. As a result, follow your instincts to use the book and each section as you see fit.

Each of the four seasonal life sections includes suggested observations and prompts for using the calendars and journaling space that are particular to that stage of life. For example, girls newly transitioning into puberty and menstruation can begin by reading the Spring section, and as they grow older, they can refer to the other seasons that address their new life stage.

Spring: Girlhood and Adolescence 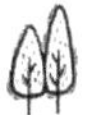

The beginning and ending of menstruation are momentous shifts in the feminine experience. Our menstrual cycle is the result of our unique hormonal balance, our own personal tidal system that pushes and pulls us toward the moments when we have energy, and when we truly need rest.

The transition of adolescence — the gradual shift from childhood to adulthood — takes place over many years. It is further complicated by the enormous pressure girls and teens experience. These pressures can be due to school and other responsibilities, social dynamics, and learning whom to trust, all while navigating changing bodies and feelings. Growing up can be exciting, and yet it can also be a confusing, overwhelming, and bumpy journey. Throughout this journey, having loving support and dedicating self-care for ourselves are essential.

Girls going through puberty must navigate a steep and winding path toward womanhood while at the same time wanting to remain in the simple, safe cocoon of childhood. And yet our hormonal symphonies propel us toward mysterious and uncomfortable changes that we must grow into, in both body and mind. It takes courage to go through the intensity of hormonal mood swings, bleeding, pain, inconvenience, bodily changes, and other challenges. Becoming comfortable with a changing body is hard at any age, but the growth from child to woman is dramatic, and deserves our great respect. Know that you are truly amazing as you navigate this journey!

We must learn to love and trust ourselves, and follow our guiding instincts. You have a long and beautiful life ahead of you. In addition to advice from your family, friends, and mentors, you have your own wit and internal wisdom that will carry you through challenges and become your north star. Developing your own love and trust for yourself can enable you to access the wisdom of your inner voice and create self-compassion and self-care rituals that contribute to your strength. *Twelve Moons* is a safe space just for you that is meant to feel nurturing, protective, and encouraging of all that you are and who you are becoming as you go through life.

Spring: When to Use *Twelve Moons*

In your book, you can write down both the big and small changes in your body. Some ideas include:

- the beginning of puberty and your body's changes, even if your period hasn't begun yet (for example: breast changes, new body hair, body odor, new and different feelings);

- your period cycle dates, including when your flow is heavy or light;

- menstrual symptoms, including: cramps, mood swings or irritability, skin changes, breast tenderness, headaches, ovulation pain, tiredness, bloating, digestive issues, food cravings, feelings of anxiety or depression;

- spotting (very light bleeding or discharge that typically does not require period products);

- noting which period products feel comfortable or don't work so well — these include reusable or disposable pads, tampons, menstrual cups, menstrual discs, and washable period underwear;

- feelings of all kinds; and

- any questions you may have, to think about later or ask a parent, mentor, teacher, doctor, or friend.

Your calendar can also be used to record the time you make for yourself to do nurturing things, exercise, spend time in nature, connect with supportive people in your life, and other choices you make that fill your soul. It's important to create habits for your well-being and overall happiness.

Make This Book Your Treasured Sacred Space

Some suggestions on how to use the calendars and journal pages:

- Circle or underline the days of your period cycle, and use the blank space next to each month to write down anything that feels important for you, or that you may want to remember in the future.

- Circle your menstrual cycle using different colors (for example, use red or purple for heavy flow, pink for light, yellow for cramps, blue for restful days, and so on). You can also draw symbols that signify things that happen each month. You can create your own fun legend or map with colors and symbols somewhere in the book to use as a guide.

- There are no rules! You can use the blank spaces to draw, make lists, write down questions, or remember certain events in your life. This book is your own, just for beautiful you.

Summer: Twenties and Thirties 

For many of us, the summer season of life is full of new freedoms, discovery, and adventure. It's often a time for finding kindred spirits and community, and cultivating other matters of the soul and heart. We experience newfound courage and a growing sense of self as we learn about ourselves and think about how we want to feel in our skin as our lives unfold. After schooling, finding ourselves in the immense real world can feel both exciting and scary. It can be complicated to keep everything together — becoming independent, trying to figure out our life's purpose or start a career, paying bills, juggling mounting responsibilities, living in new environments, and adjusting to interacting or living with our families as adult versions of ourselves.

Figuring out who we want to be as women now that we have overcome adolescence is a beautiful but complex process. This life stage of our twenties and thirties, often termed the reproductive or child-bearing years, are rife with expectations about who we are and who we are becoming. Not everyone fits into the various assumptions for us and our lives that we are confronted with by others and within our own culture. Neatly crafted societal expectations about our choice of partner, decisions about parenthood, and/or our working life often result in our having to defend our choices or explain our lifestyles, which can be exhausting. There is pressure in this stage of life across cultures, much of it having to do with our bodies and what they are capable of, which is a deeply personal matter.

We are the best guardians of our own health and the protectors of our time. In juggling busy life and trying to become the greatest versions of ourselves as women in the world, it's easy to forget our needs or overlook our body's signals. By recording our own stories in these or other sacred pages, we honor ourselves, knowing that our bodies and their accompanying sea changes matter deeply to the whole picture of who we are and what comes next for us. There is more than enough space for all of us to evolve into different versions of ourselves and love every single one of them.

Summer: When to Use *Twelve Moons*

Some ideas of what to record include:

- your period cycle dates or spotting, including when your flow is heavy or light;
- menstrual symptoms, including: cramps, mood swings, skin changes, breast tenderness, headaches, ovulation pain, tiredness, bloating, digestive issues, food cravings, feelings of anxiety or depression;
- irregular or unpredictable periods, as the absence of a period is something to investigate;
- symptoms related to chronic disease and chronic pain, endometriosis, adenomyosis, polycystic ovary syndrome (PCOS), fibroids, cysts, mood disorders, premenstrual disorder or syndrome, and other conditions and difficult diagnoses;
- decisions made related to fertility, the use of birth control and contraception, family planning, and whether or not to have children;
- observations about ovulation, fertility challenges, pregnancy, childbirth, breastfeeding, weaning, or postpartum life;
- significant physical experiences such as pregnancy, childbirth, pregnancy loss and other traumas, health interventions, surgeries such as a hysterectomy or an oophorectomy, accidents, and recovery;
- visible changes in your breasts, or soreness or sensitivity that give you pause;
- the use of and side effects related to any prescribed medications or supplements;
- sleep patterns, travel (especially over multiple time zones);

- sweeping life changes that affect our mind-body state and biorhythms, such as the loss of a loved one, long-held dreams that we've had to let go of, or other sources of considerable grief, all of which are integral to our life experience and well-being;

- reflections on ways our perspectives have changed or things we have learned, ways we have overcome stress or transformed challenging experiences; and

- feelings or small observations if you feel intuitively that they are worth recording; these are often the important moments we will want to remember years later.

Take up space in your own life and in your heart. Yours are the twinkling lights illuminating your starry sky. With these calendar pages, you can record the time you make for yourself to do nurturing things, exercise, spend time in nature, connect with supportive people in your life, and other choices you make that fill your soul. Your entries are like letters to yourself that can help you feel rooted into your innate strength and support your ongoing process of becoming.

Fall: Forties and Fifties 

In midlife, even though our responsibilities have greatly increased, our life experiences have gifted us with a stronger sense of self-worth, and hopefully, intolerance for what we aren't willing to put up with anymore, or add onto our plate. We often realize we need to create more space for joy and laughter with friends, and to experience the restorative power of nature in new ways. We finally have a chance to catch our breath and truly consider our own needs for the first time after the whirlwind of establishing our careers or beginning to care for our families or perhaps our aging parents. Such assertiveness comes in handy when we are forced to focus on our increasing physical, mental, and emotional needs that result from our shifting into the momentous transition of menopause.

Women going through the menopause transition encounter a formidable rollercoaster that is sometimes described as puberty in reverse. Not all women have a challenging time with the menopause transition, but for most it can be accompanied by a long list of symptoms for which most women need medical, nutritional, emotional, and mental health support. Our hormones are still figuring themselves out, which means we must prioritize our well-being and self-compassion while we adjust to our new normal.

The *pause* in menopause calls upon us to rest and reflect on the courage and sheer force of will and strength that we have drawn upon until now. We may want to go inward and be meditative during this time, or we may need to fling the doors wide open in our lives and let ourselves experience the world in ways we haven't had a chance to or felt brave enough to before. This is especially true for women whose menopause has commenced due to a medical condition and has taken place earlier than their psyche may have been prepared for. We may experience grief as we undergo transitions, which must be honored and given space.

Fall: When to Use *Twelve Moons*

During this time of transition, changes can sometimes be hardly perceptible, but they are nonetheless significant and are evidence of our need for support. Some ideas of notations to record during this stage of life include:

- your period cycle dates, flow, or spotting — even if they may be waning — will help signal when the twelve months without a period have transpired, indicating that menopause has occurred;

- symptoms of menopause, including: hot flashes or night sweats, sleep disturbances or sleeplessness, fatigue, irregular or heavy periods, cramps, mood swings, irritability, changes in libido, vaginal dryness and/or painful sex, weight gain, skin and nail changes, thinning hair, breast tenderness, body odor, headaches, dizziness, tiredness, bloating, digestive issues, food cravings, heart palpitations, joint pain and muscle aches, osteopenia and osteoporosis, itchy skin, stress incontinence and other bladder and urinary tract issues, pelvic floor concerns, difficulty concentrating or remembering things, and feelings of anxiety or depression, among others;

- visible changes in your breasts, or soreness or sensitivity that give you pause;

- symptoms related to chronic disease and chronic pain, endometriosis, adenomyosis, polycystic ovary syndrome (PCOS), fibroids, cysts, fertility challenges, mood disorders, premenstrual disorder or syndrome, other conditions and difficult diagnoses, and symptoms related to procedures or surgeries, such as a hysterectomy or an oophorectomy;

- observations about ovulation, fertility challenges, pregnancy, childbirth, breastfeeding, or weaning, postpartum life;

- significant physical experiences such as pregnancy, childbirth, pregnancy loss and other traumas, health interventions, surgeries, accidents, and recovery;

- the use of and side effects related to any prescribed medications or supplements;

- sleep patterns, travel (especially over multiple time zones);

- sweeping life changes that affect our mind-body state and biorhythms, such as the loss of a loved one, long-held dreams that we've had to let go of, or other sources of considerable grief, all of which are integral to our life experience and well-being;

- reflections on ways our perspectives have changed or things we have learned, ways we have overcome stress or transformed challenging experiences; and

- feelings or small observations if you feel intuitively that they are worth recording; these are often the important moments we will want to remember years later.

As our bodies change, we often need to learn how to adapt to and care for them. What worked for us once may no longer serve us, and tuning in to our new normal and our body's ebbs and flows can help us learn what we need as we mature over the years. Your calendar can be used to record the time you make for yourself to do nurturing things, exercise, spend time in nature, connect with supportive people in your life, and other choices you make that fill your soul. Our bodies' evolving needs urge us to care for ourselves in new ways and affirm the guiding wisdom of our bodies.

Winter: Sixties and Beyond 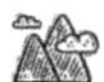

Women in the postmenopausal life stage continue to have their own unique biological rhythms as their hormone levels are dropping and/or they no longer have a period. Tuning in to the changes in our bodies is paramount as we age further, including caring for our cardiovascular, brain, bone, breast, and sexual health. One of the ways we can build a foundation of wellness is to establish healthy lifestyle habits right away, as it's never too late to start taking care of our health, and such changes can have immeasurable effects on the current and future state of our health.

For postmenopausal women in their fifties, sixties, seventies, eighties, nineties, and beyond, life can feel extraordinarily beautiful and peaceful, free from the challenges and constraints of menstruation, birth control, parental responsibility, and the hard work of establishing oneself in life. Living with confidence and being able to live more fully in joy and gratitude can feel like a tremendous gift. Being guided by the wisdom that comes with having lived through different stages of womanhood, women elders are often better able to fully grasp what it means to truly care for ourselves, perhaps for the first time in our lives, after nurturing others in our families and communities for decades.

In this life stage, we may feel profound relief along with some unexpected grief as our menstruating and childbearing life stages have come to an end. In addition, many postmenopausal women find that they observe their body cycles and rhythms in new and illuminating ways, just as we all experience internal shifts as we welcome new seasons of the year.

Winter: When to Use *Twelve Moons*

The postmenopausal stage of life is accompanied by freedom from menstruation and some newly found gifts, yet women still need to pay attention to their bodies more than ever in order to protect their health. Some ideas of what to record include:

- changes in your body, mood, sleep patterns, and energy levels;

- symptoms of menopause or postmenopause, including: hot flashes or night sweats, sleep disturbances or sleeplessness, fatigue, mood swings, irritability, changes in libido, vaginal dryness and/or painful sex, weight gain, skin and nail changes, thinning hair, breast tenderness, body odor, headaches, dizziness, tiredness, bloating, digestive issues, food cravings, heart palpitations, joint pain and muscle aches, osteopenia and osteoporosis, itchy skin, stress incontinence and other bladder and urinary tract issues, pelvic floor concerns, difficulty concentrating or remembering things, and feelings of anxiety or depression, among others;

- spotting or other notable vaginal discharge;

- visible changes in your breasts, or soreness or sensitivity that give you pause;

- observations about strength, mobility, coordination, balance, and agility; memory and concentration;

- symptoms related to chronic disease and chronic pain, polycystic ovary syndrome (PCOS), fibroids, cysts, mood disorders, and other conditions and difficult diagnoses;

- surgeries such as a hysterectomy or an oophorectomy, or any other medical procedures, head to toe;

- the use of and side effects related to any prescribed medications or supplements;

- sleep patterns, travel (especially over multiple time zones);

- sweeping life changes that affect our mind-body state and biorhythms, such as the loss of a loved one, long-held dreams that we've had to let go of, or other sources of considerable grief, all of which are integral to our life experience and well-being;

- reflections on ways our perspectives have changed or things we have learned, ways we have overcome stress or transformed challenging experiences; and

- feelings or small observations if you feel intuitively that they are worth recording; these are often the important moments we will want to remember years later.

We must be the historians of and advocates for our own health, and we can use the information we gather as a protective tool to enable us to live not just longer, but more healthy and vibrant lives. In addition to the suggestions above, you can also use your calendar to record the time you make for yourself to do nurturing things, exercise, spend time in nature, connect with supportive people in your life, and other choices you make that fill your soul and support your journey of joy and health.

PART 3: CALENDARS 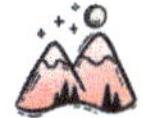

The calendars begin on the following pages. 

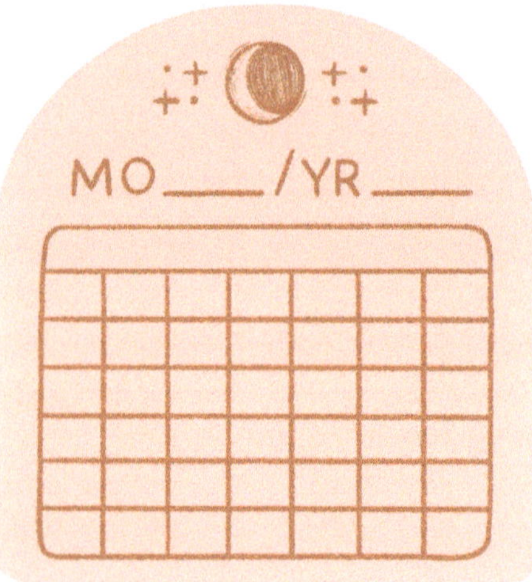

MO____/YR____

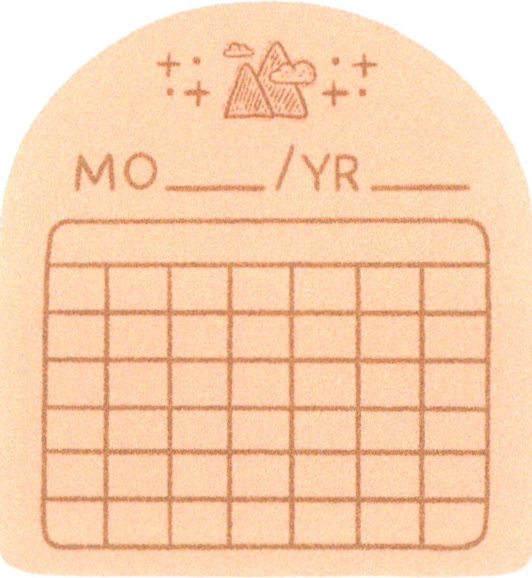

MO____/YR____

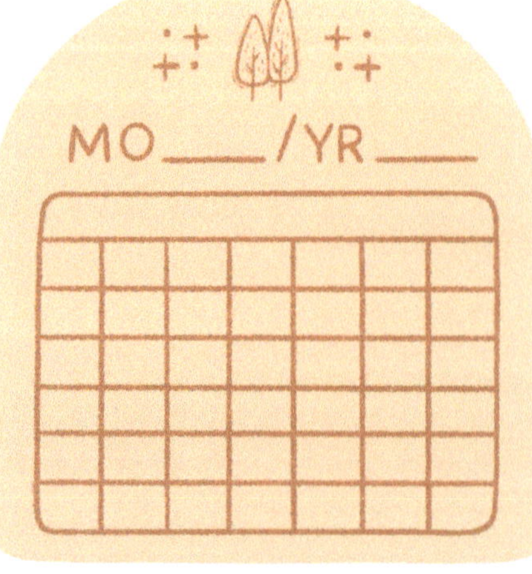

MO____/YR____

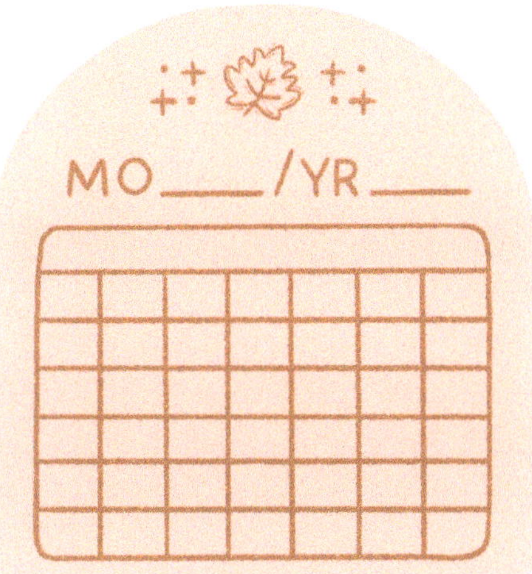
MO____/YR____

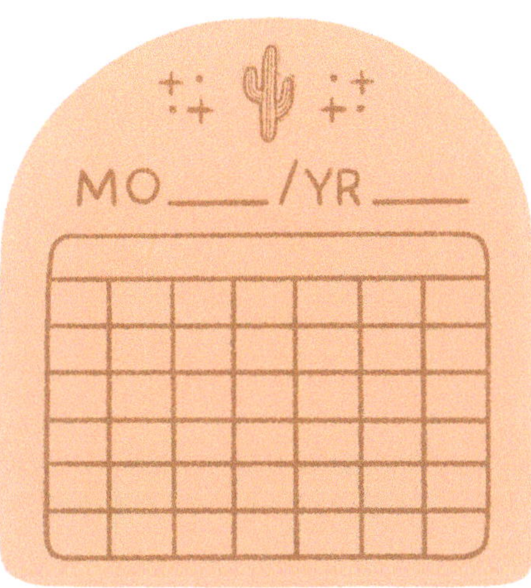
MO____/YR____

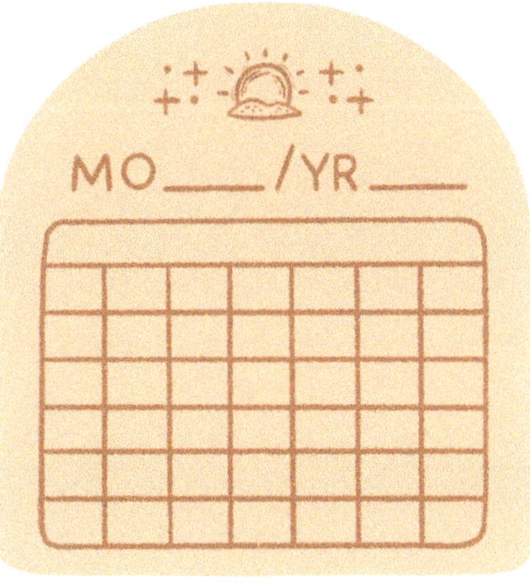
MO____/YR____

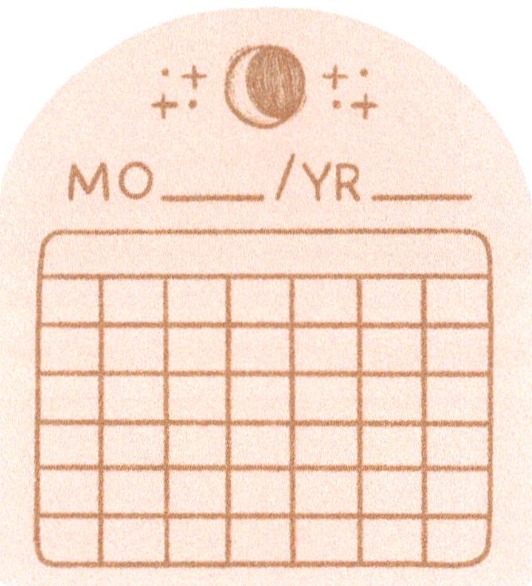

MO____/YR____

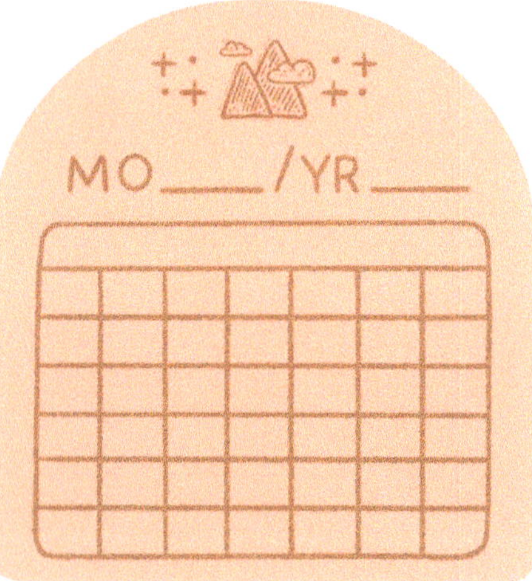

MO____/YR____

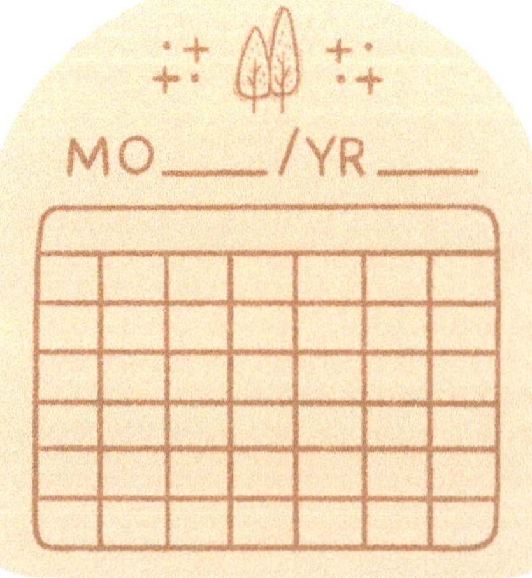

MO____/YR____

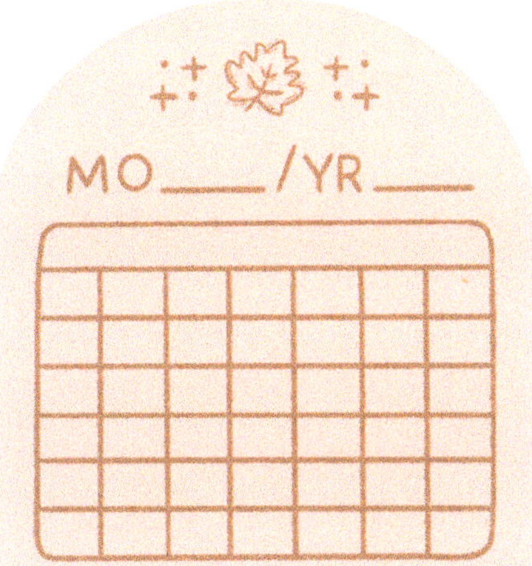

MO____/YR____

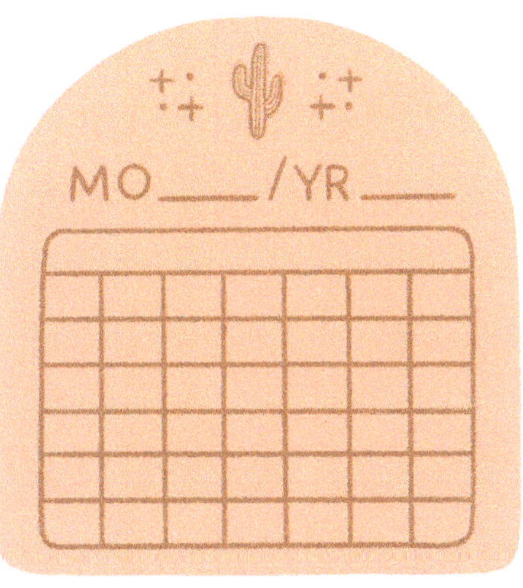

MO____/YR____

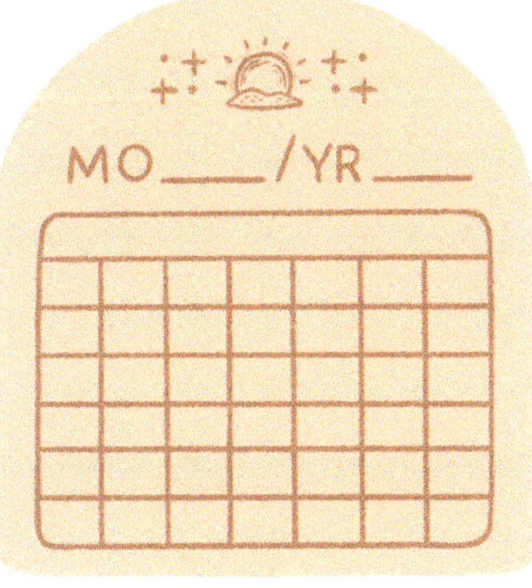

MO____/YR____

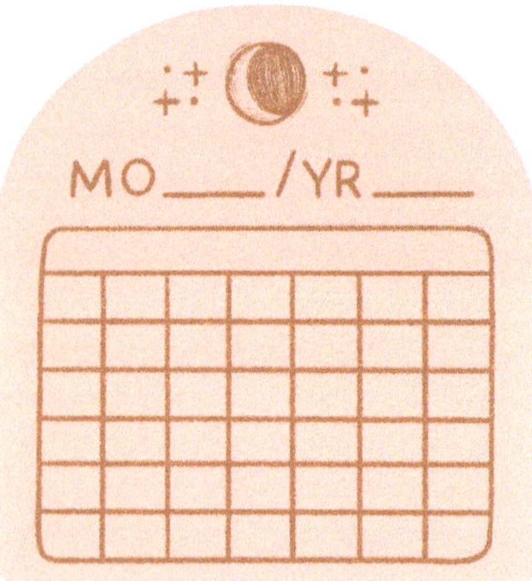
MO____/YR____

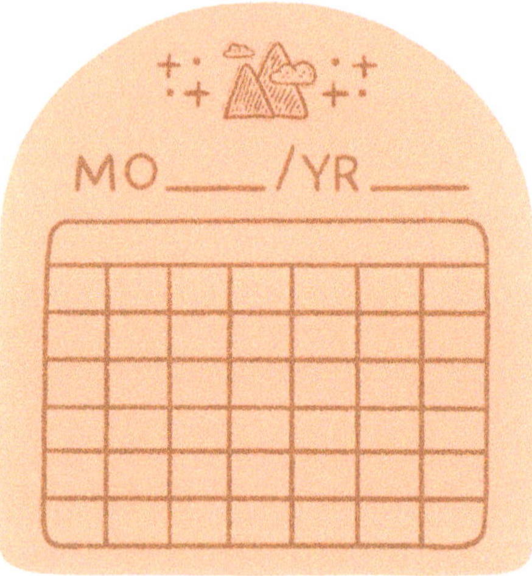
MO____/YR____

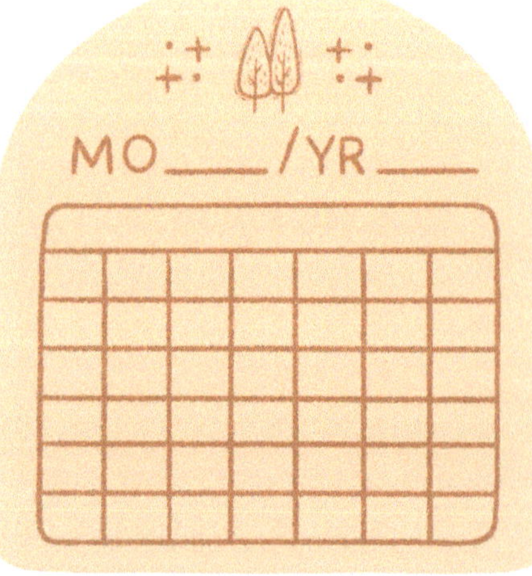
MO____/YR____

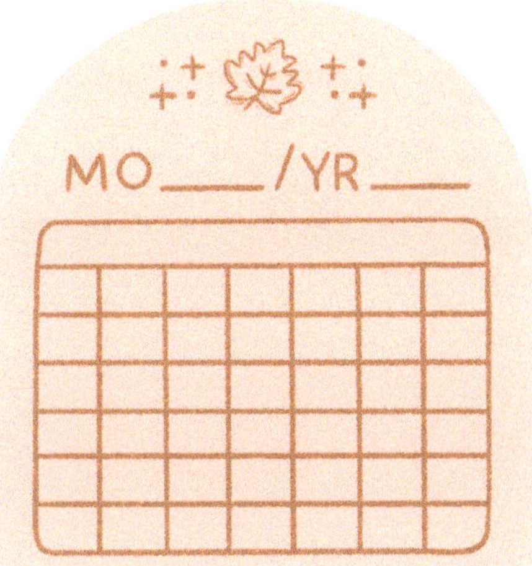
MO____/YR____

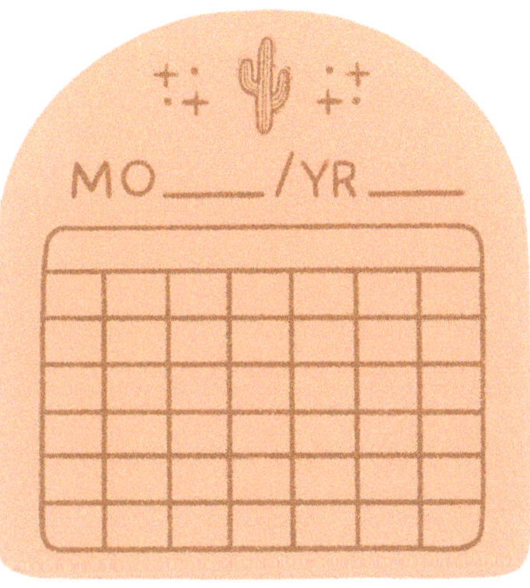
MO____/YR____

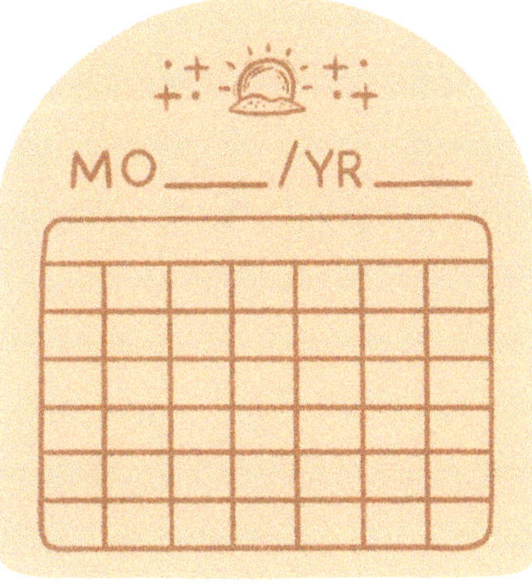
MO____/YR____

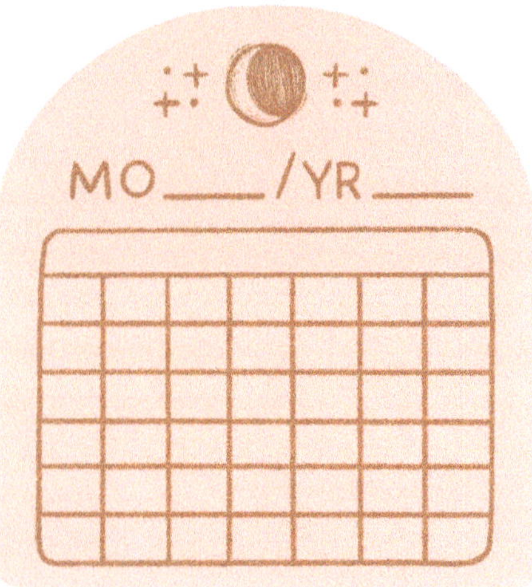
MO____/YR____

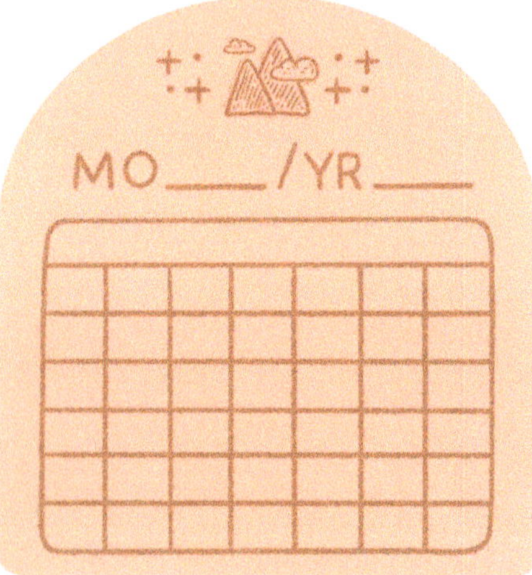
MO____/YR____

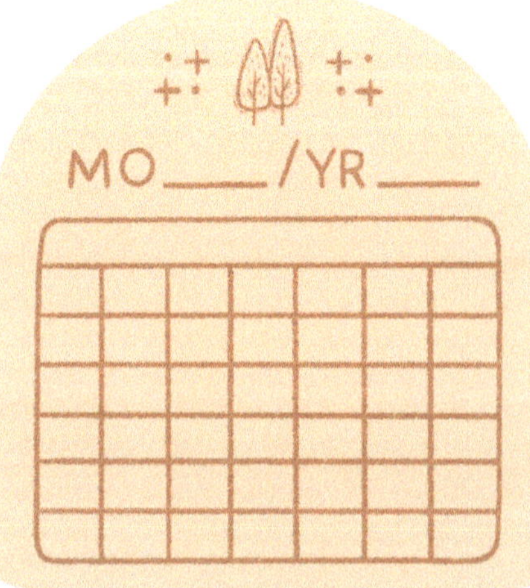
MO____/YR____

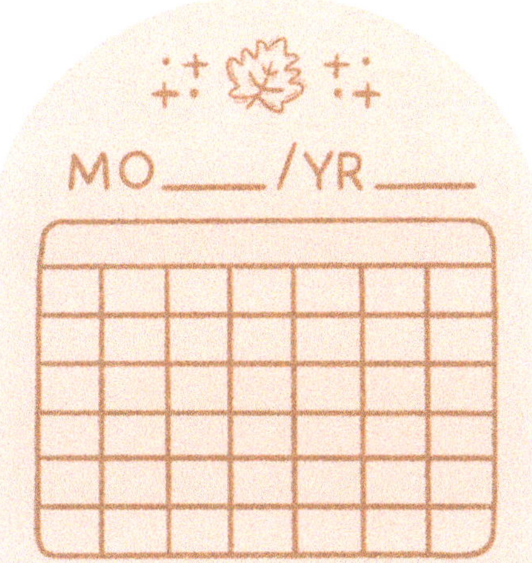

MO____/YR____

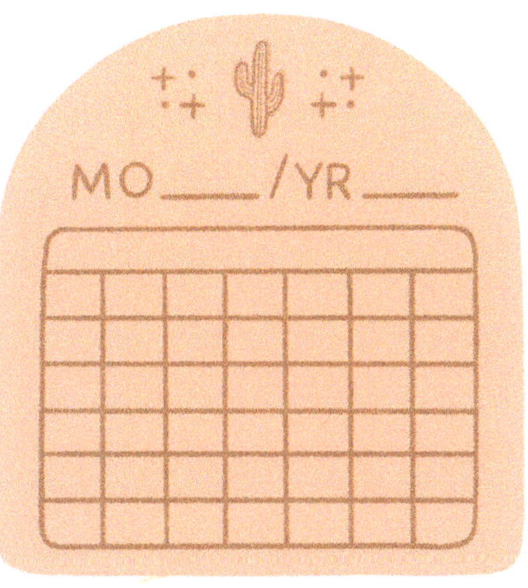

MO____/YR____

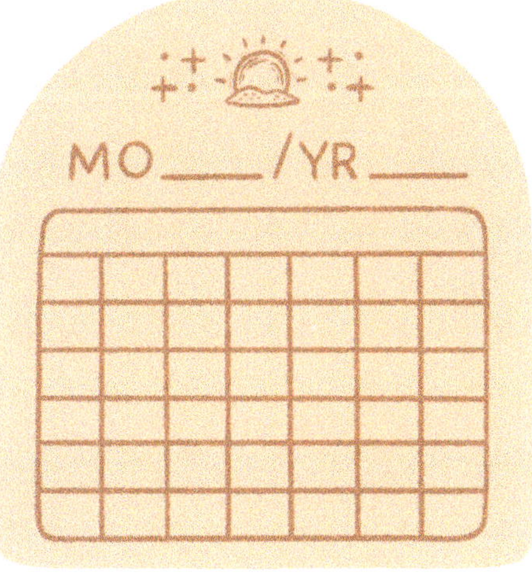

MO____/YR____

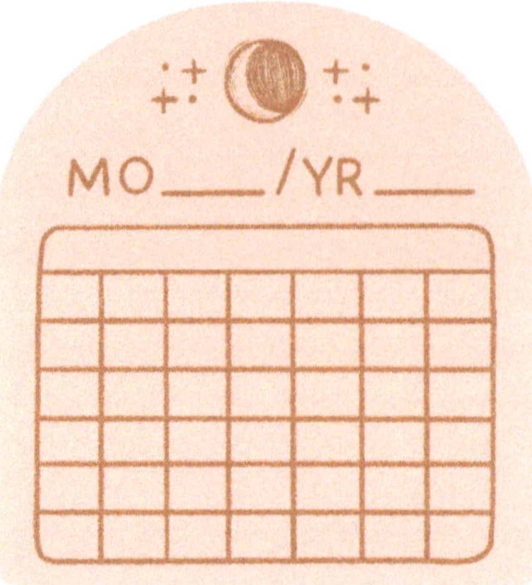

MO______/YR______

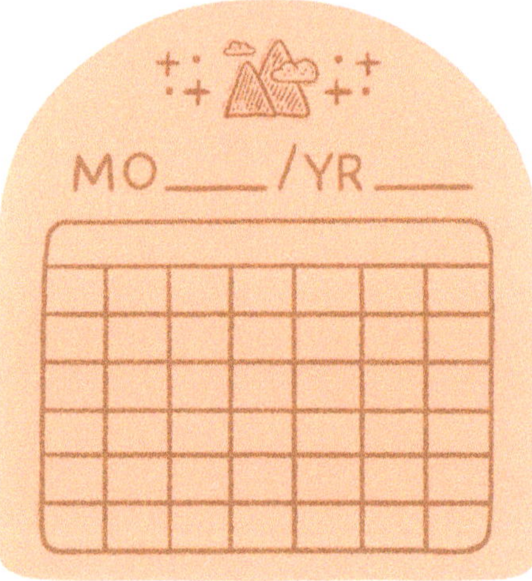

MO______/YR______

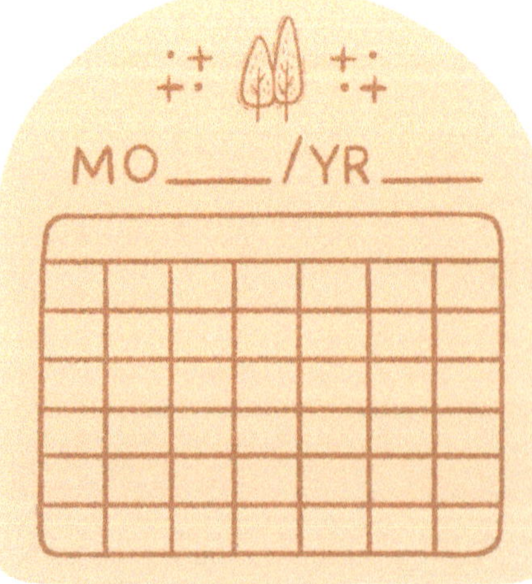

MO______/YR______

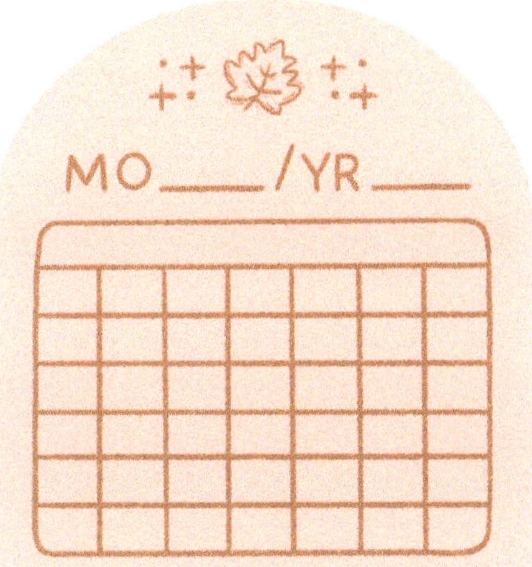

MO____/YR____

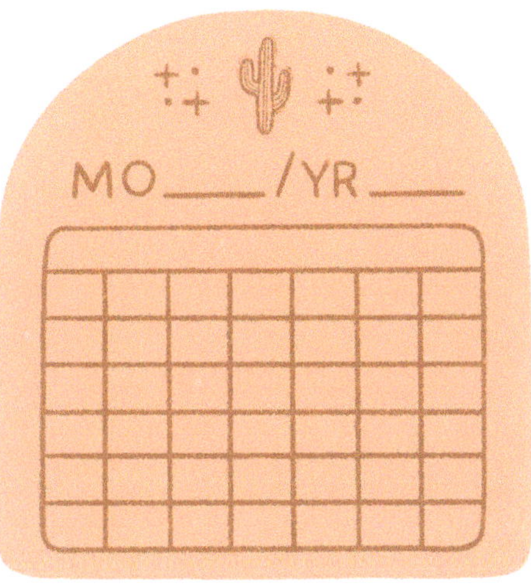

MO____/YR____

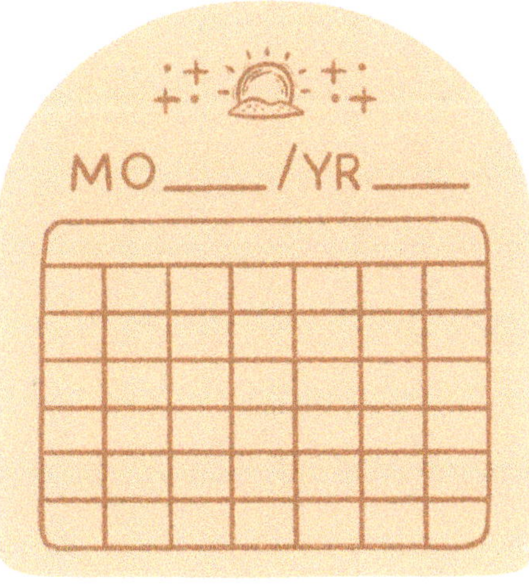

MO____/YR____

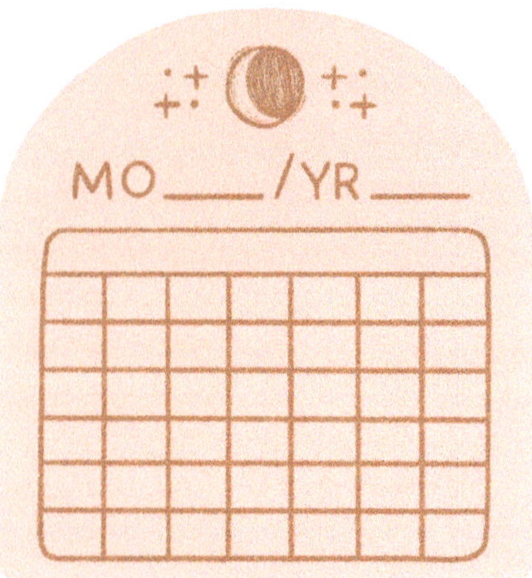

MO____/YR____

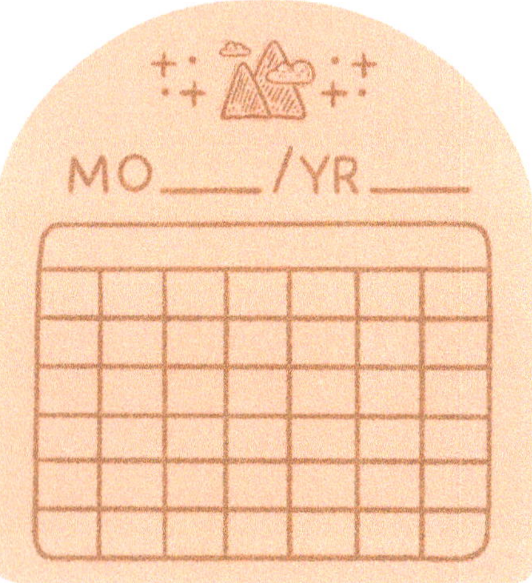

MO____/YR____

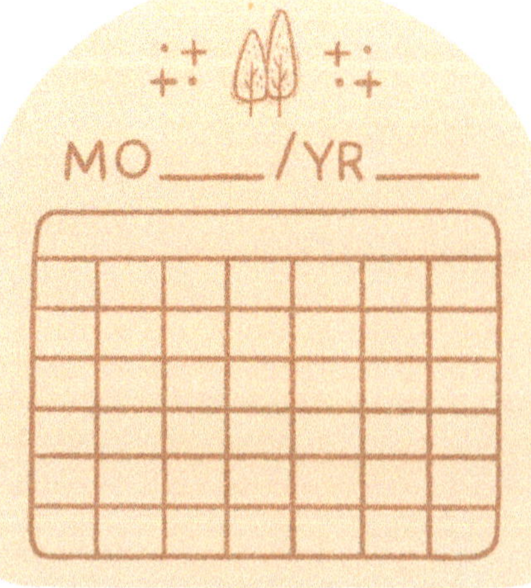

MO____/YR____

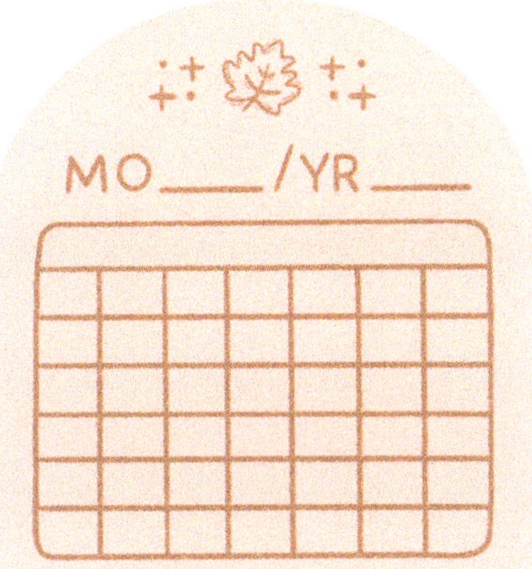

MO____/YR____

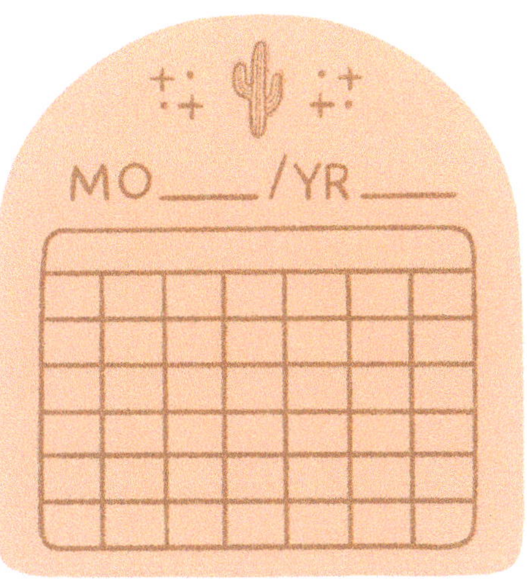

MO____/YR____

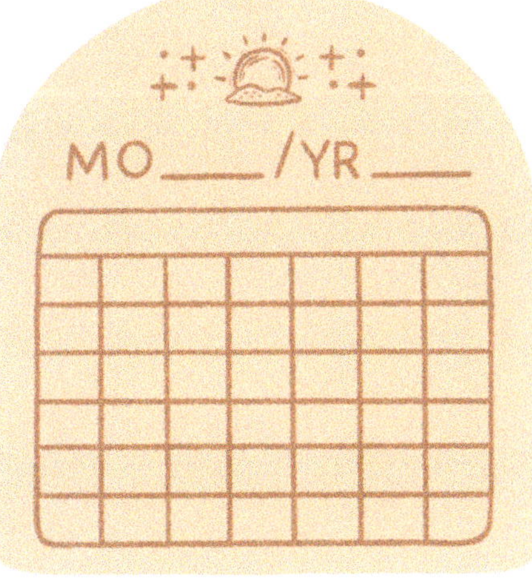

MO____/YR____

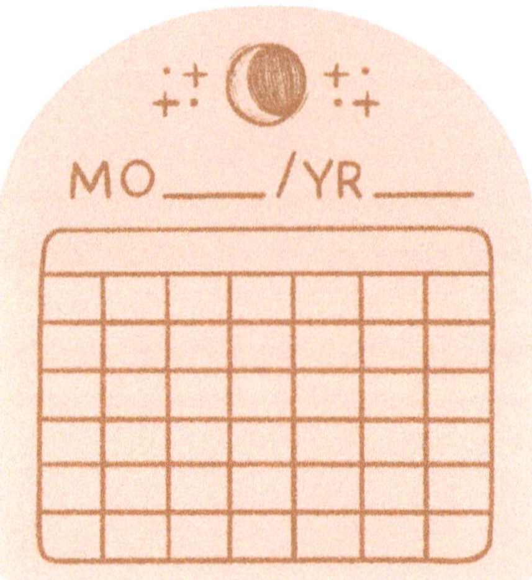
MO_____/YR_____

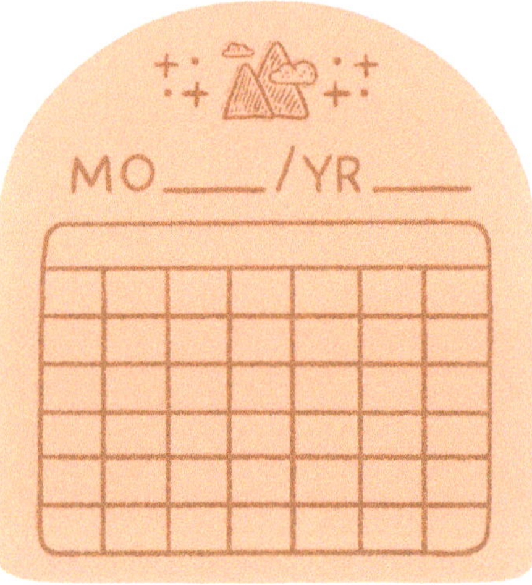
MO_____/YR_____

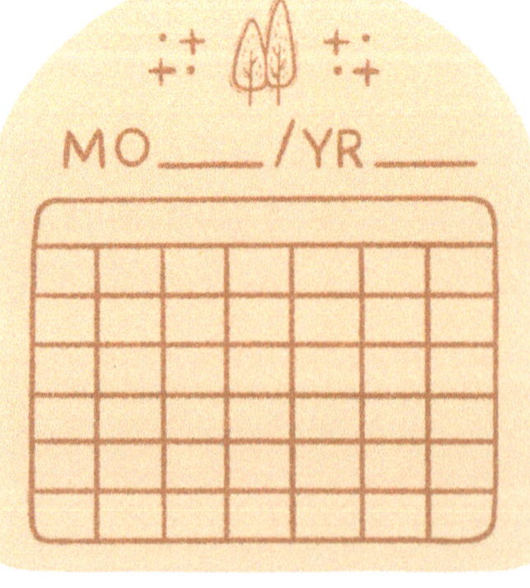
MO_____/YR_____

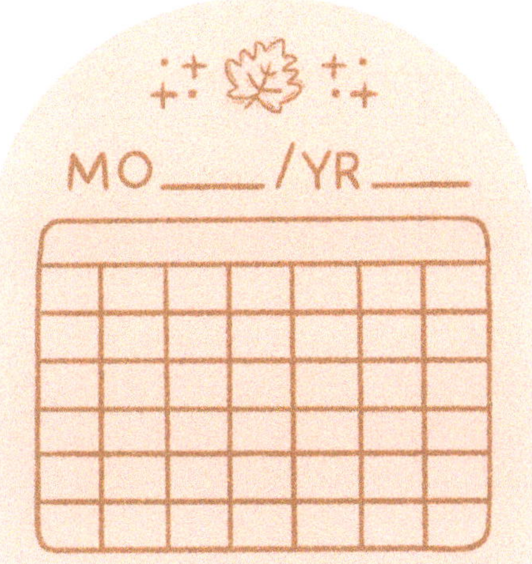

MO___/YR___

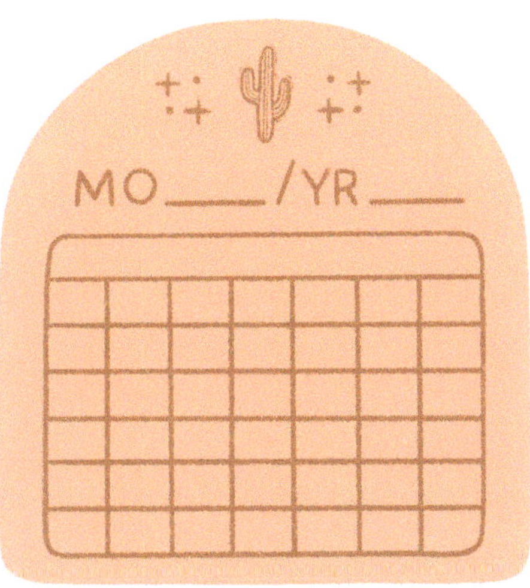

MO___/YR___

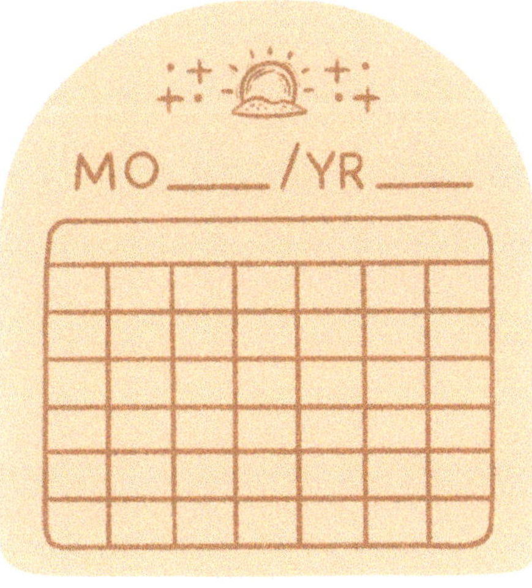

MO___/YR___

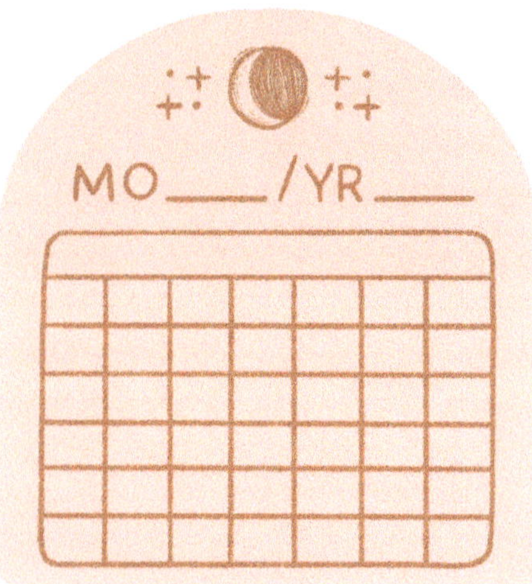
MO____/YR____

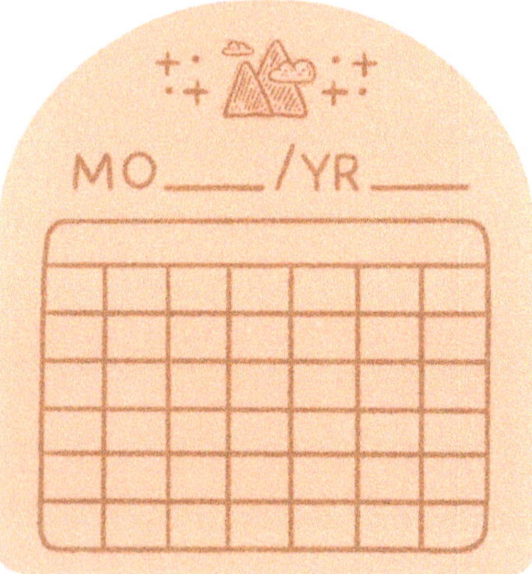
MO____/YR____

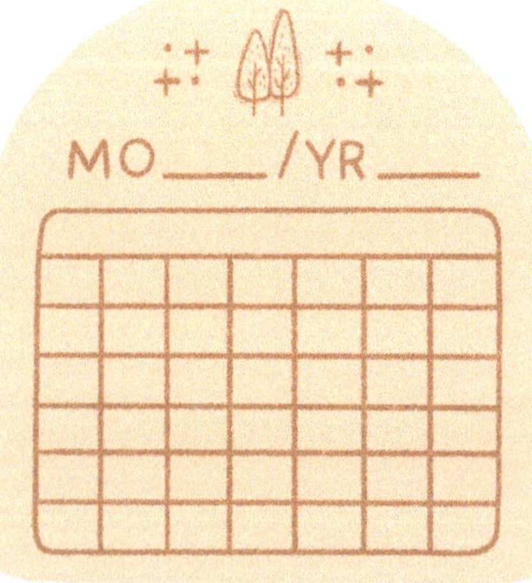
MO____/YR____

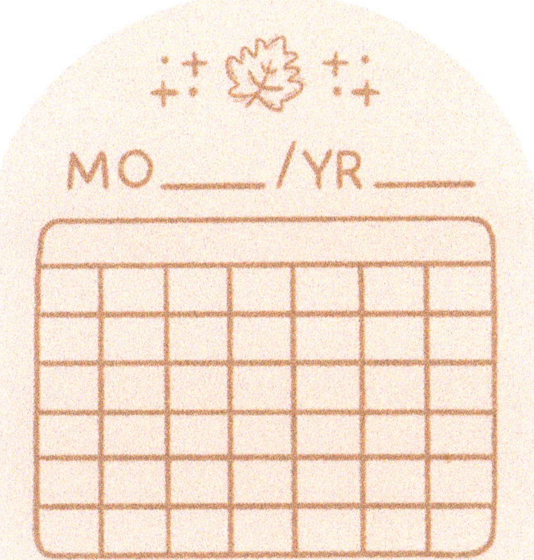

MO____/YR____

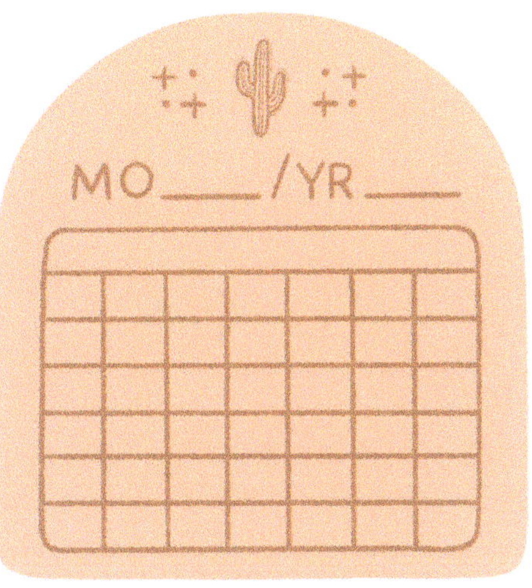

MO____/YR____

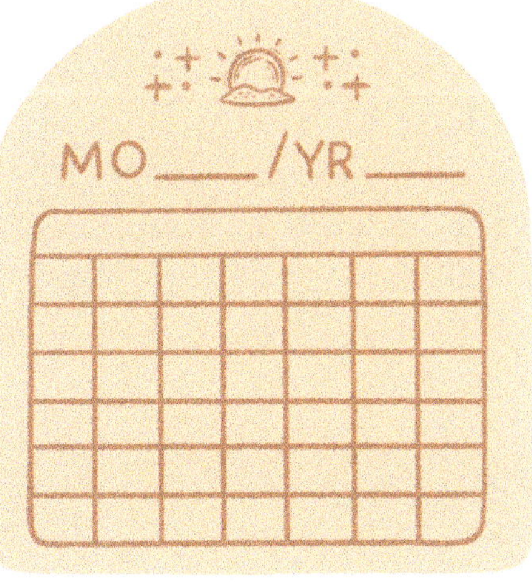

MO____/YR____

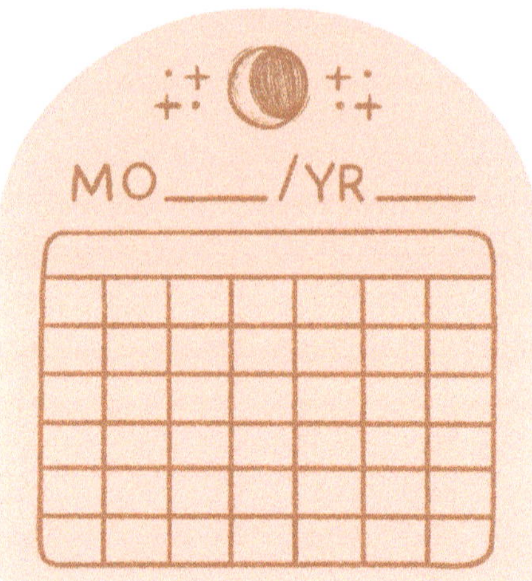
MO____/YR____

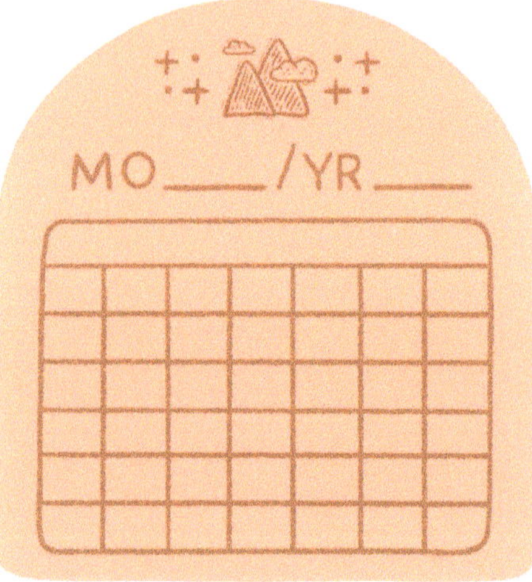
MO____/YR____

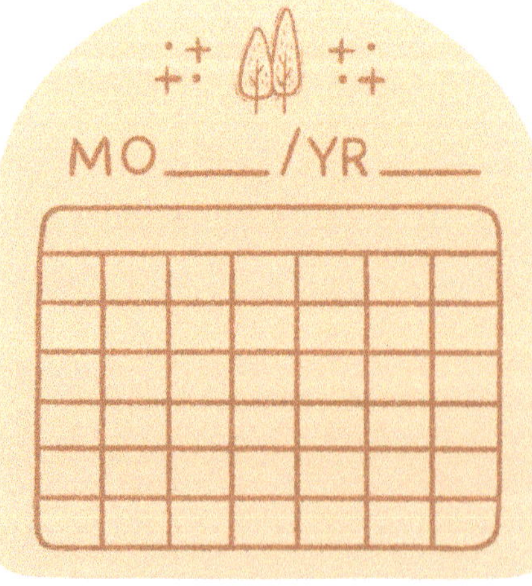
MO____/YR____

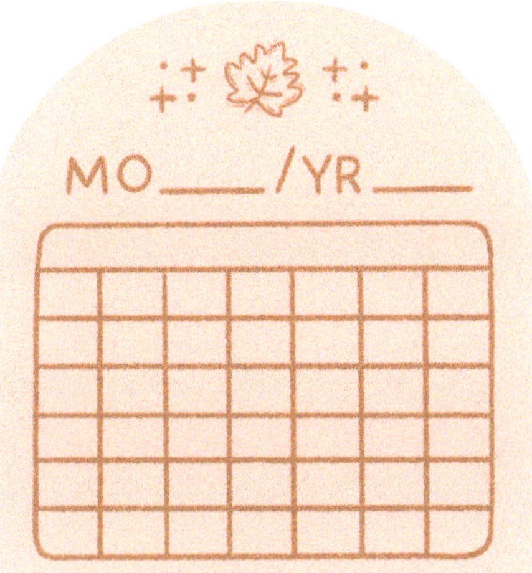
MO____/YR____

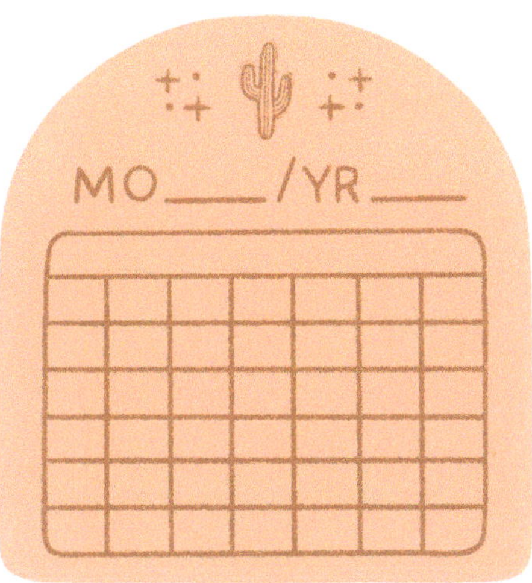
MO____/YR____

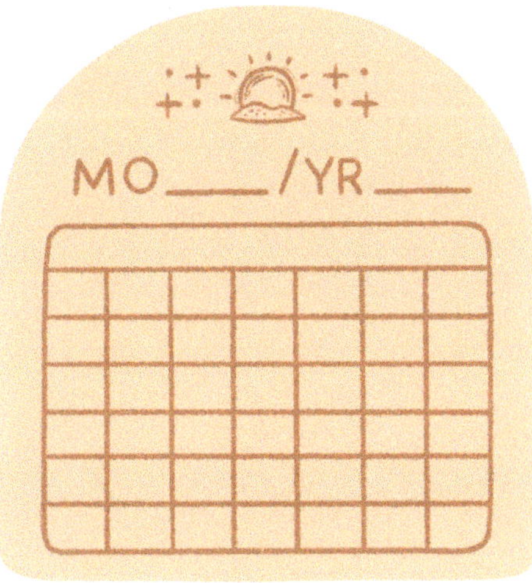
MO____/YR____

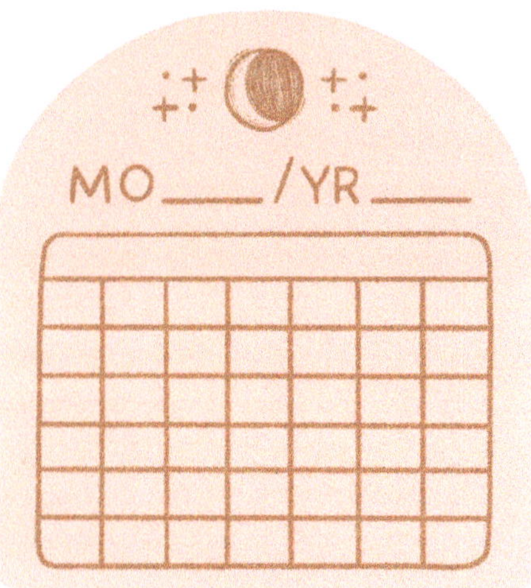

MO_____/YR_____

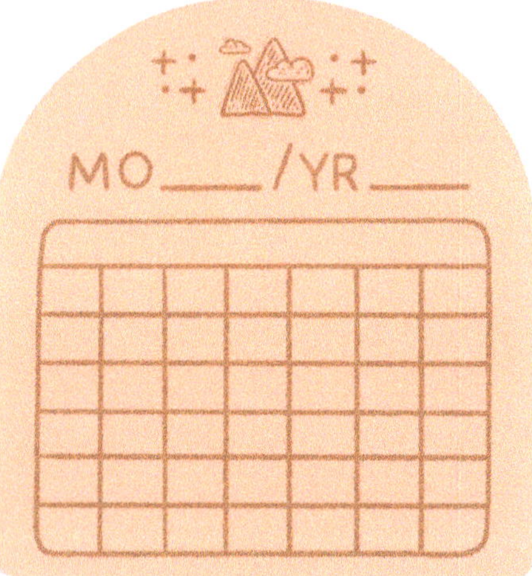

MO_____/YR_____

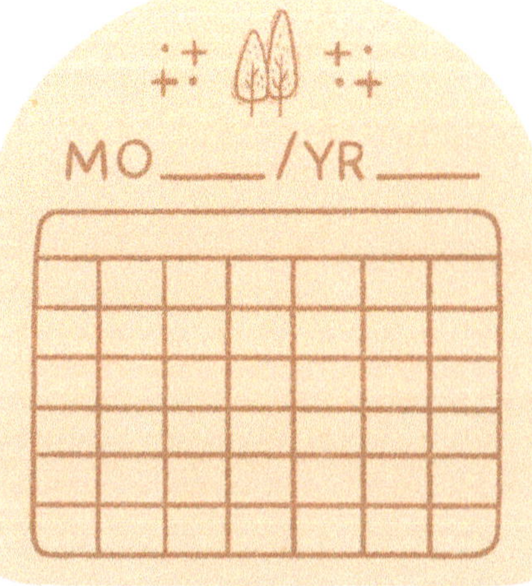

MO_____/YR_____

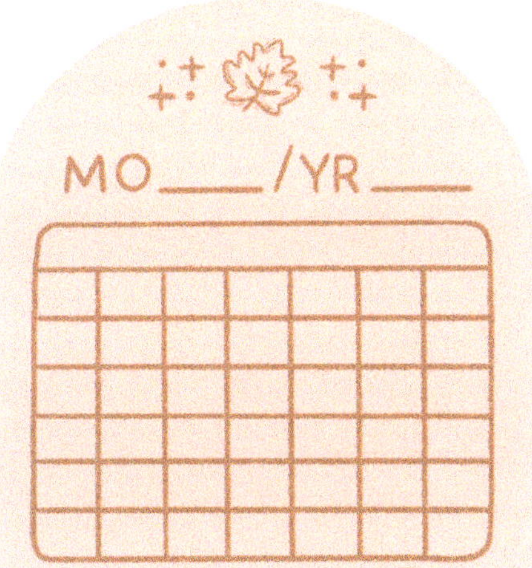
MO____/YR____

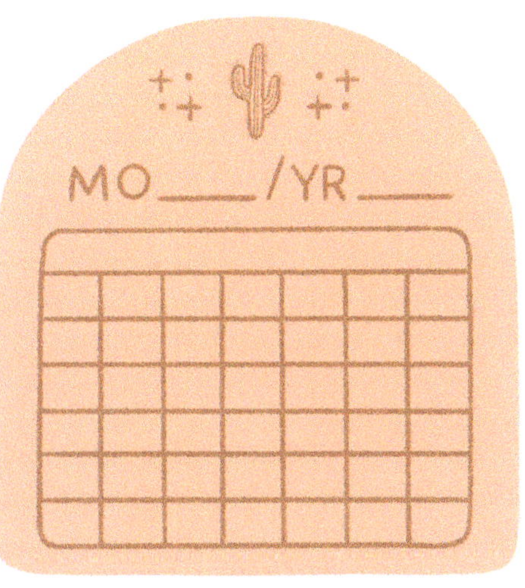
MO____/YR____

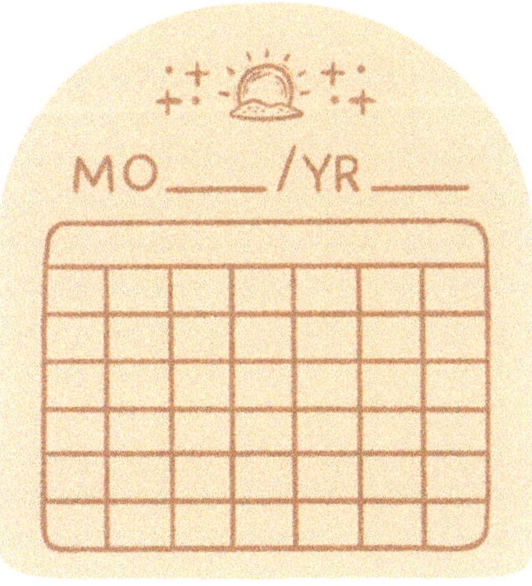
MO____/YR____

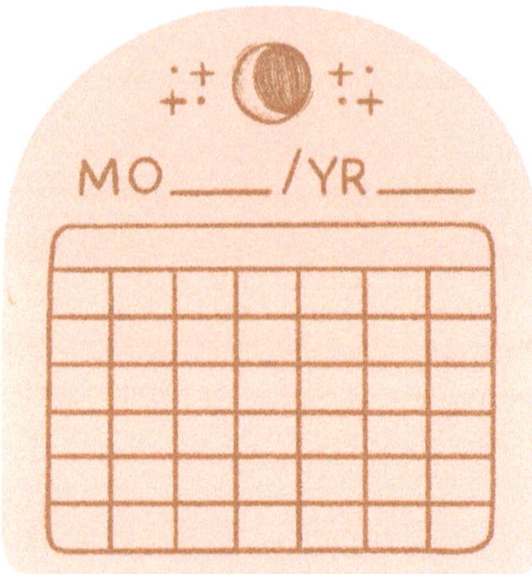

MO____/YR____

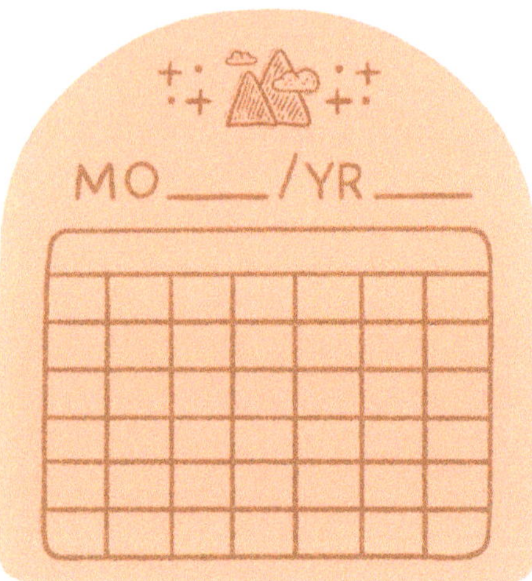

MO____/YR____

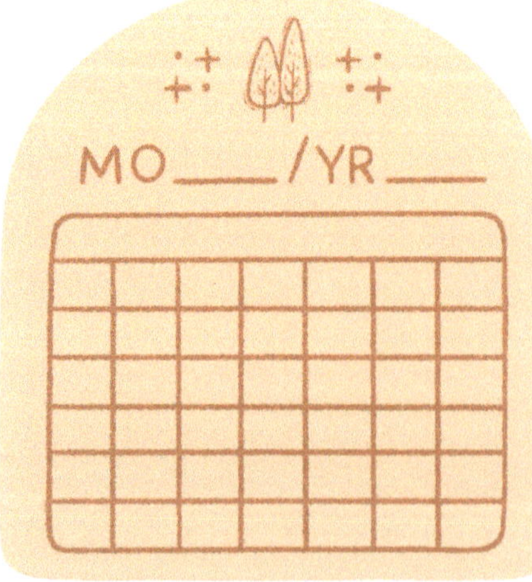

MO____/YR____

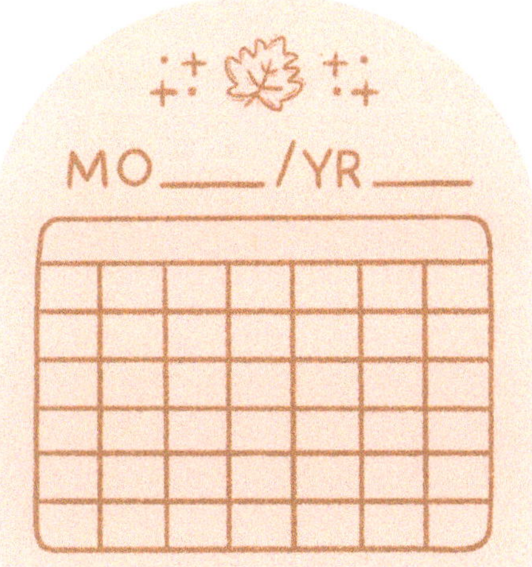

MO____/YR____

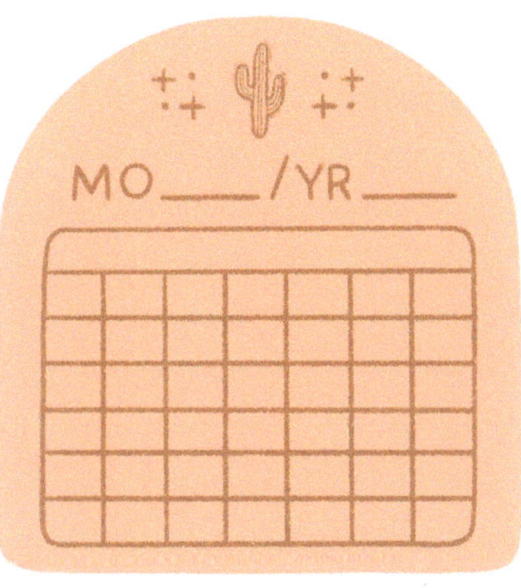

MO____/YR____

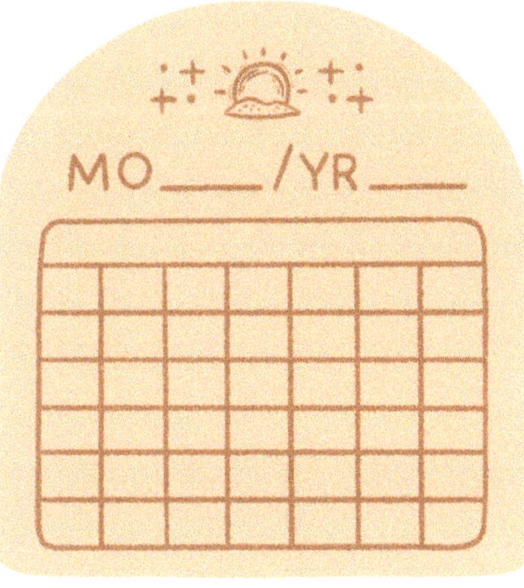

MO____/YR____

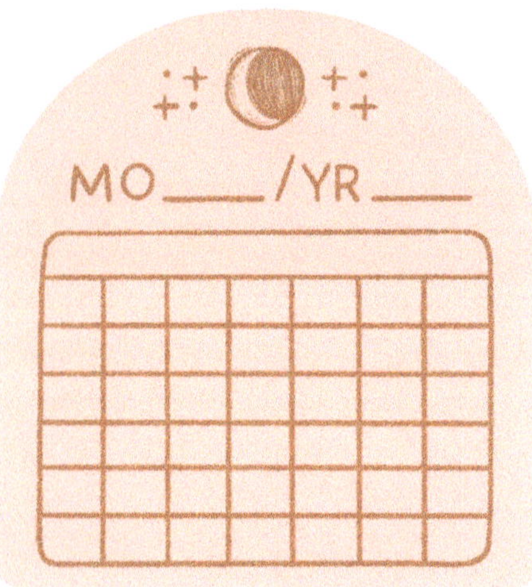
MO____/YR____

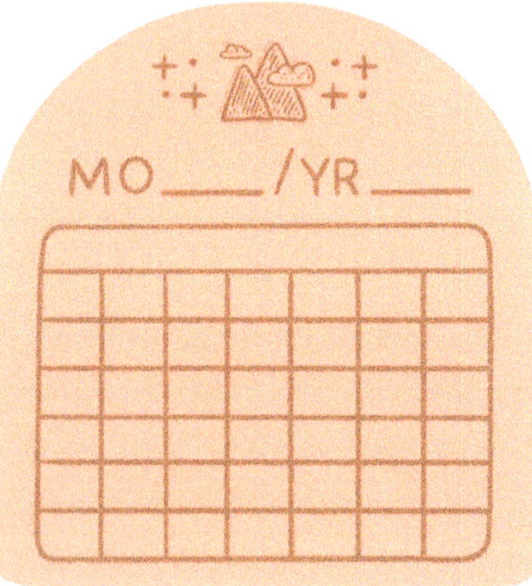
MO____/YR____

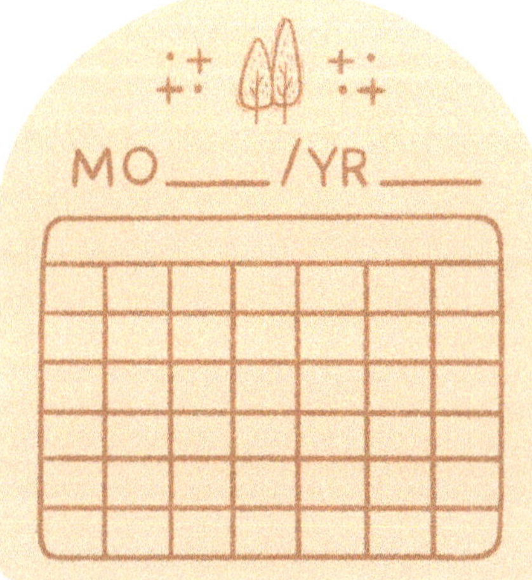
MO____/YR____

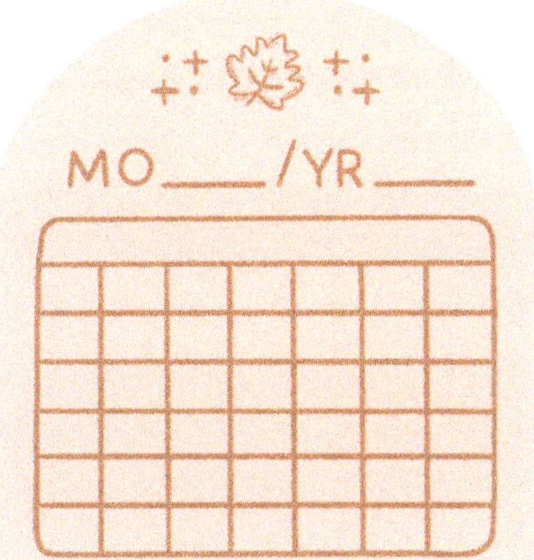
MO____/YR____

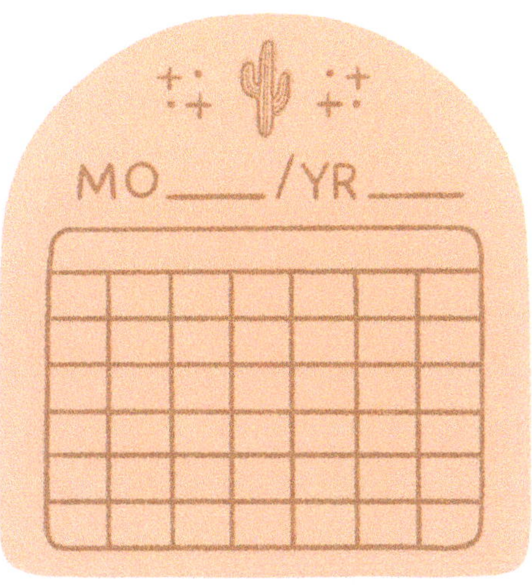
MO____/YR____

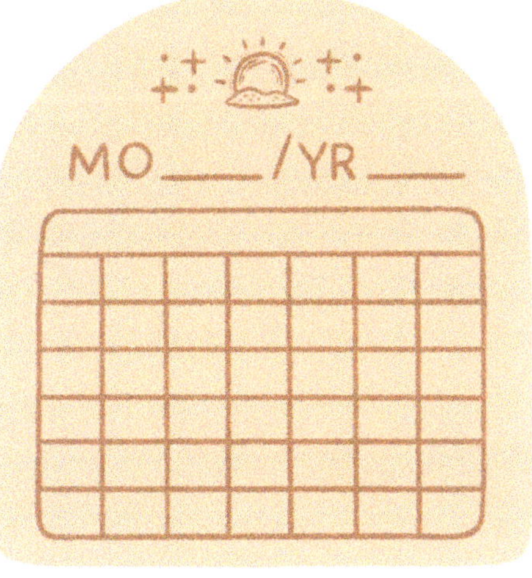
MO____/YR____

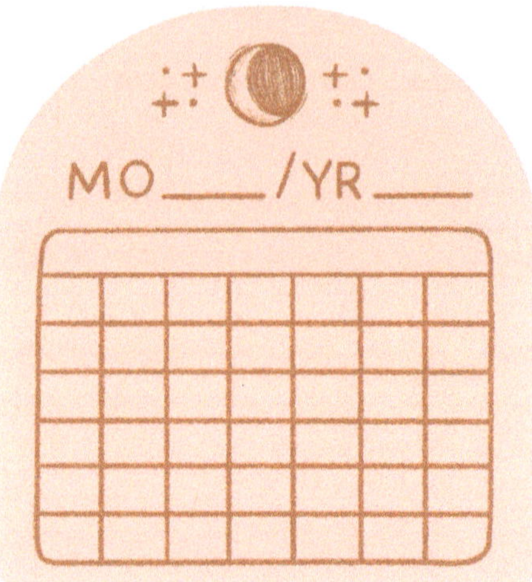
MO____/YR____

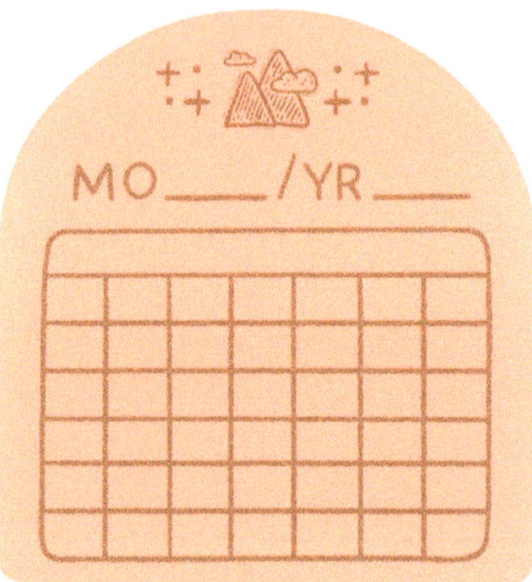
MO____/YR____

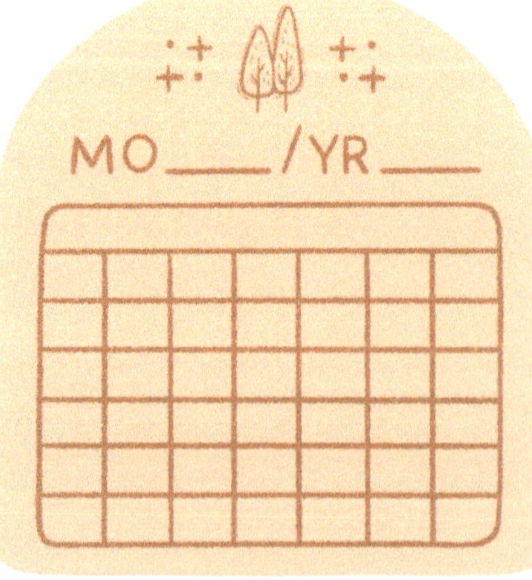
MO____/YR____

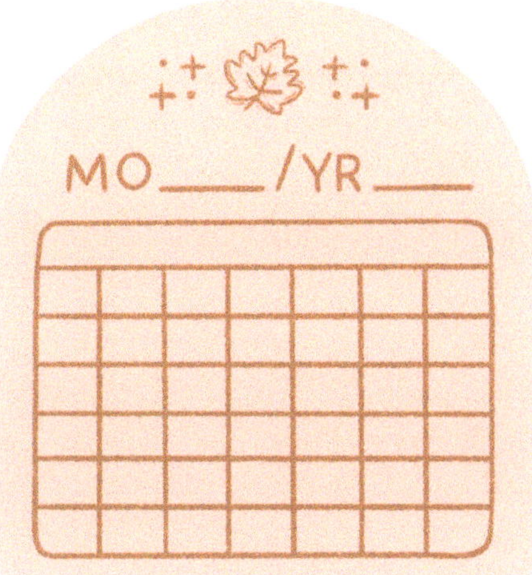

MO____/YR____

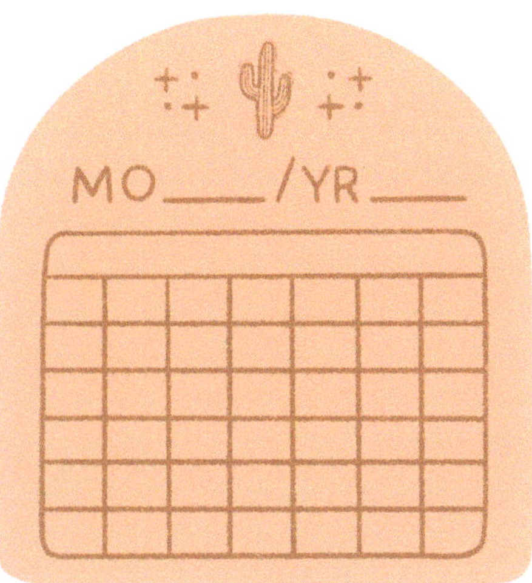

MO____/YR____

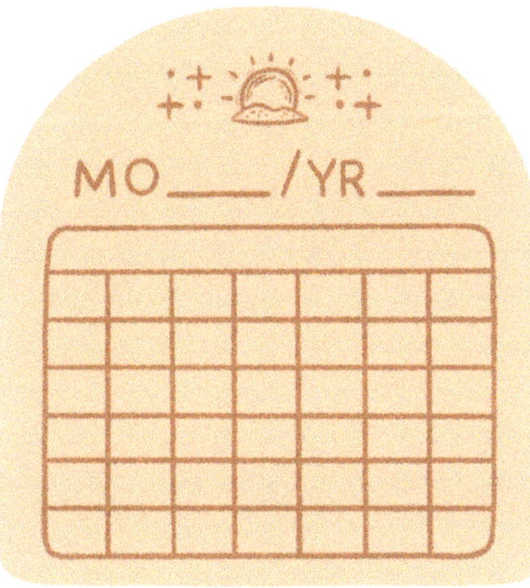

MO____/YR____

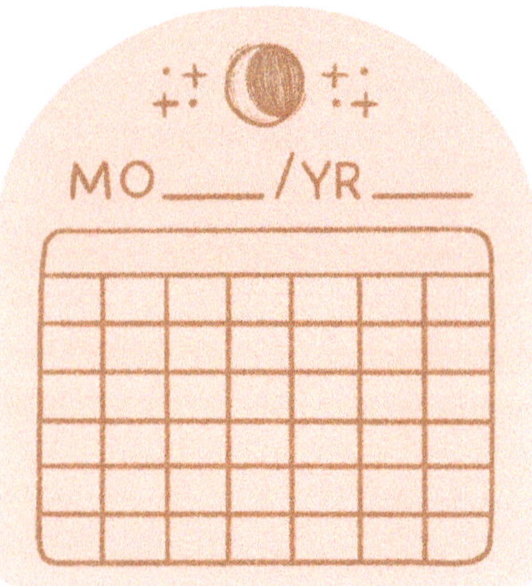

MO____/YR____

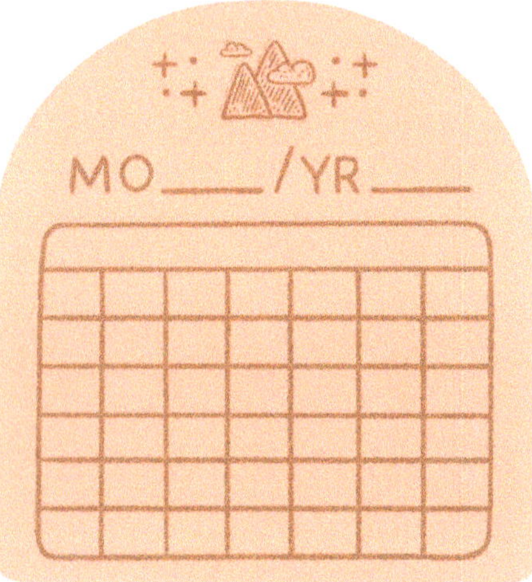

MO____/YR____

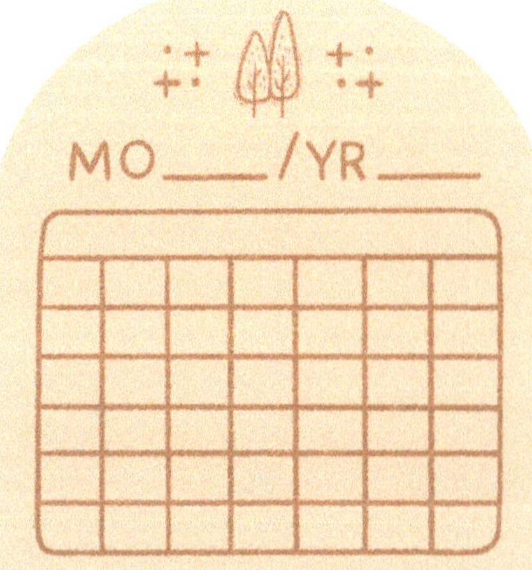

MO____/YR____

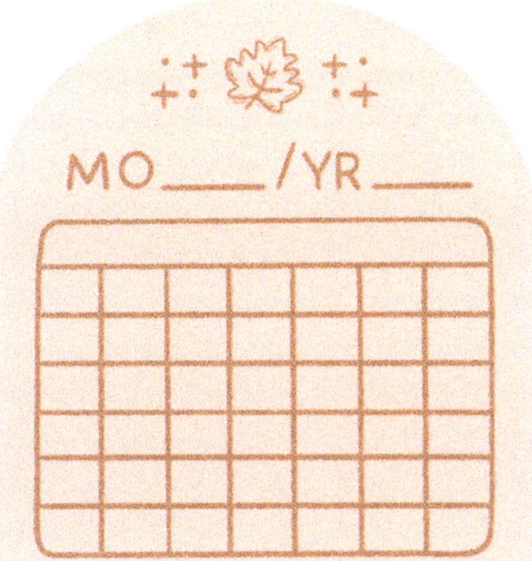
MO____/YR____

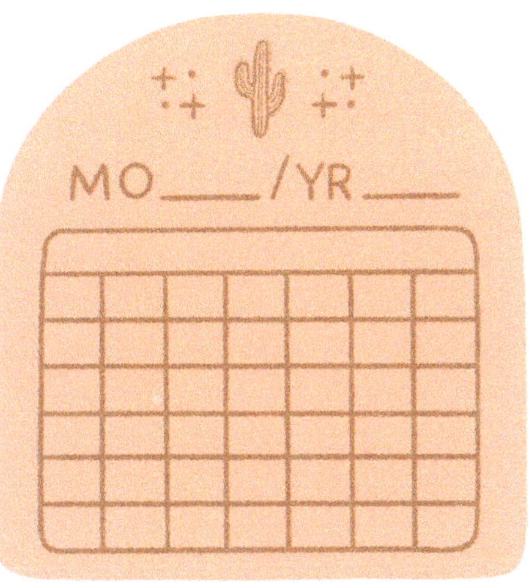
MO____/YR____

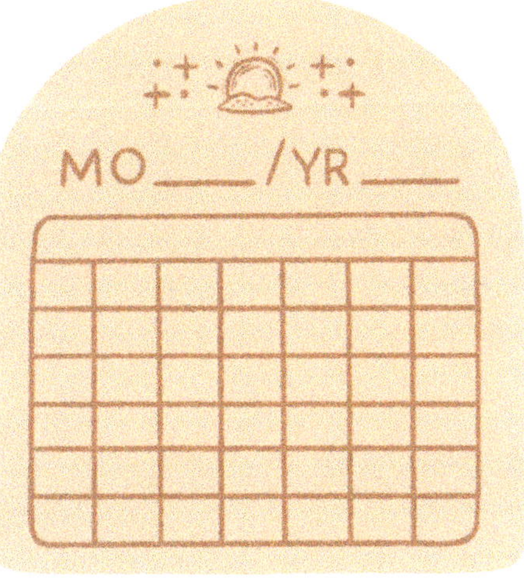
MO____/YR____

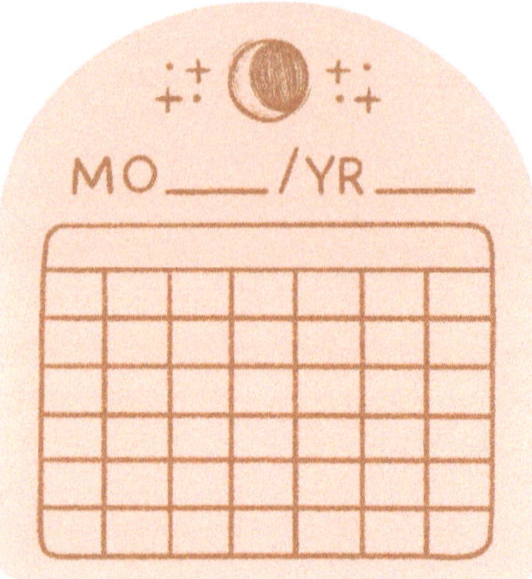

MO____/YR____

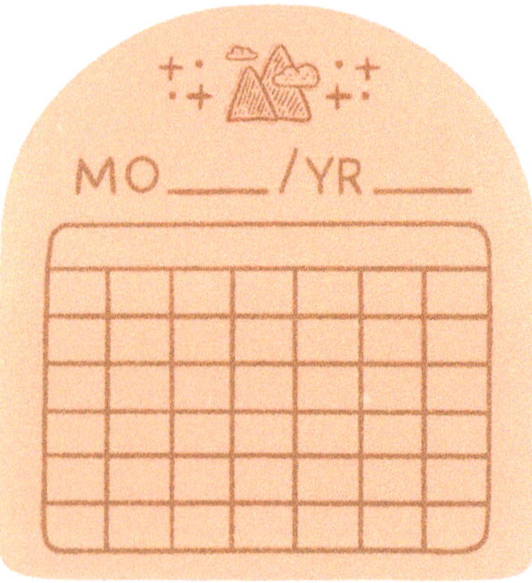

MO____/YR____

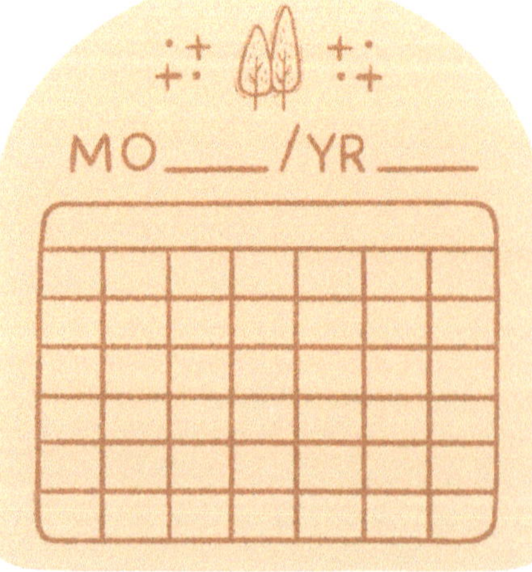

MO____/YR____

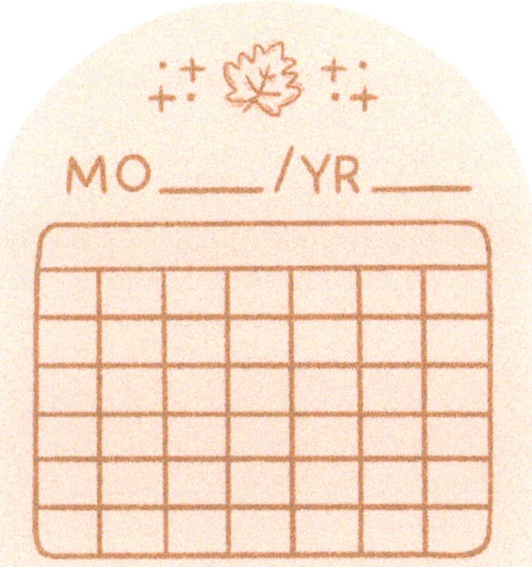

MO____/YR____

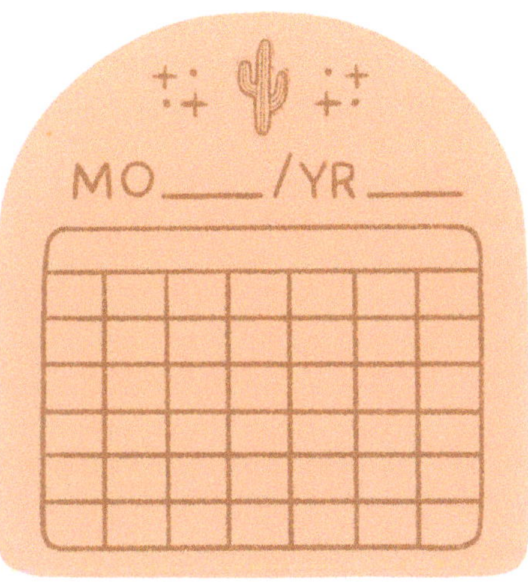

MO____/YR____

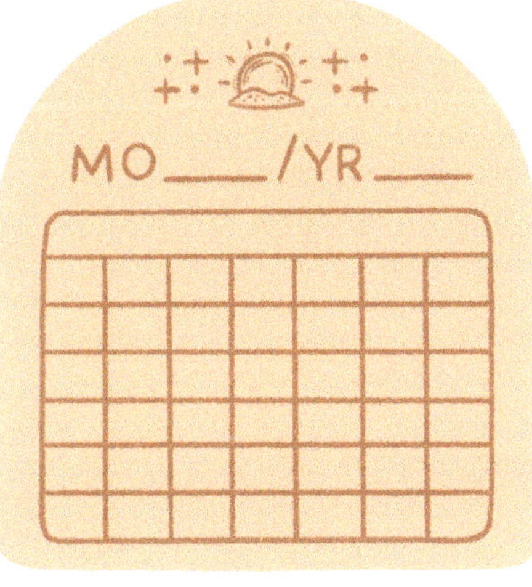

MO____/YR____

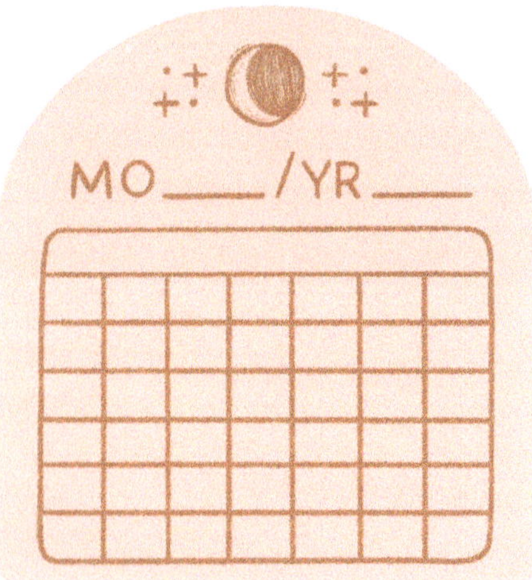

MO____ /YR____

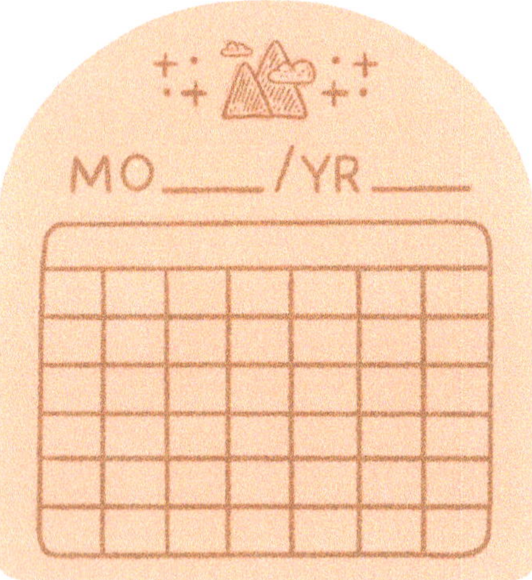

MO____ /YR____

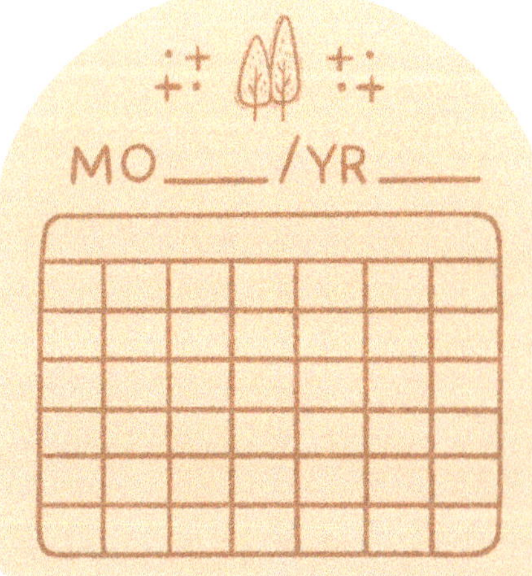

MO____ /YR____

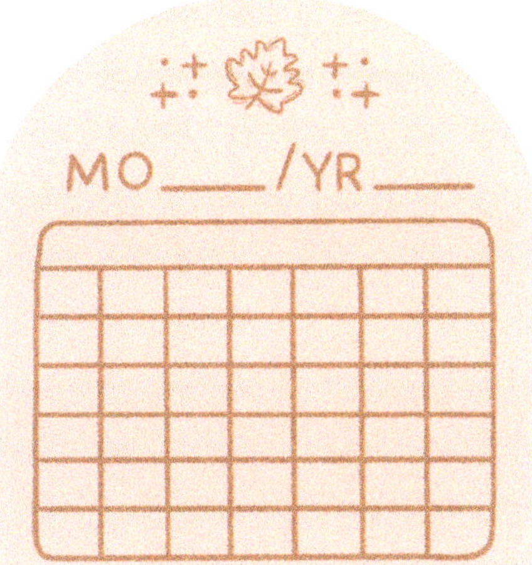
MO____/YR____

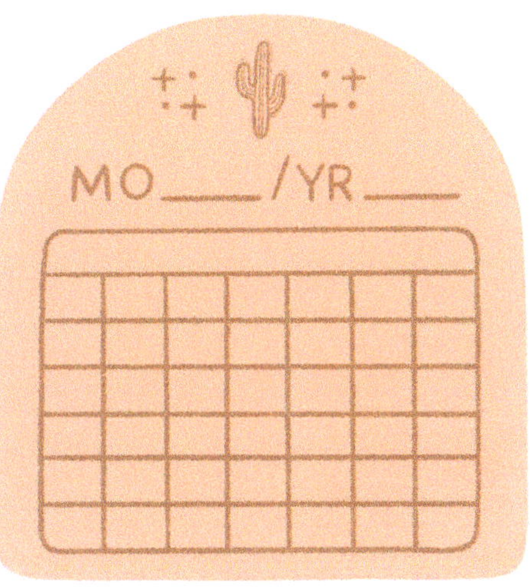
MO____/YR____

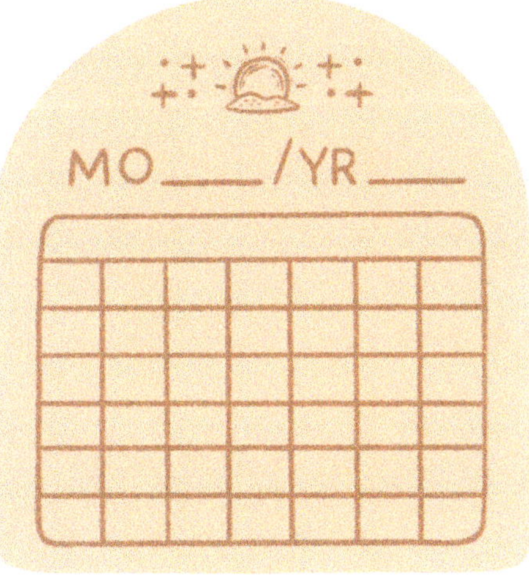
MO____/YR____

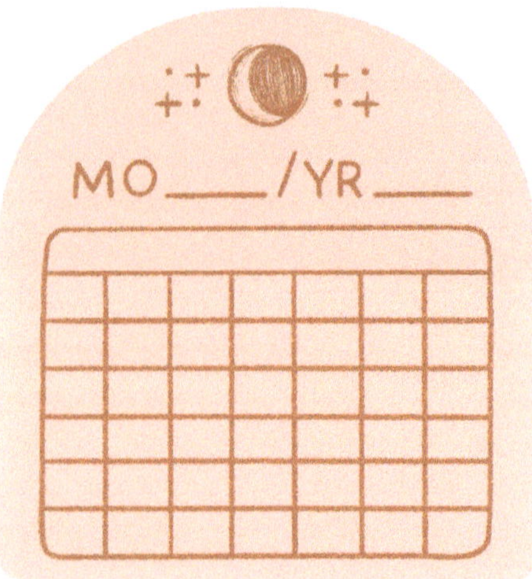
MO____/YR____

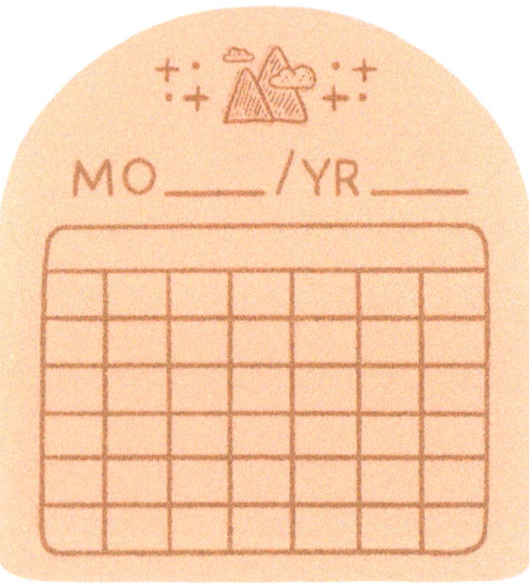
MO____/YR____

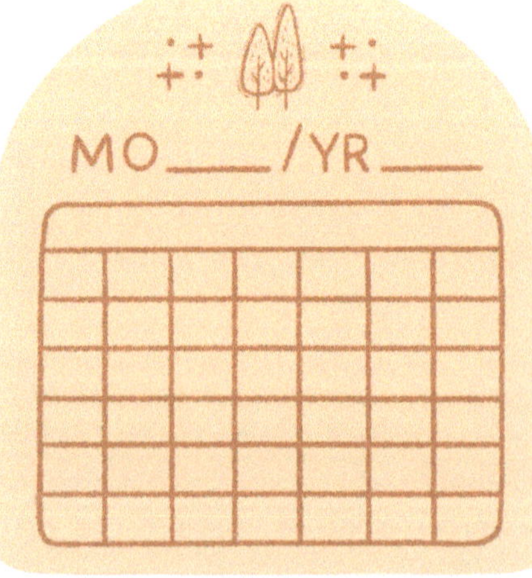
MO____/YR____

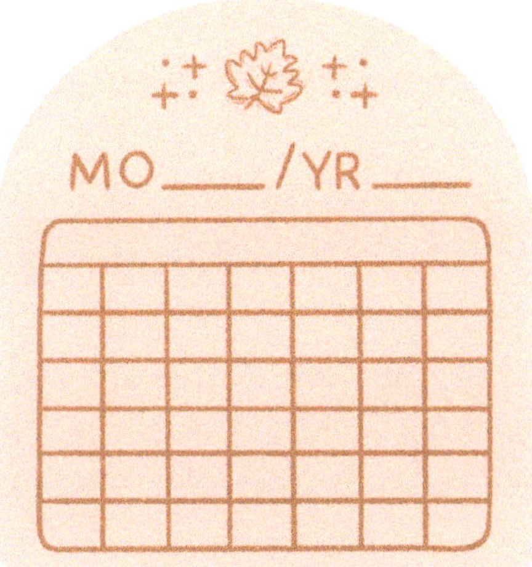
MO____/YR____

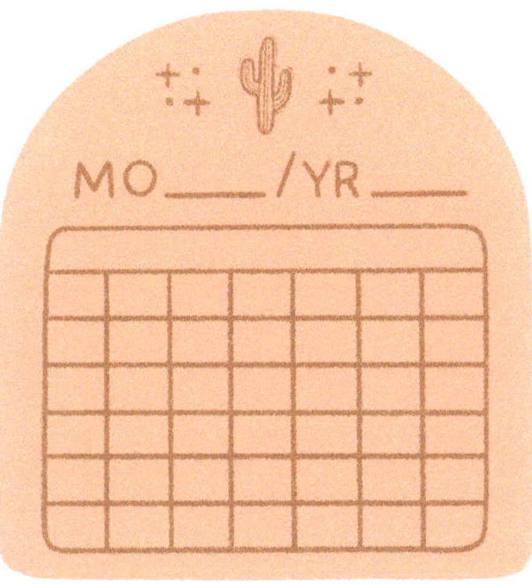
MO____/YR____

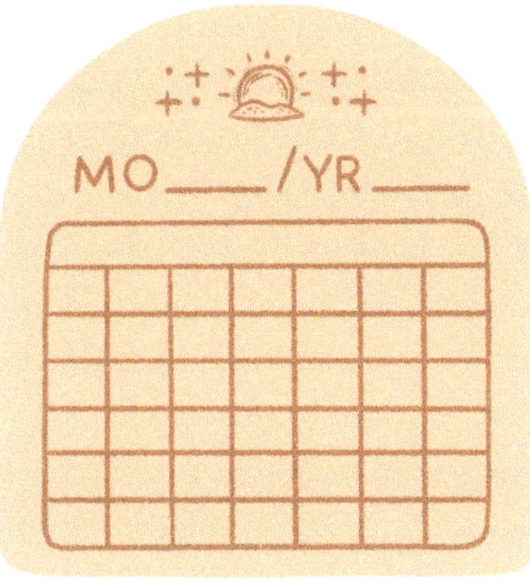
MO____/YR____

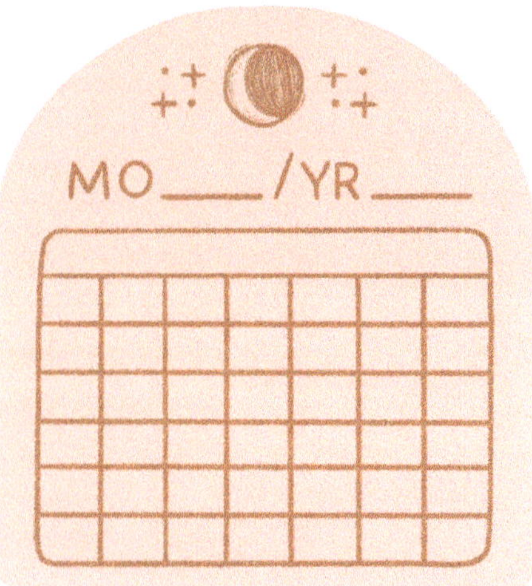
MO____/YR____

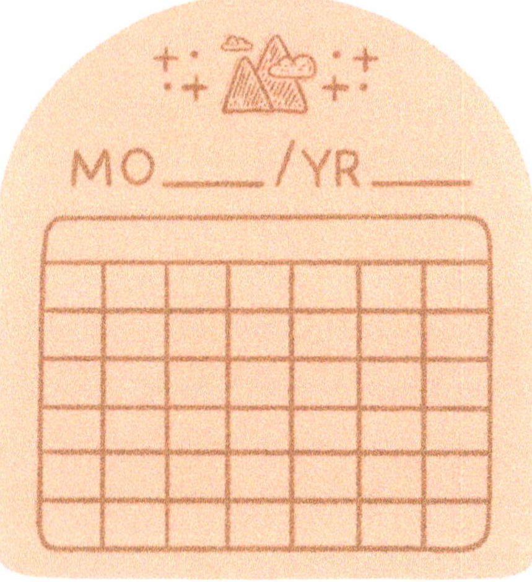
MO____/YR____

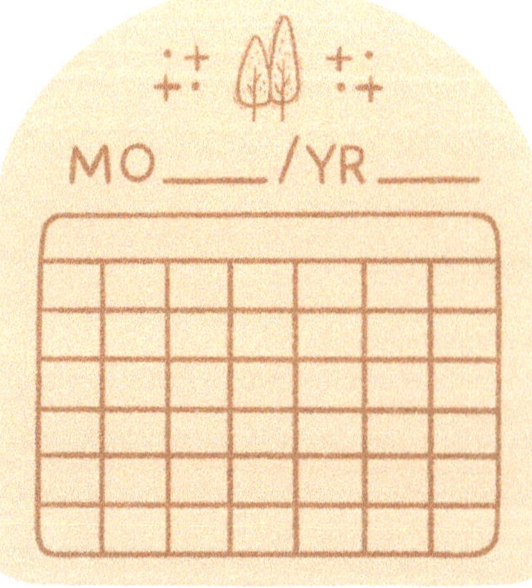
MO____/YR____

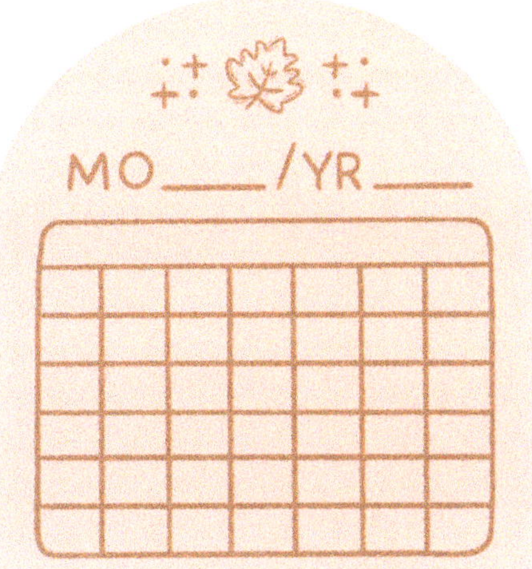

MO____/YR____

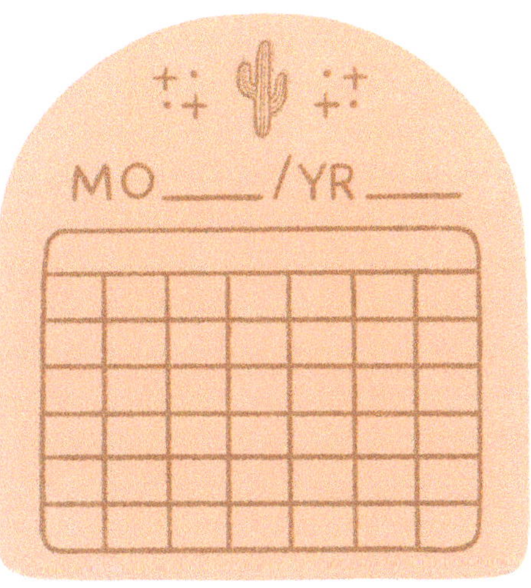

MO____/YR____

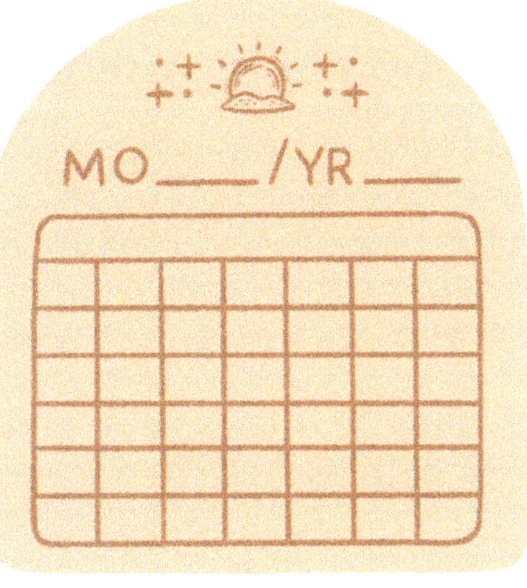

MO____/YR____

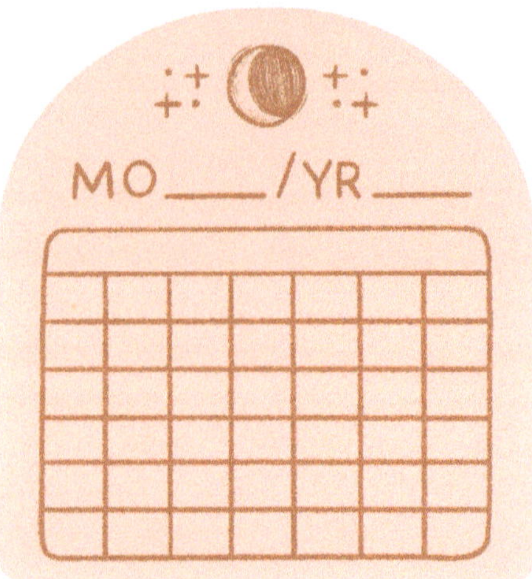

MO____/YR____

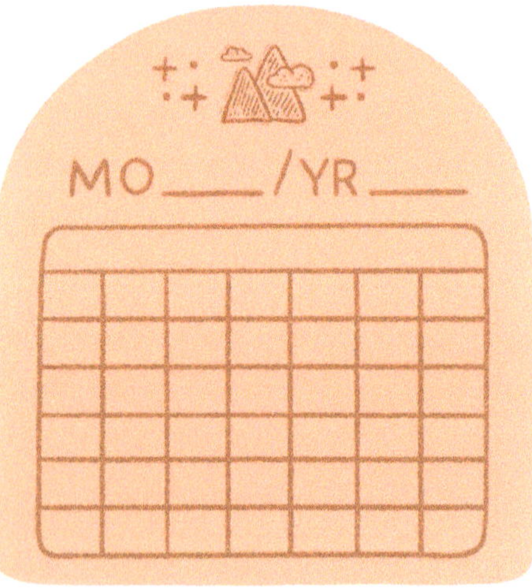

MO____/YR____

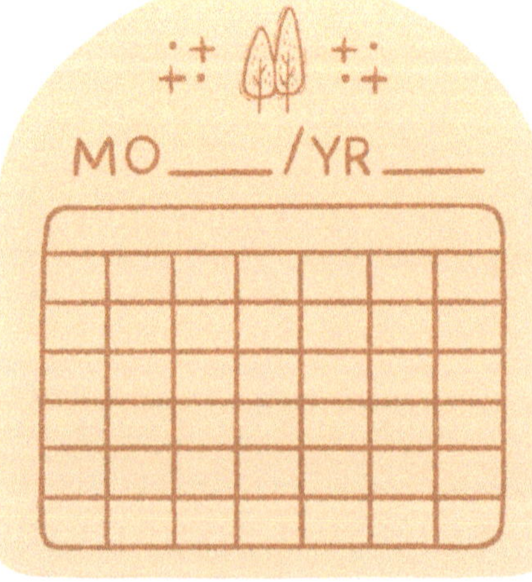

MO____/YR____

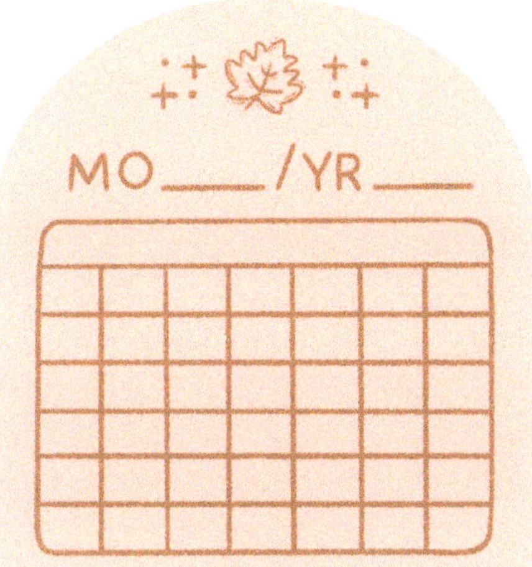
MO____/YR____

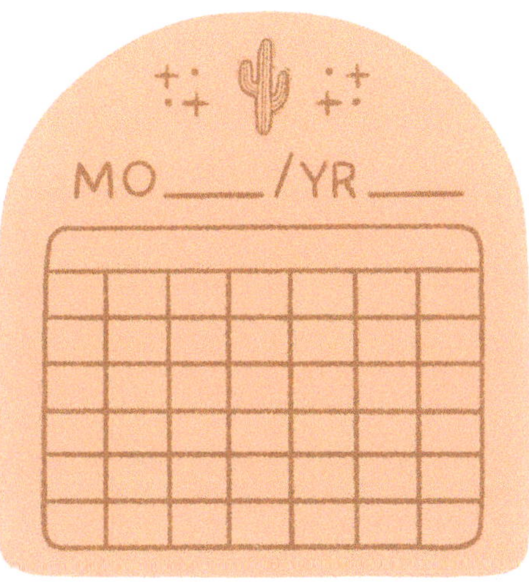
MO____/YR____

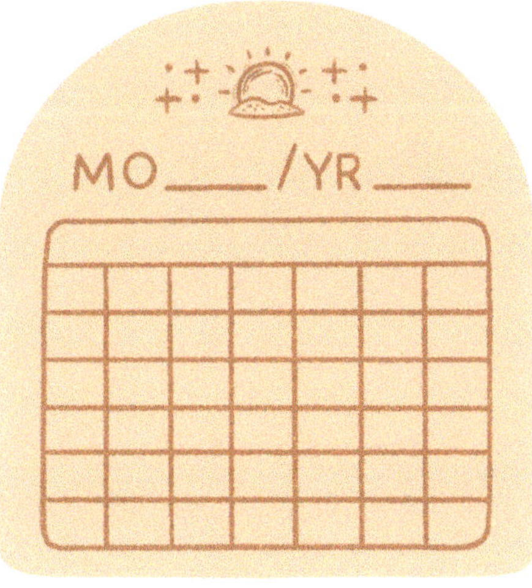
MO____/YR____

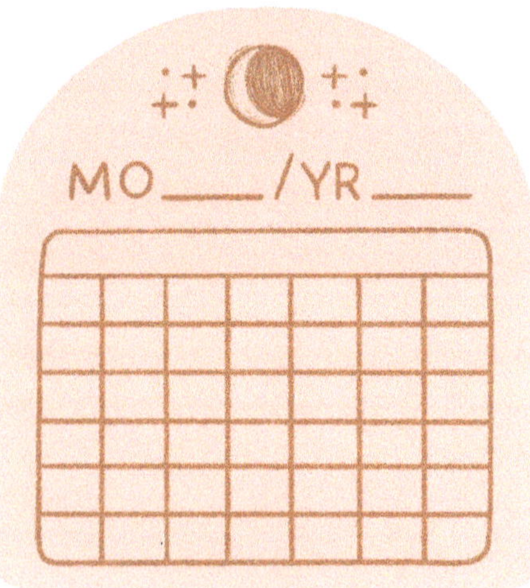
MO_____ /YR_____

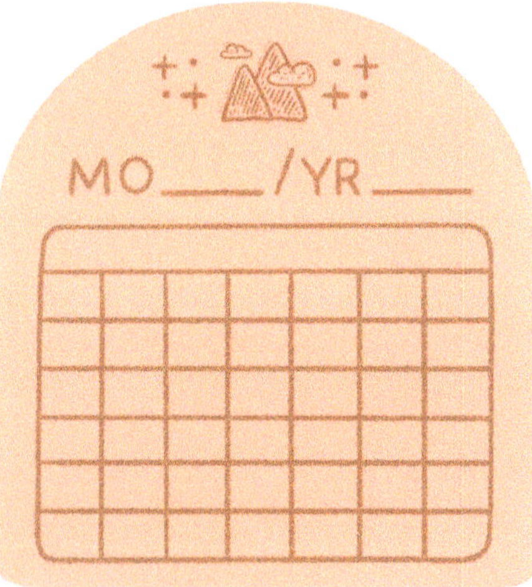
MO_____ /YR_____

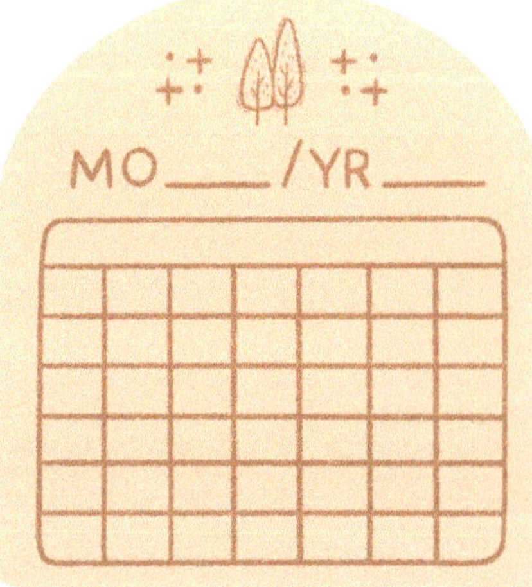
MO_____ /YR_____

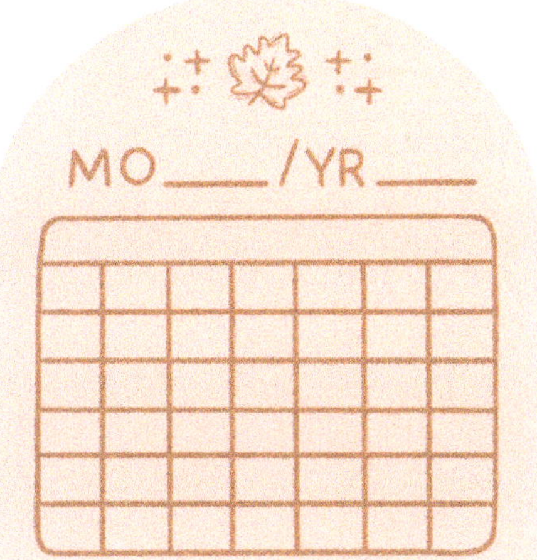
MO____/YR____

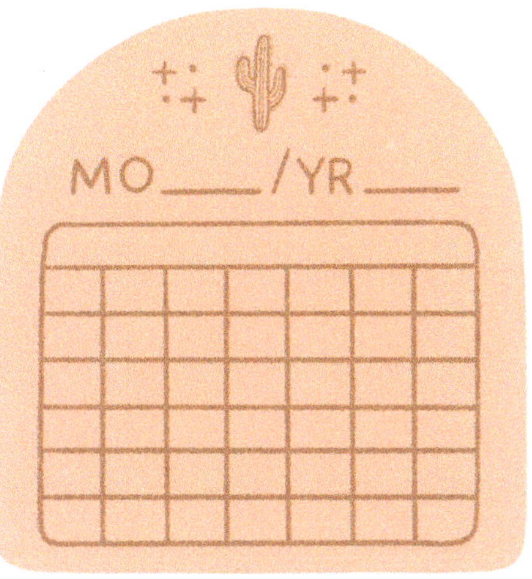
MO____/YR____

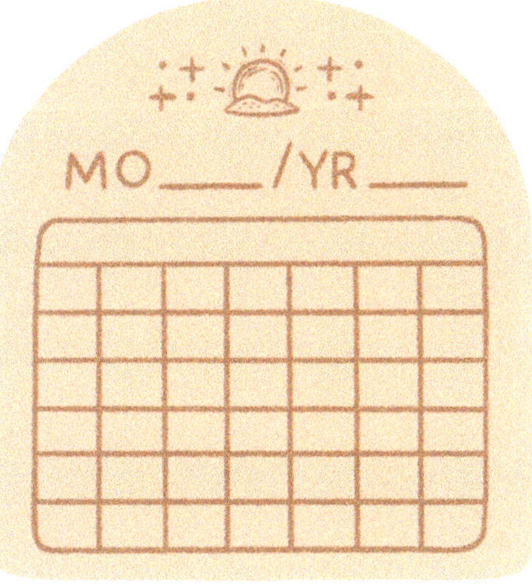
MO____/YR____

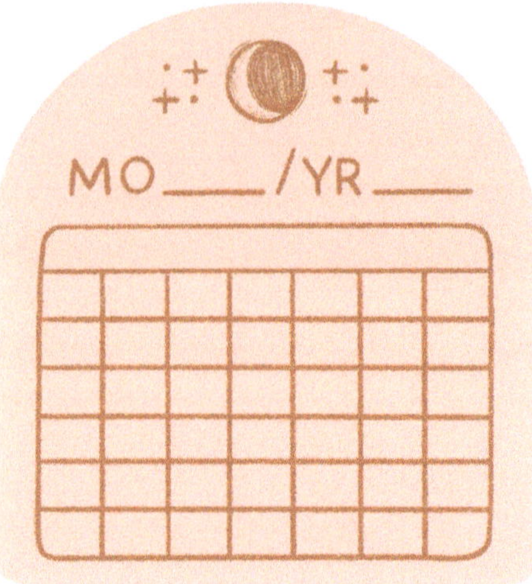
MO____/YR____

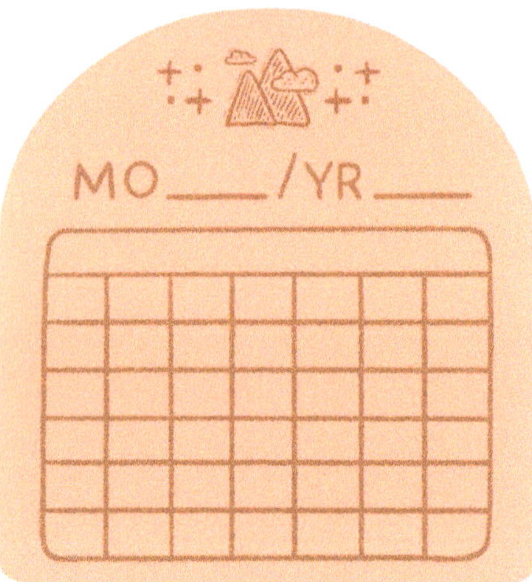
MO____/YR____

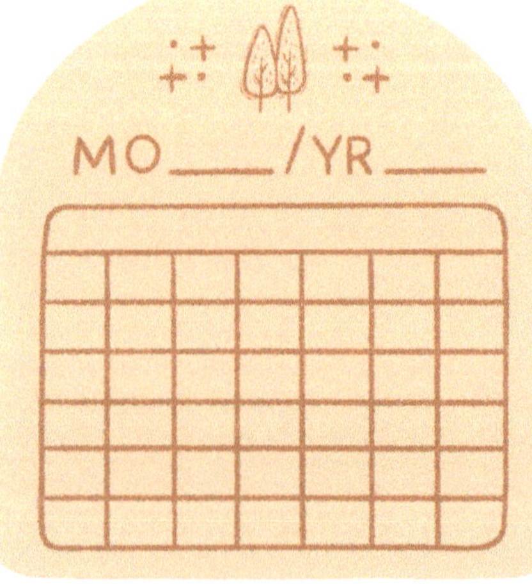
MO____/YR____

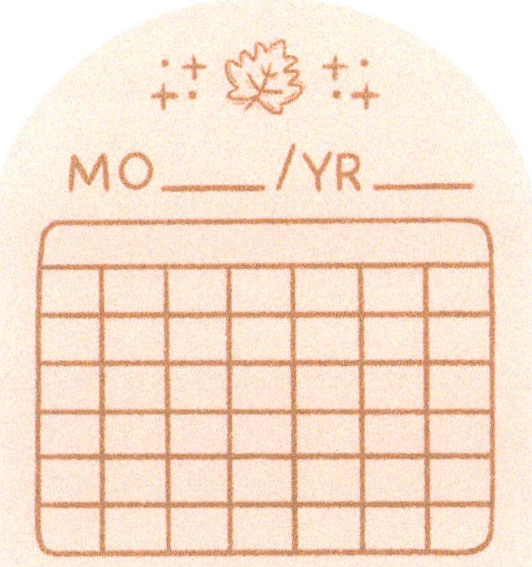

MO____/YR____

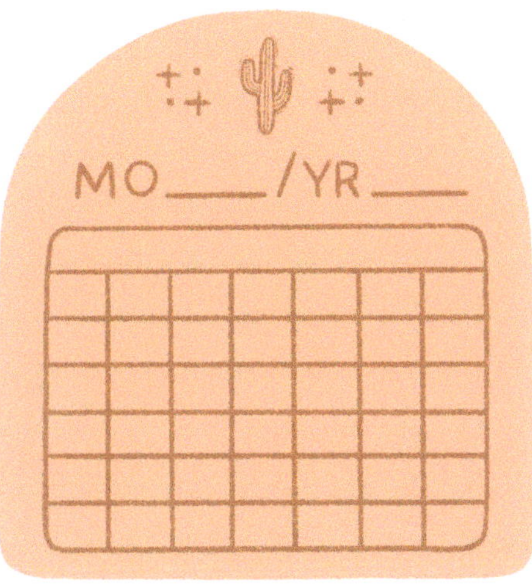

MO____/YR____

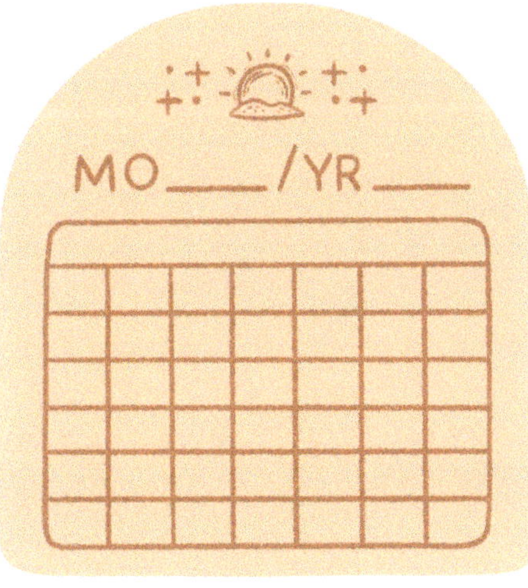

MO____/YR____

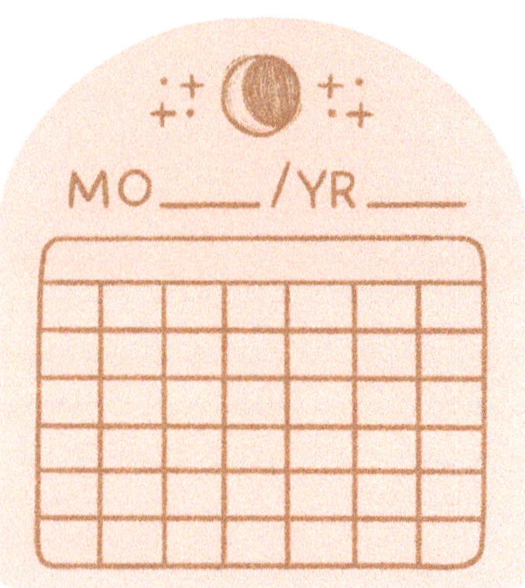
MO____/YR____

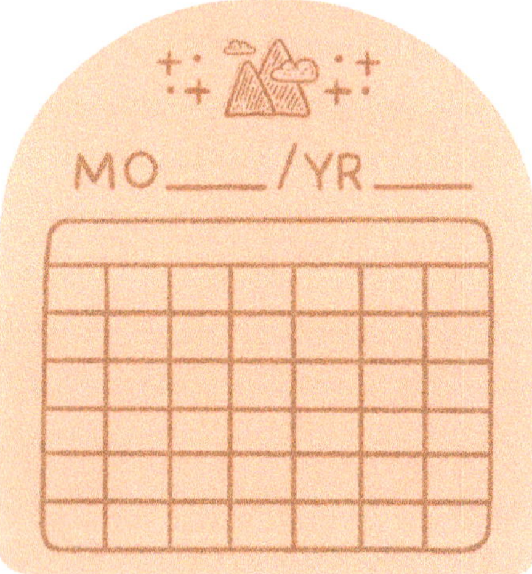
MO____/YR____

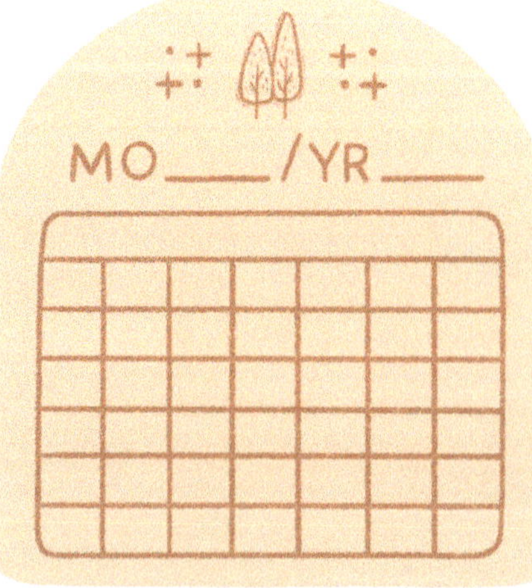
MO____/YR____

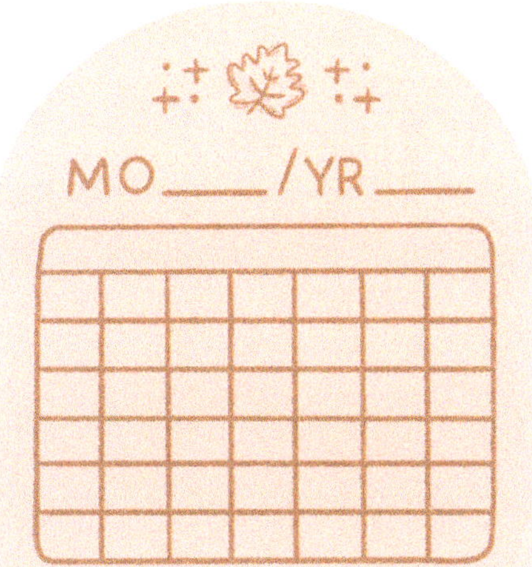

MO____/YR____

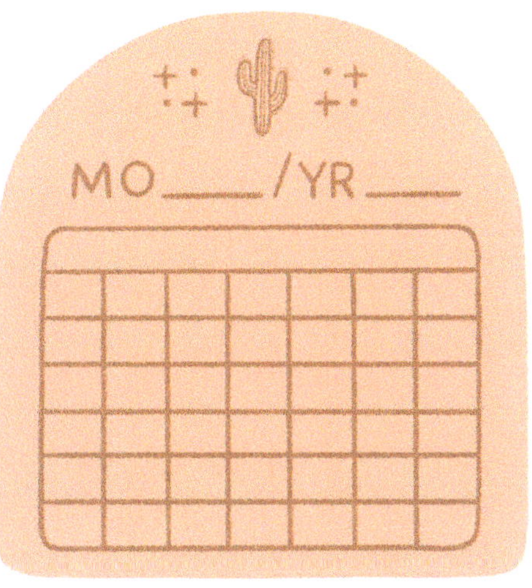

MO____/YR____

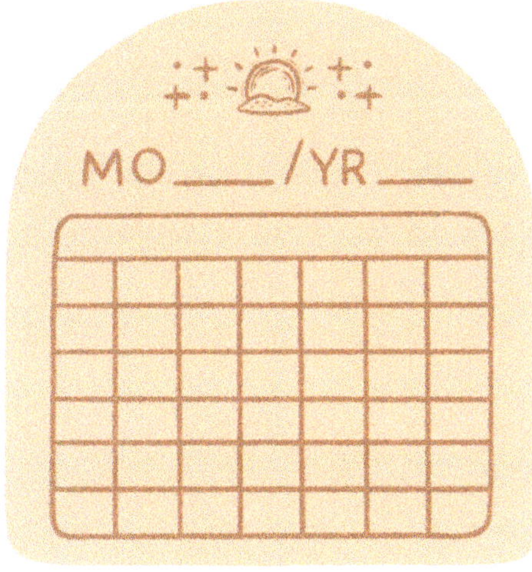

MO____/YR____

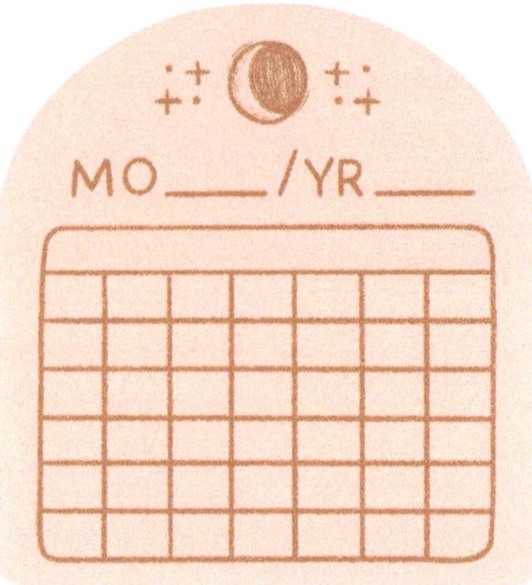

MO ___/YR ___

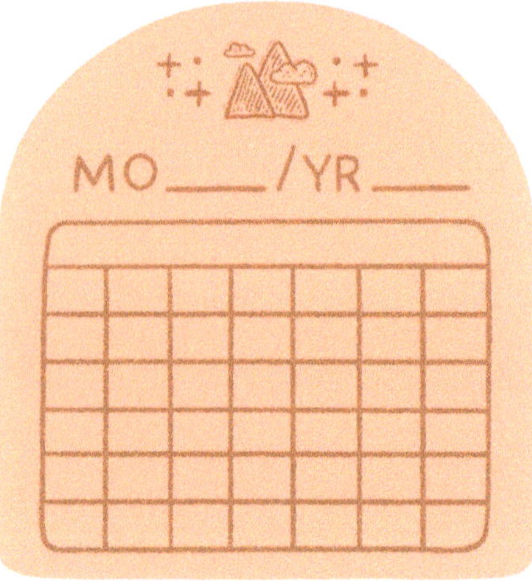

MO ___/YR ___

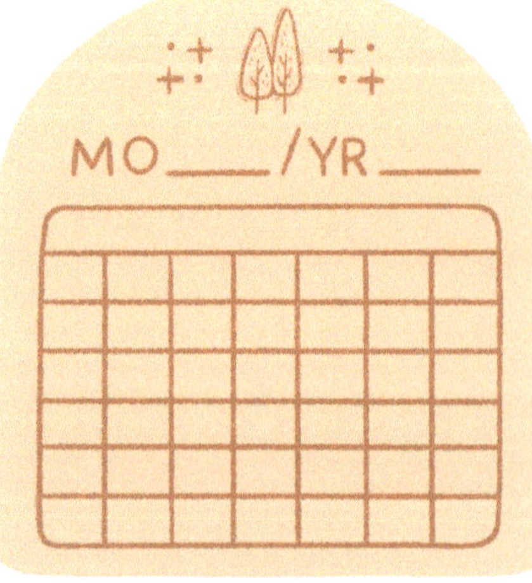

MO ___/YR ___

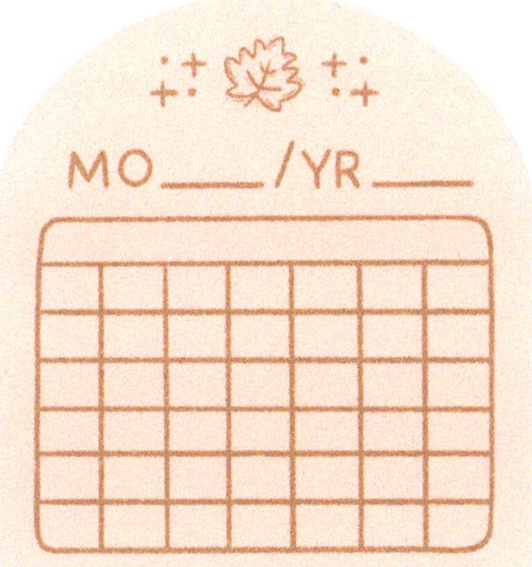
MO____/YR____

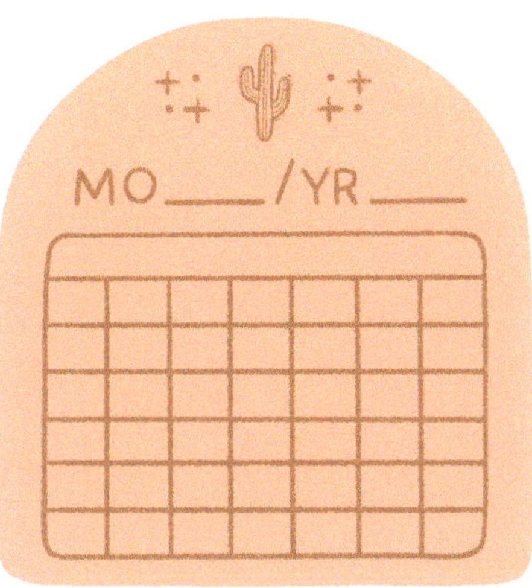
MO____/YR____

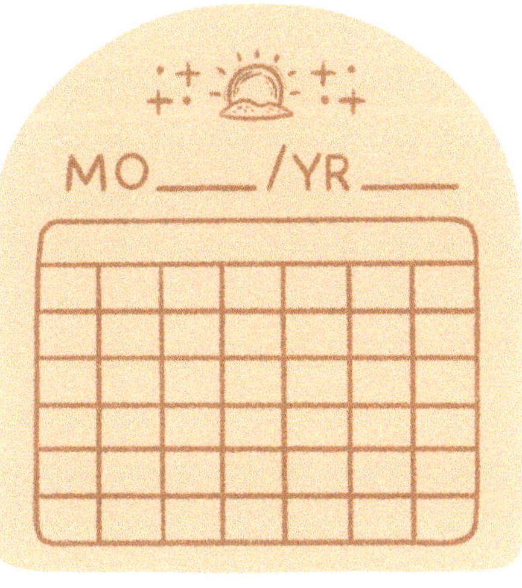
MO____/YR____

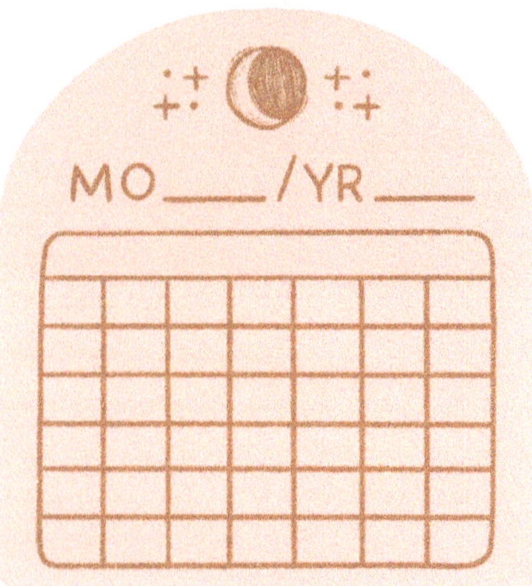
MO____/YR____

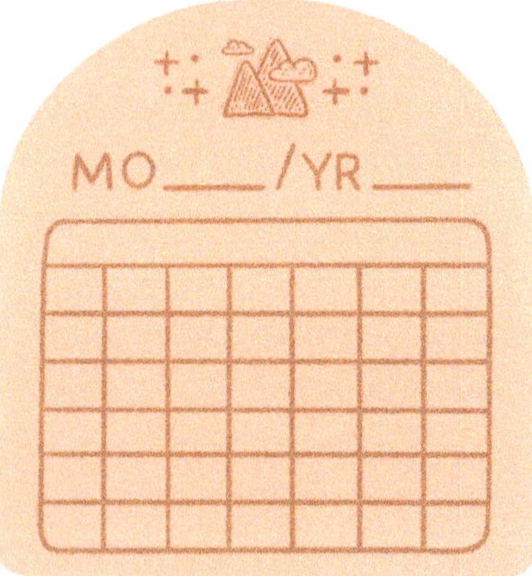
MO____/YR____

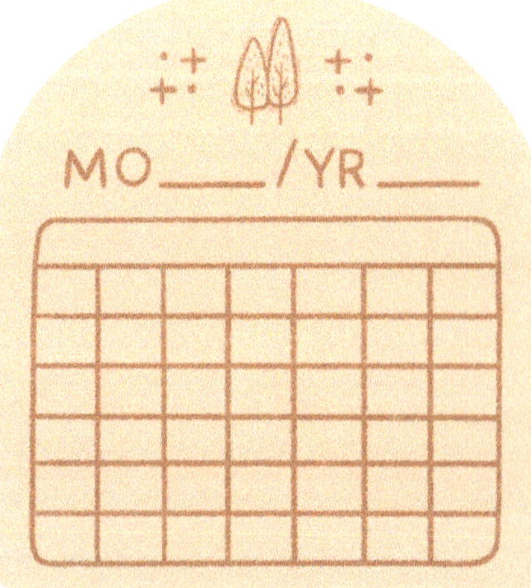
MO____/YR____

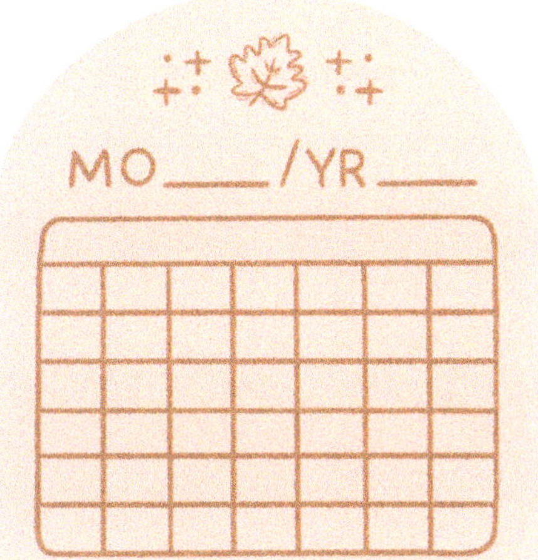
MO____/YR____

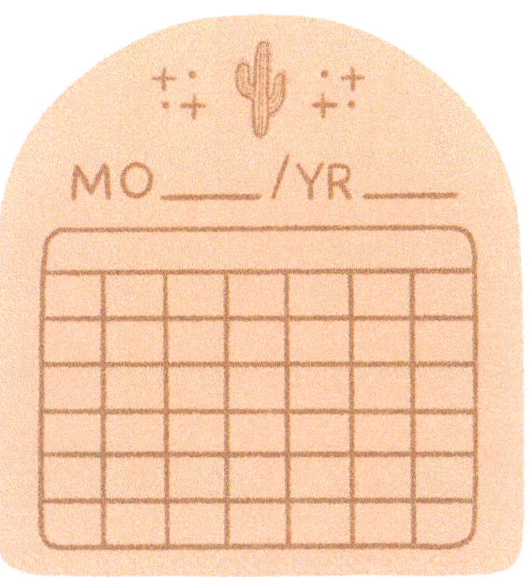
MO____/YR____

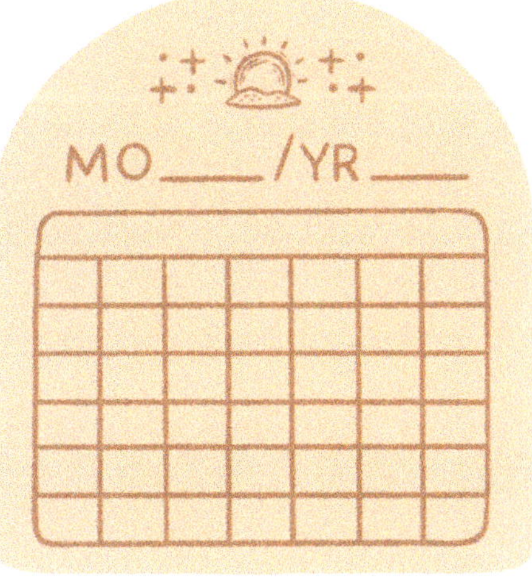
MO____/YR____

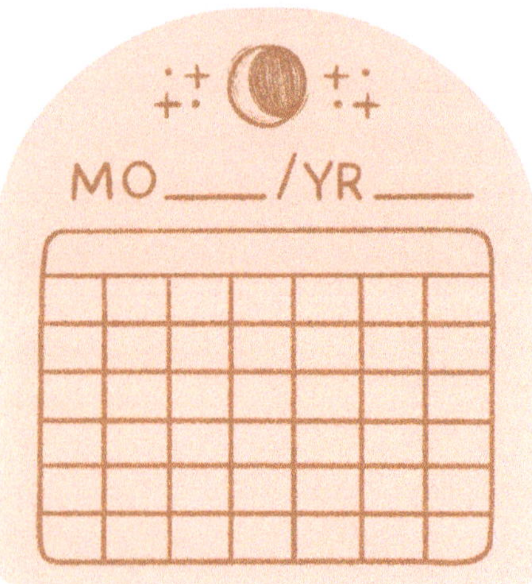

MO____/YR____

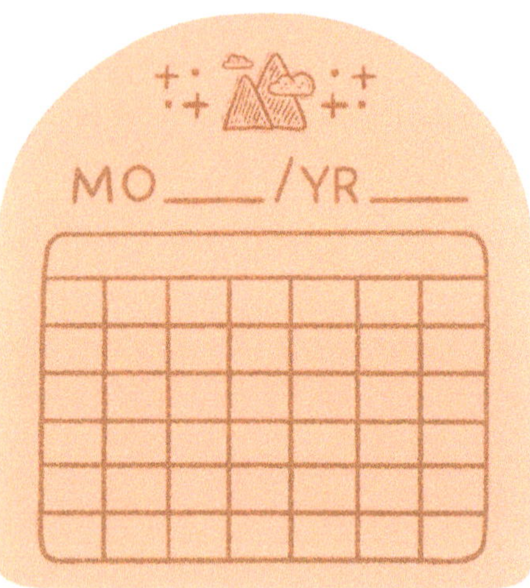

MO____/YR____

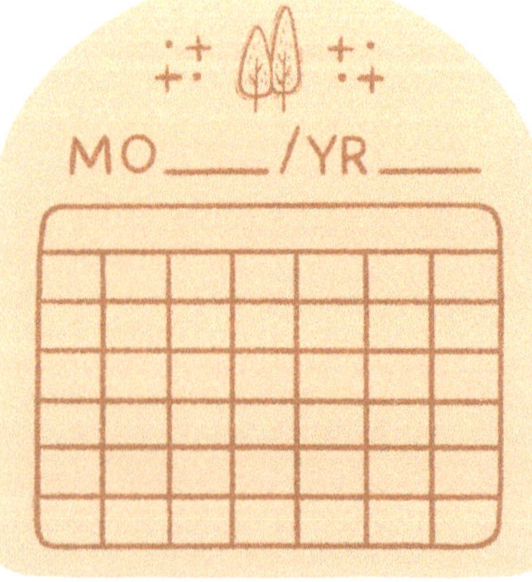

MO____/YR____

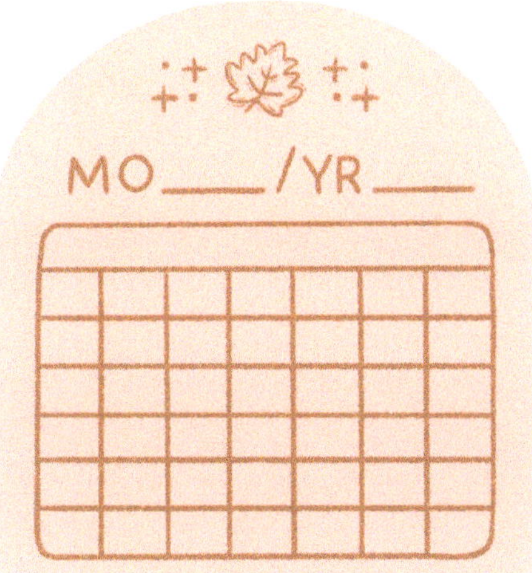

MO____/YR____

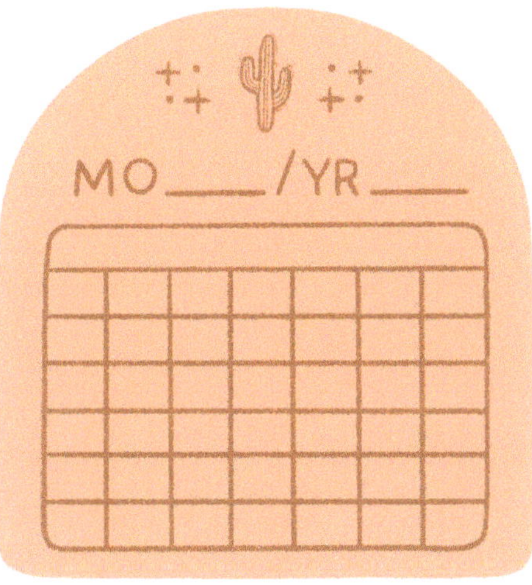

MO____/YR____

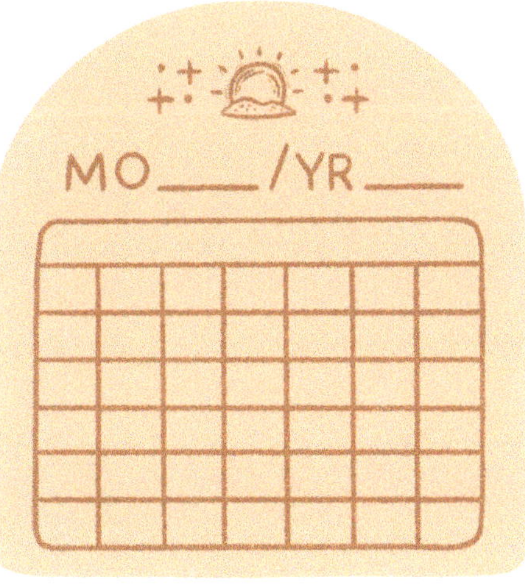

MO____/YR____

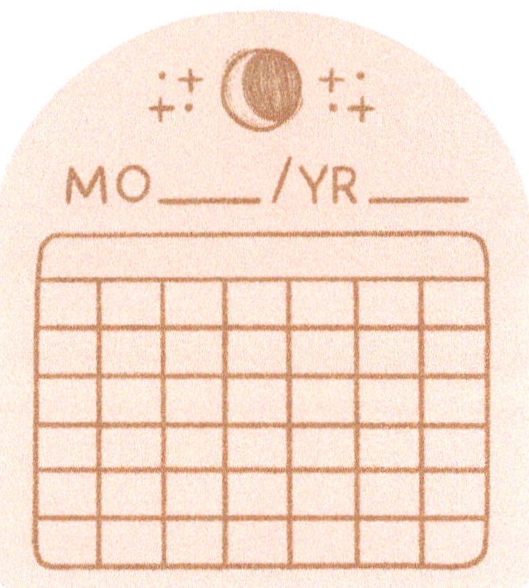
MO____/YR____

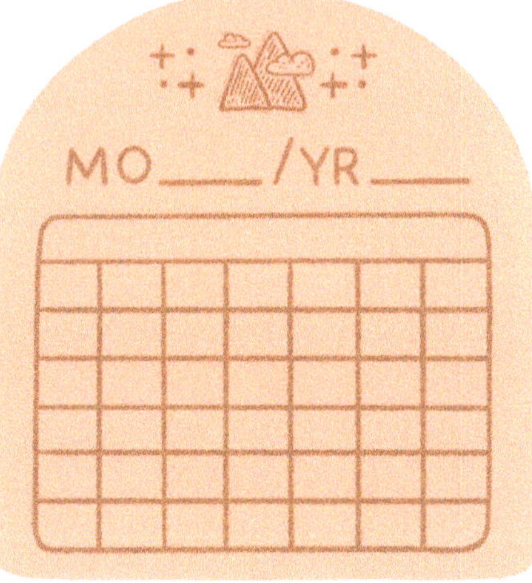
MO____/YR____

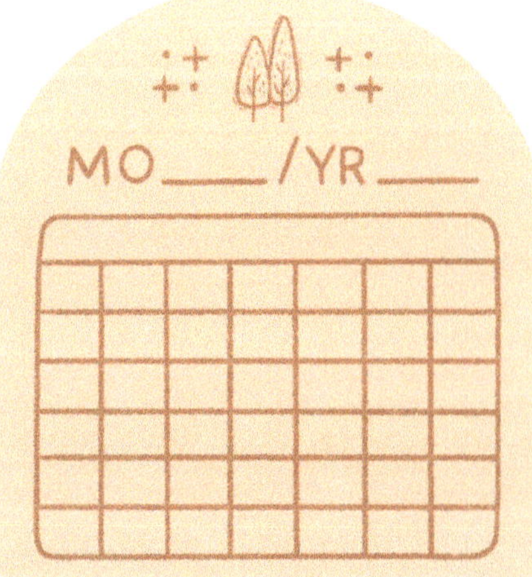
MO____/YR____

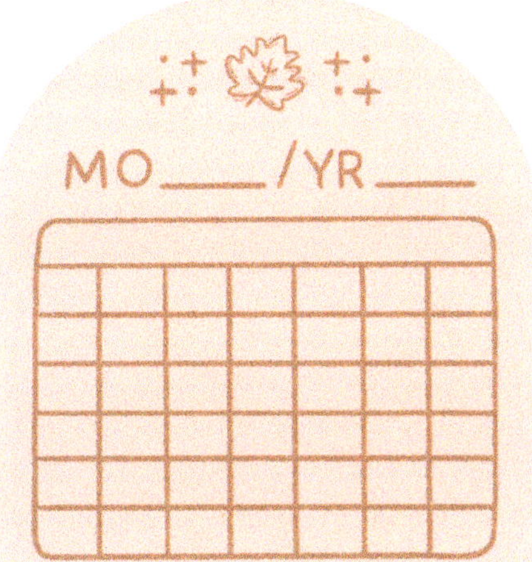
MO____/YR____

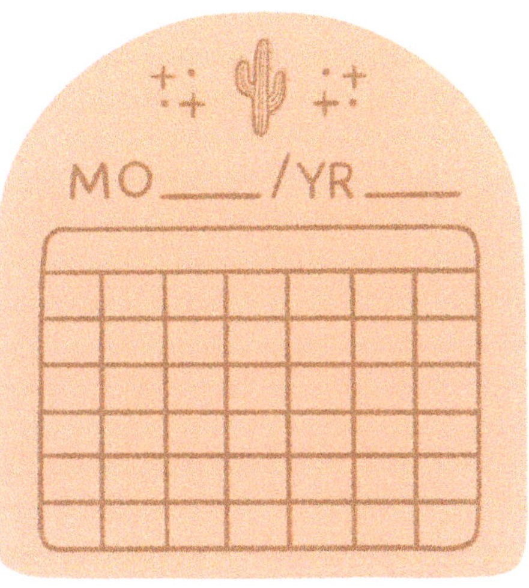
MO____/YR____

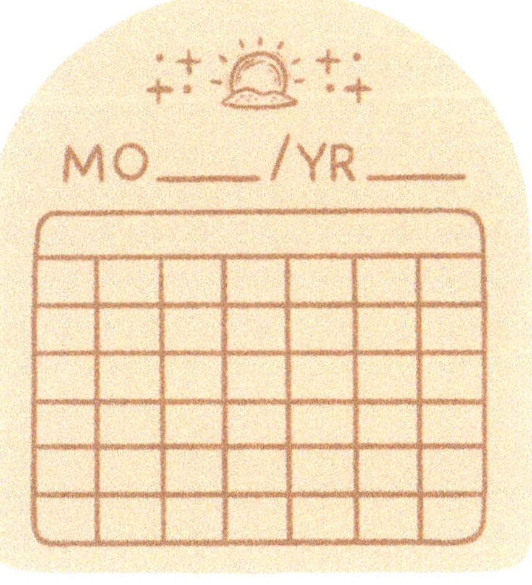
MO____/YR____

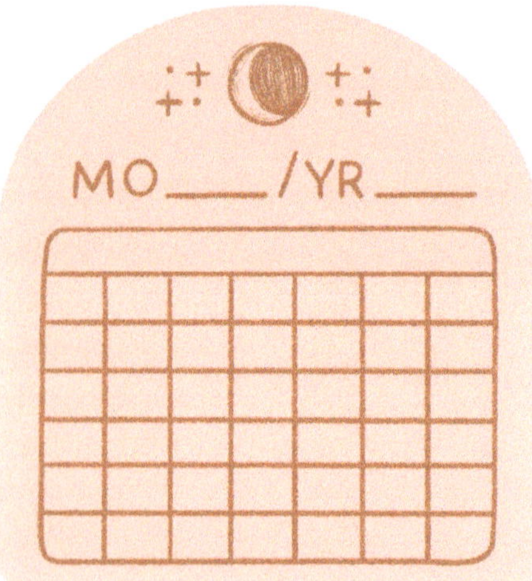
MO____/YR____

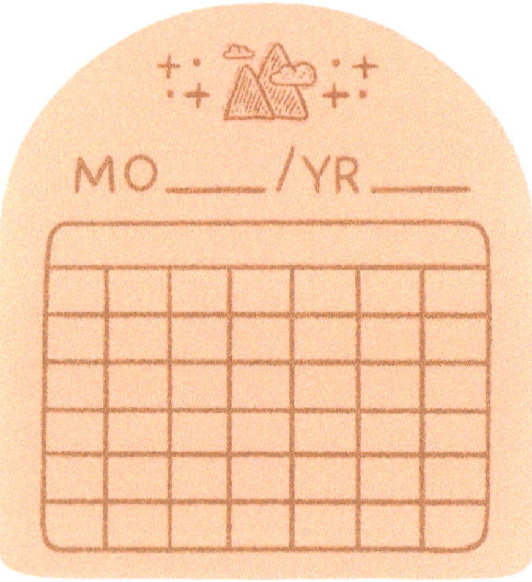
MO____/YR____

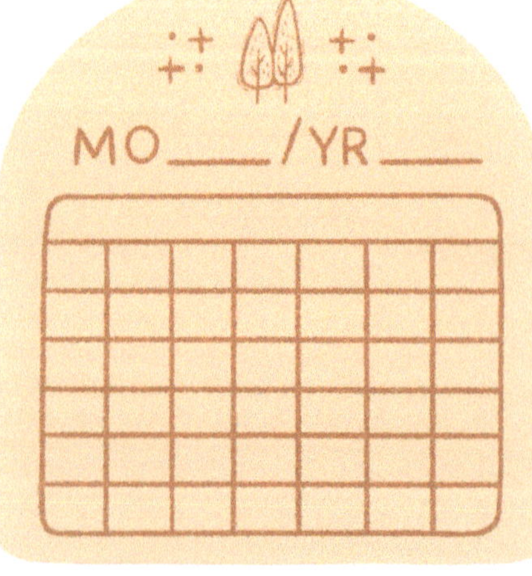
MO____/YR____

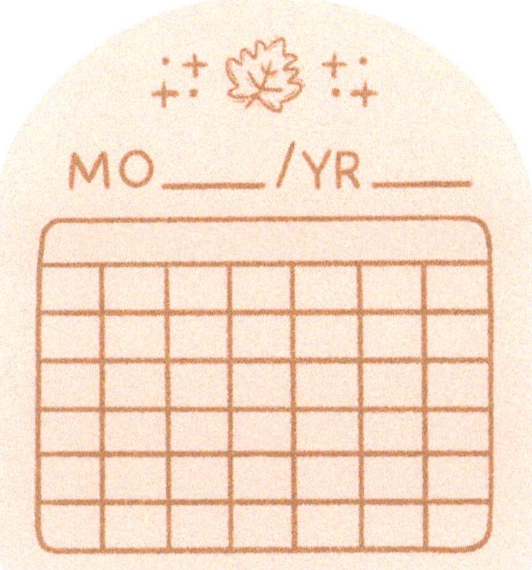
MO___/YR___

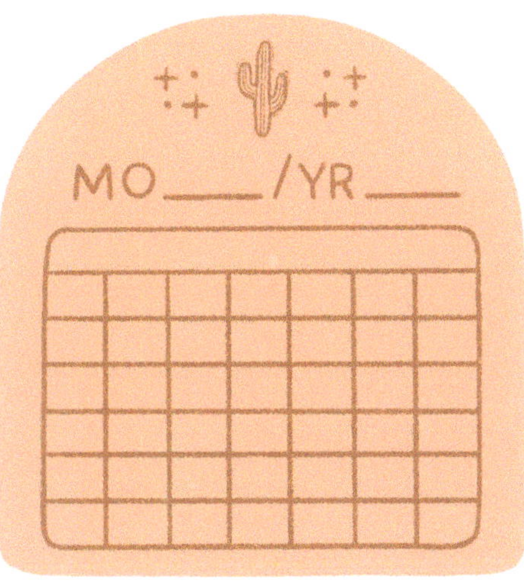
MO___/YR___

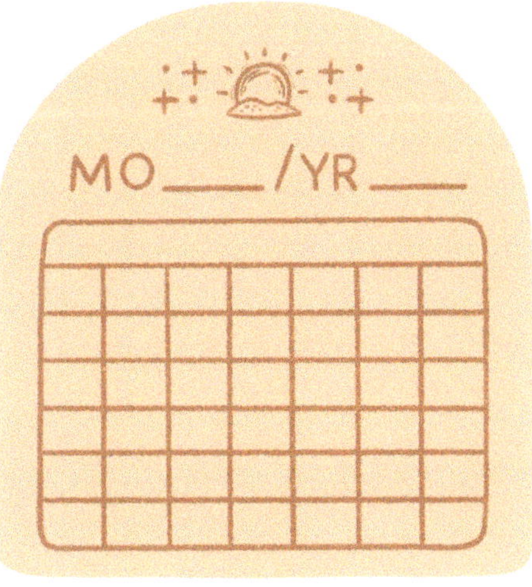
MO___/YR___

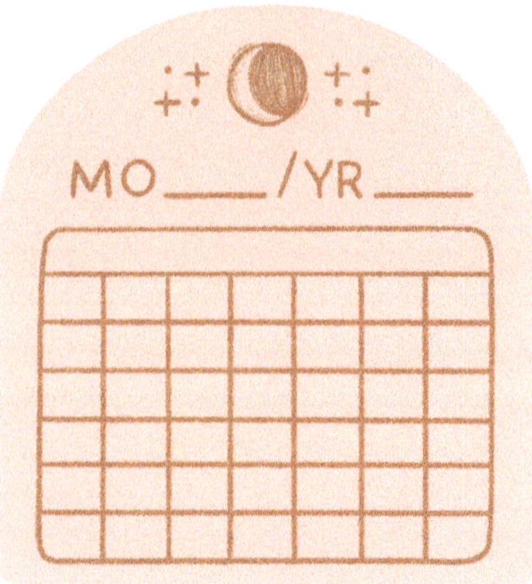

MO____/YR____

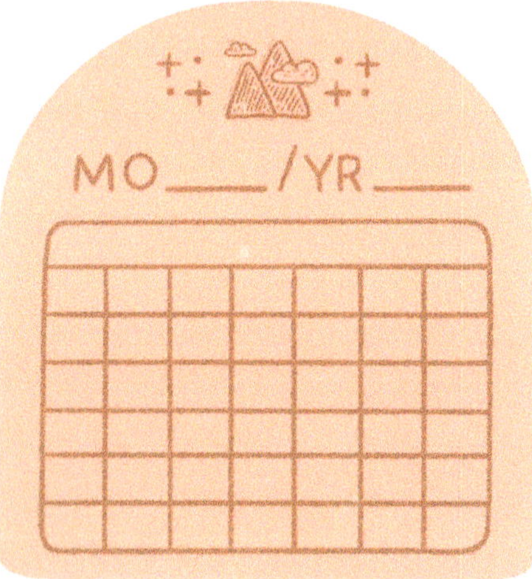

MO____/YR____

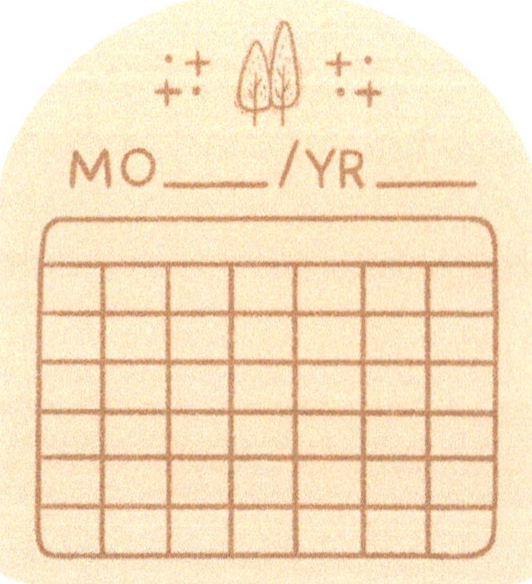

MO____/YR____

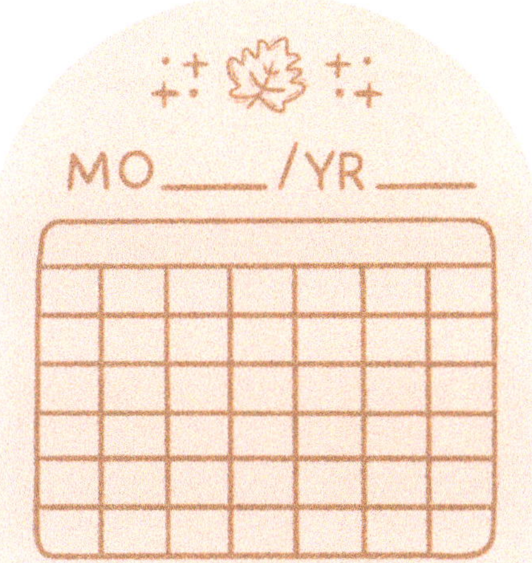

MO____/YR____

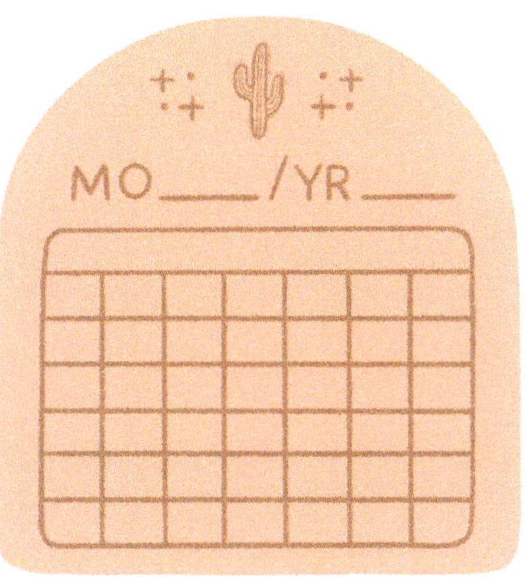

MO____/YR____

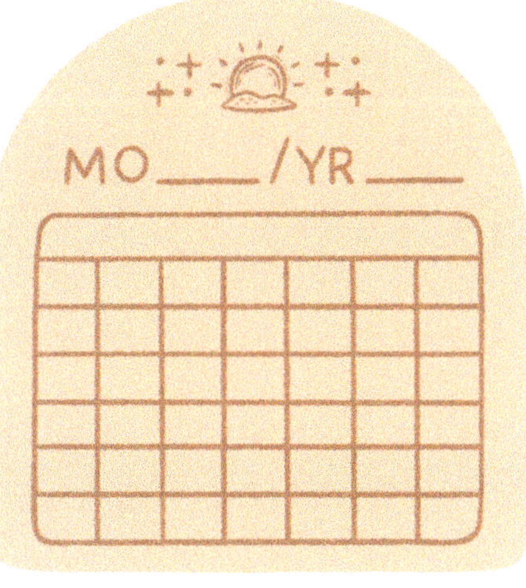

MO____/YR____

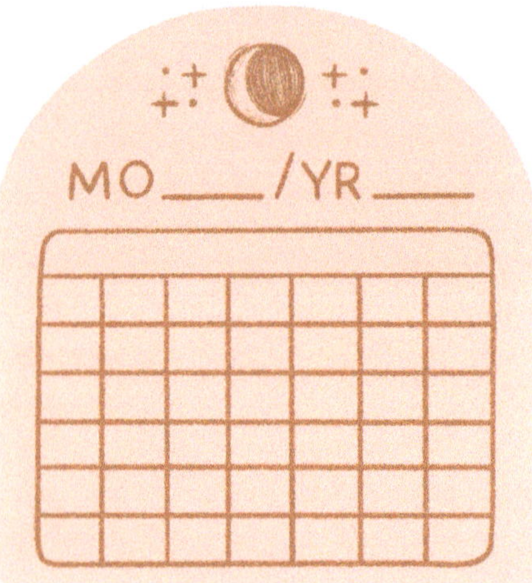
MO____/YR____

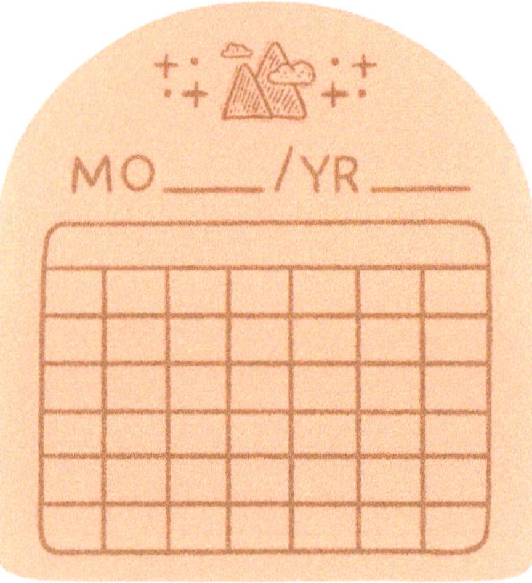
MO____/YR____

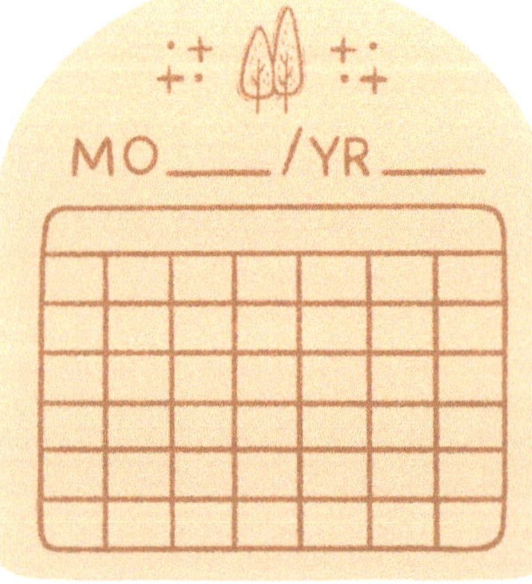
MO____/YR____

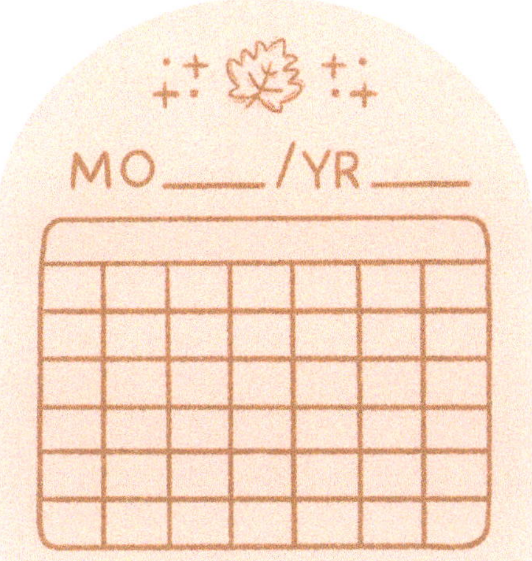

MO ____ / YR ____

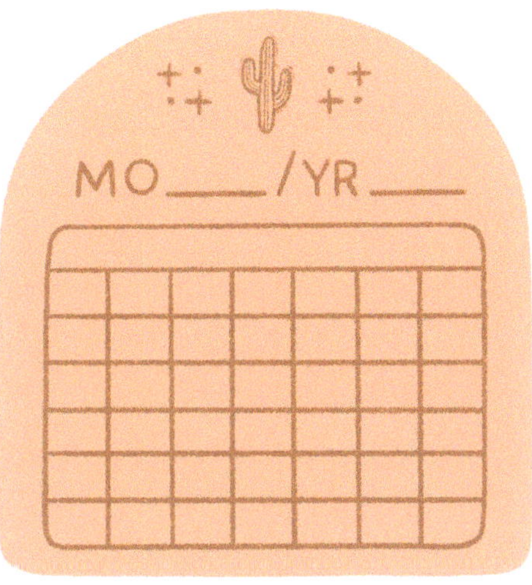

MO ____ / YR ____

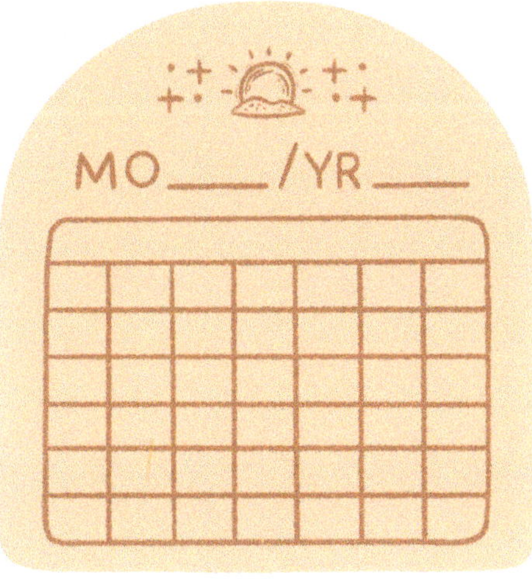

MO ____ / YR ____

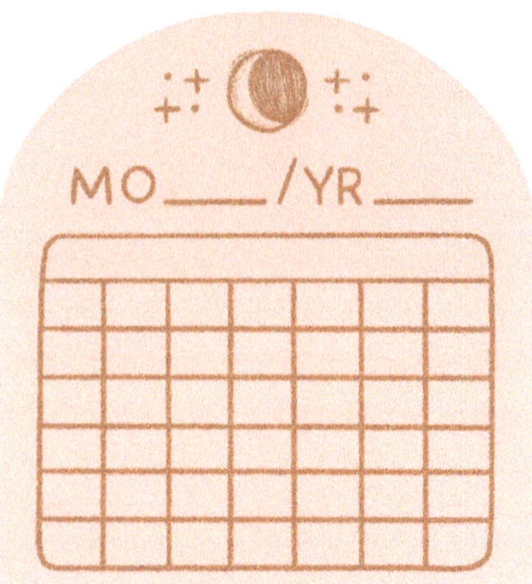

MO____ / YR____

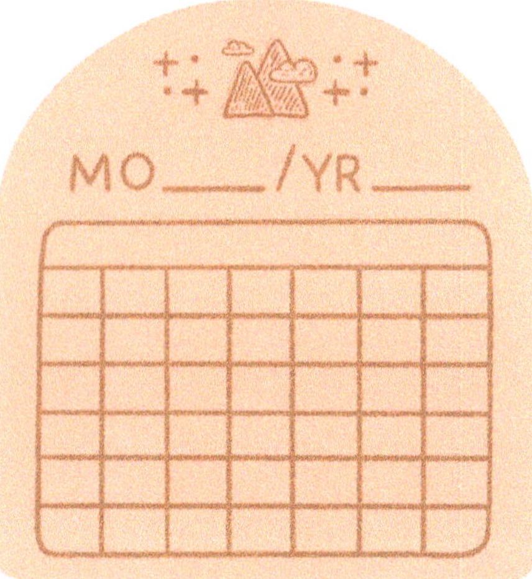

MO____ / YR____

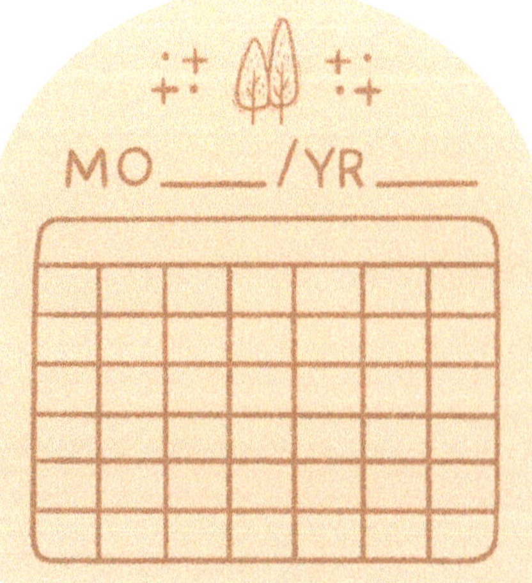

MO____ / YR____

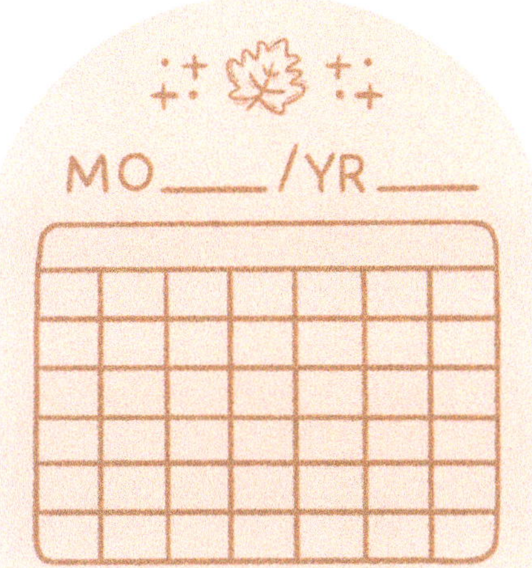
MO____/YR____

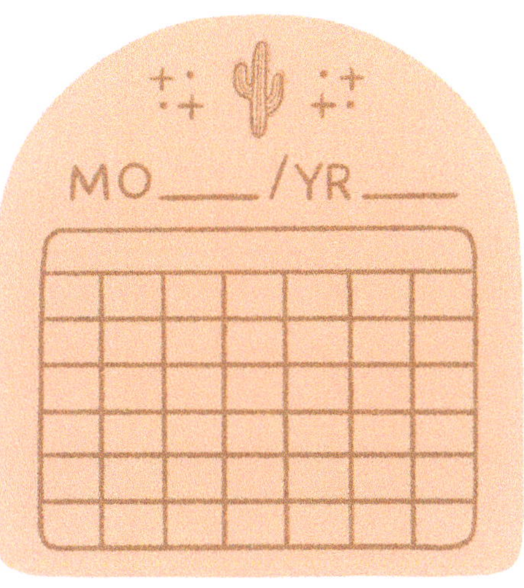
MO____/YR____

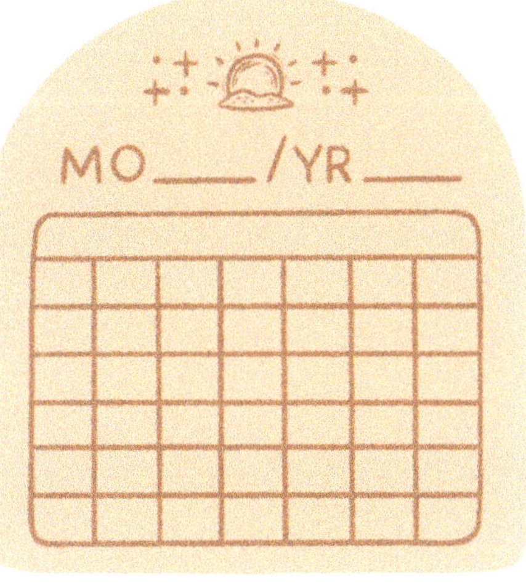
MO____/YR____

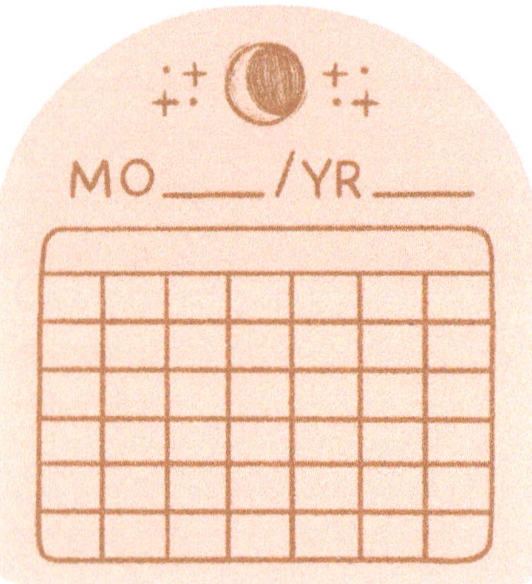

MO____/YR____

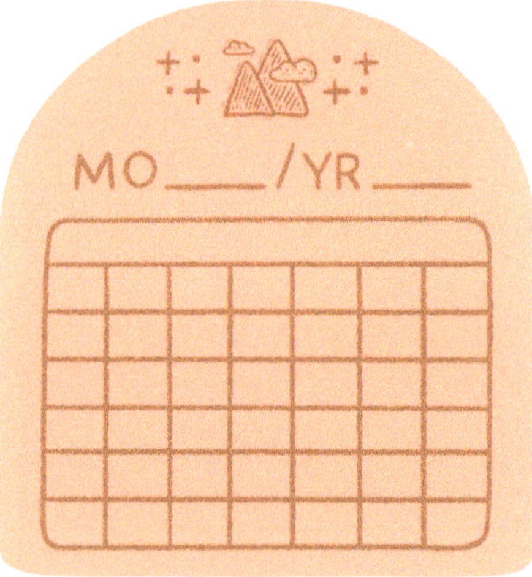

MO____/YR____

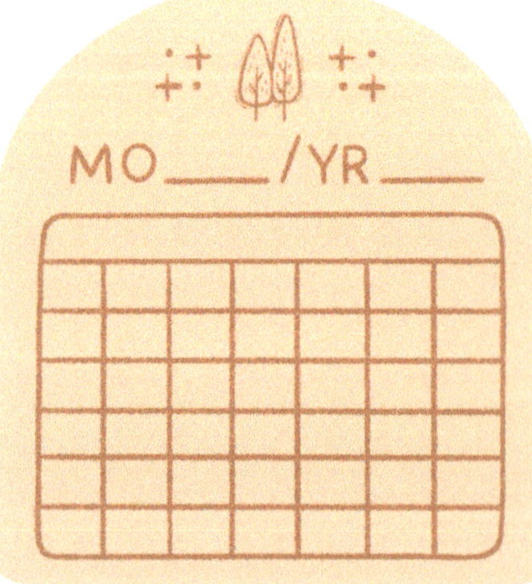

MO____/YR____

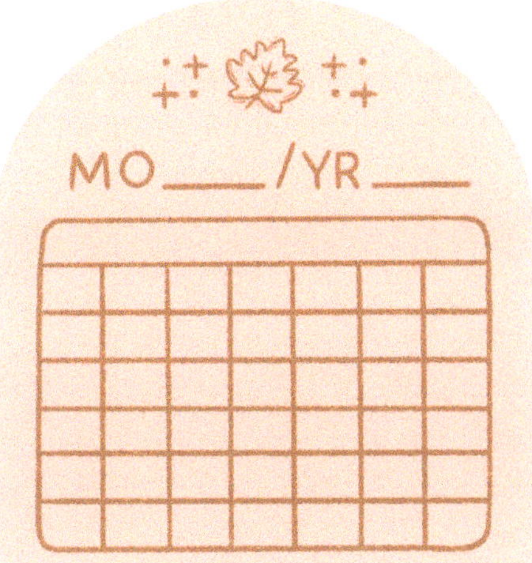

MO____/YR____

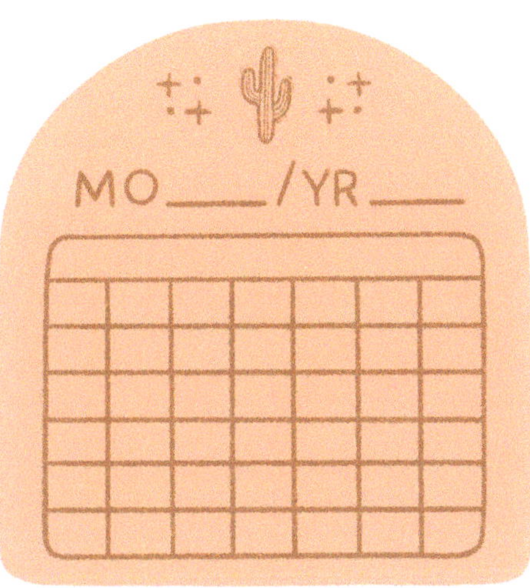

MO____/YR____

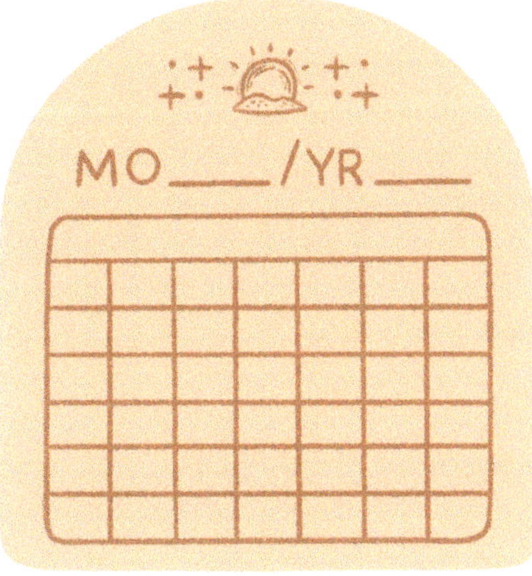

MO____/YR____

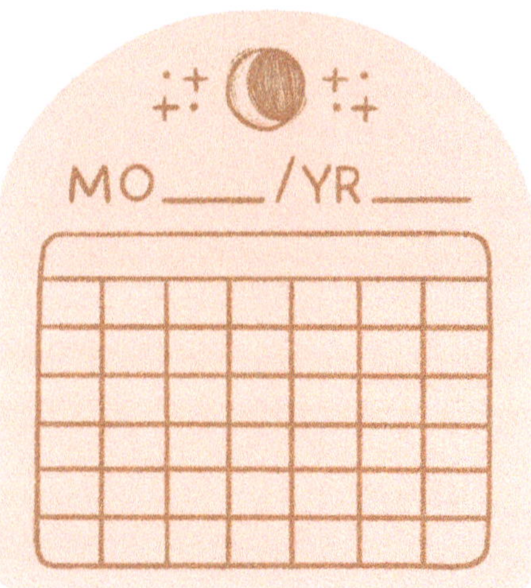

MO____/YR____

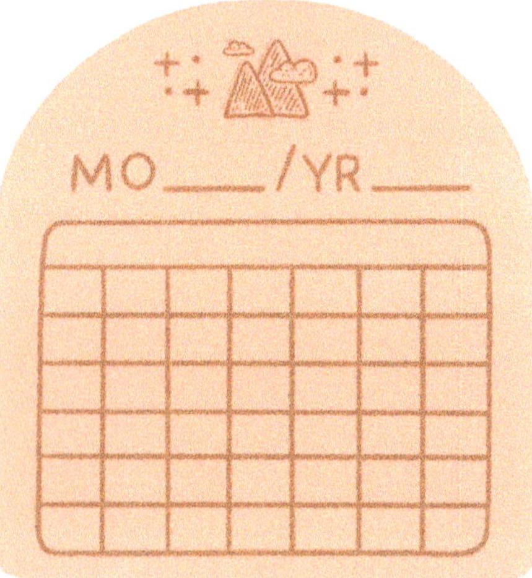

MO____/YR____

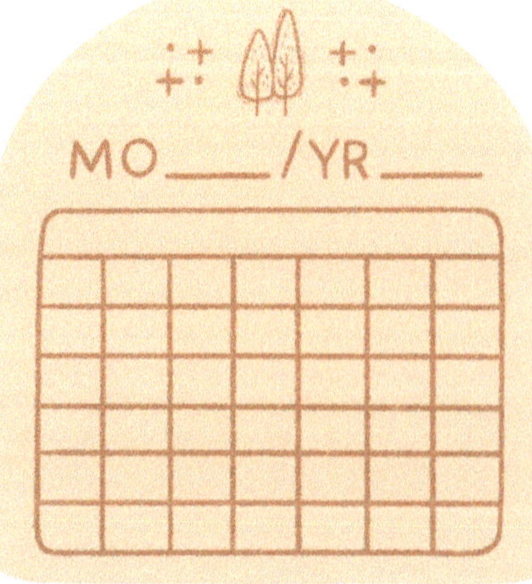

MO____/YR____

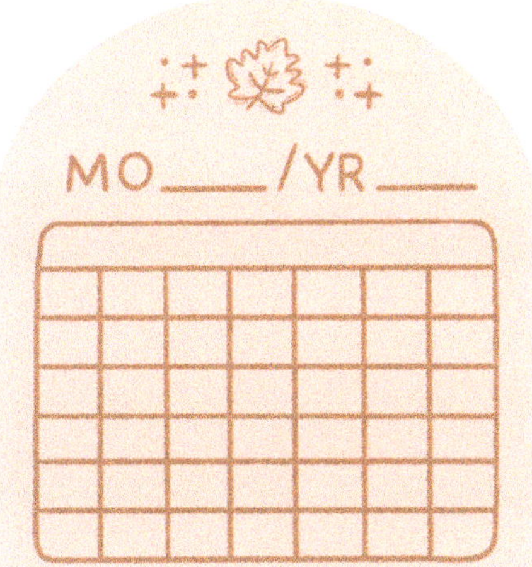
MO____/YR____

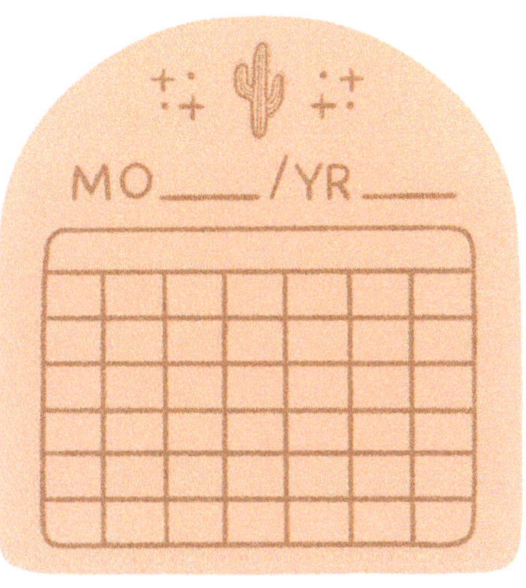
MO____/YR____

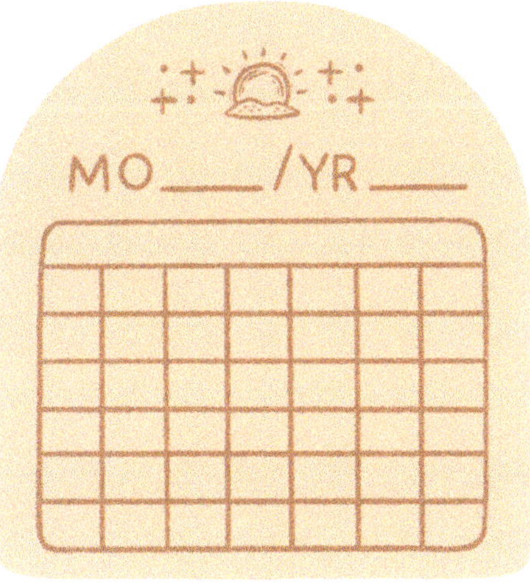
MO____/YR____

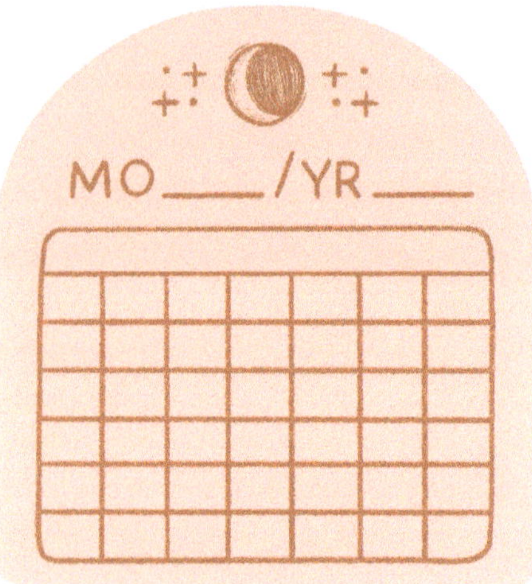

MO____/YR____

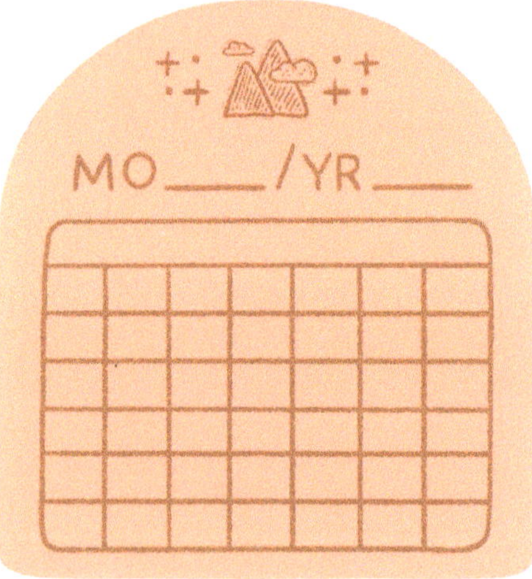

MO____/YR____

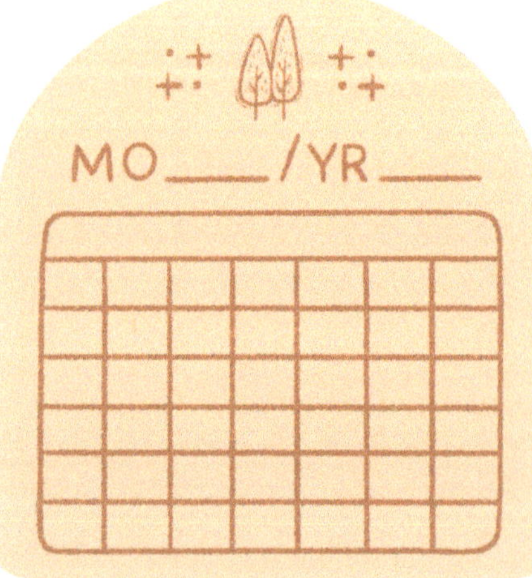

MO____/YR____

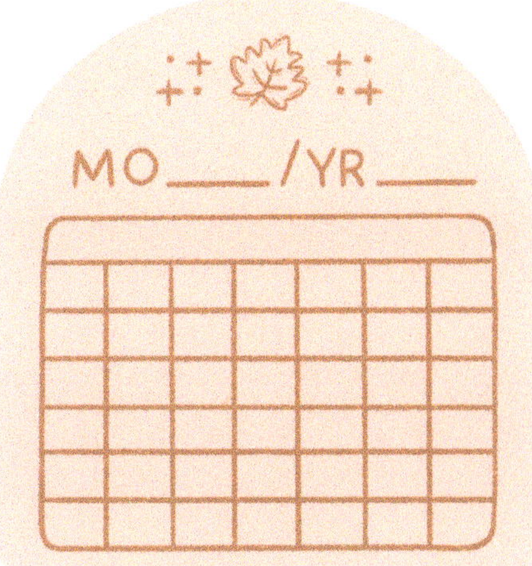
MO____/YR____

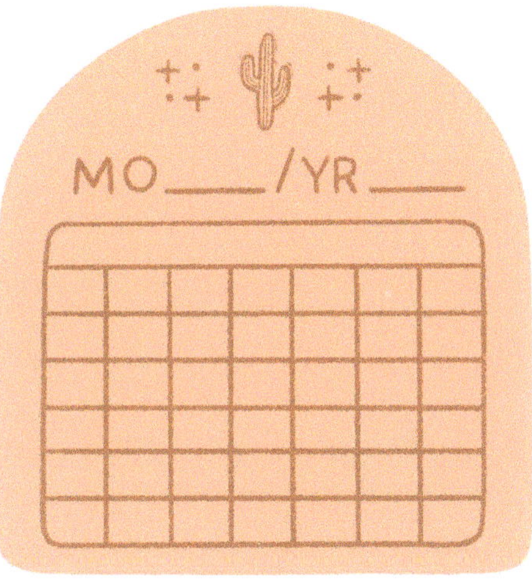
MO____/YR____

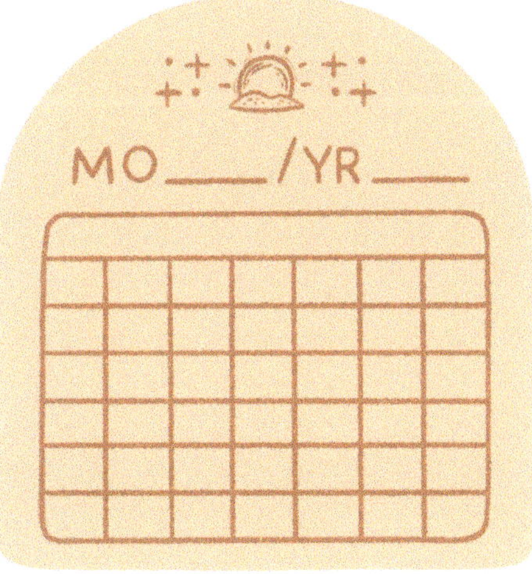
MO____/YR____

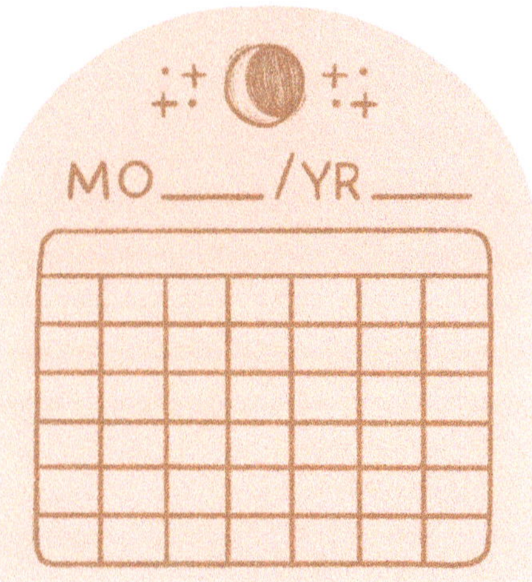

MO____/YR____

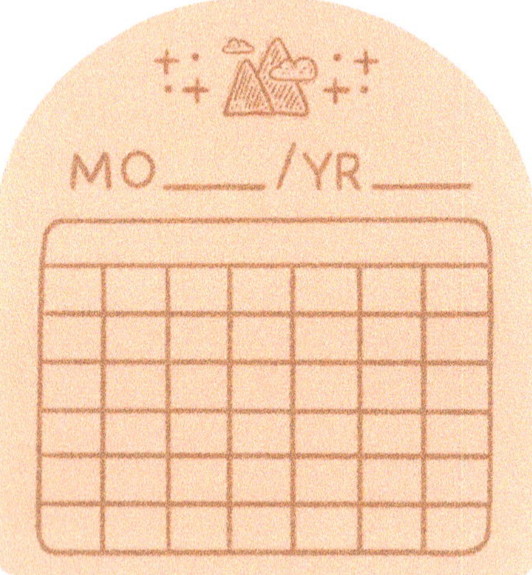

MO____/YR____

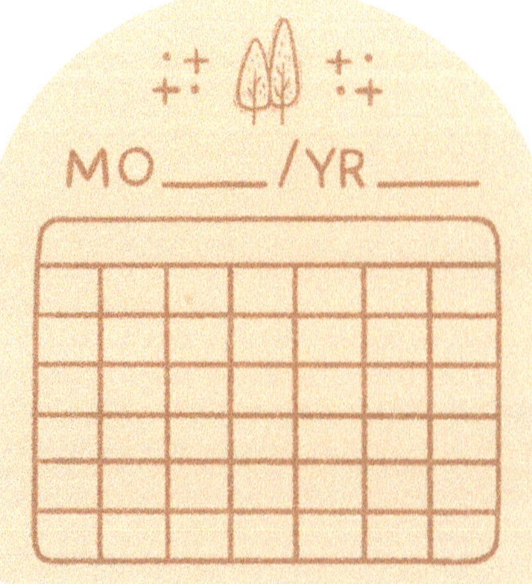

MO____/YR____

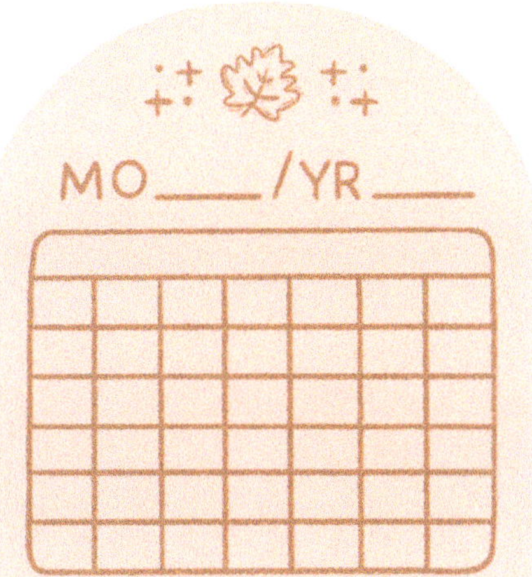

MO____/YR____

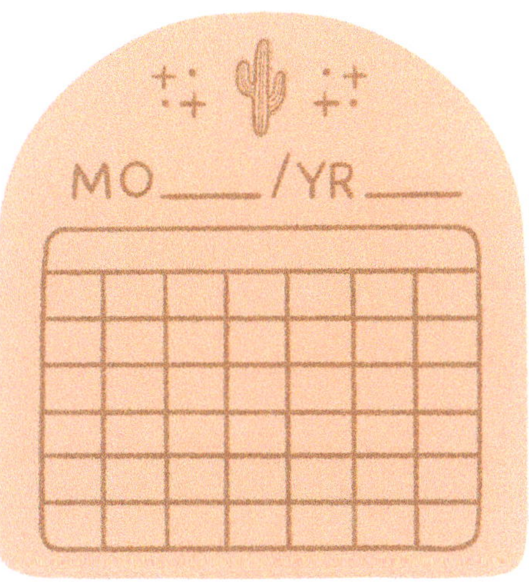

MO____/YR____

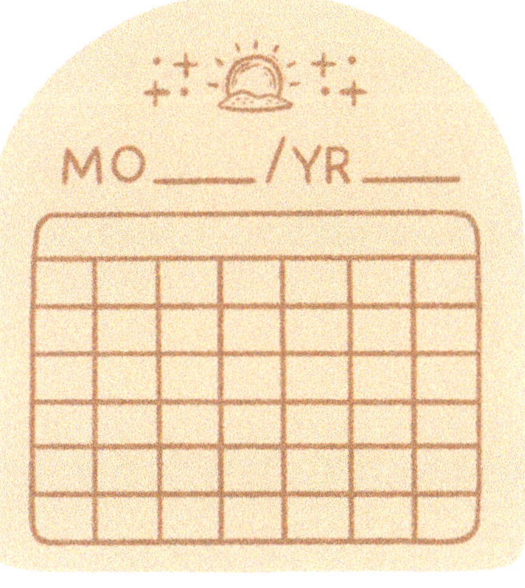

MO____/YR____

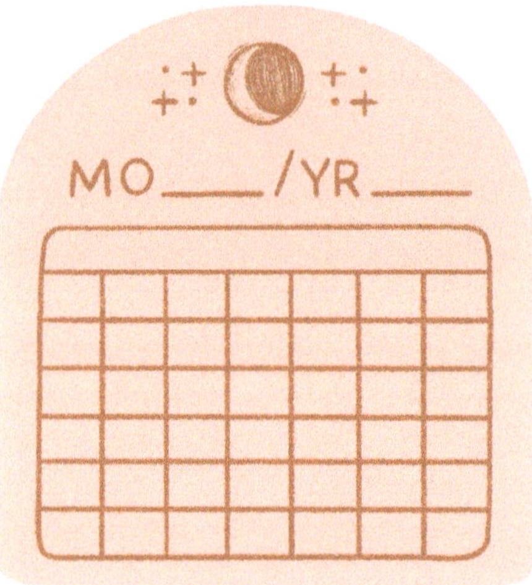

MO____/YR____

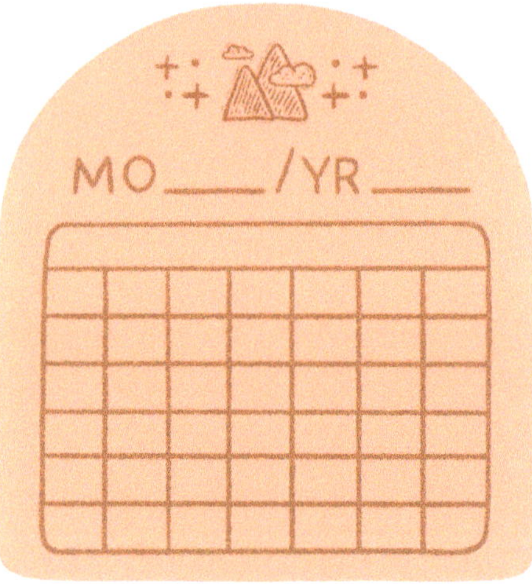

MO____/YR____

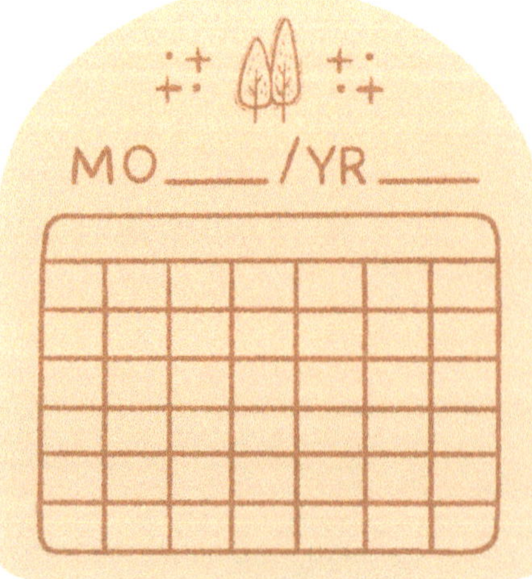

MO____/YR____

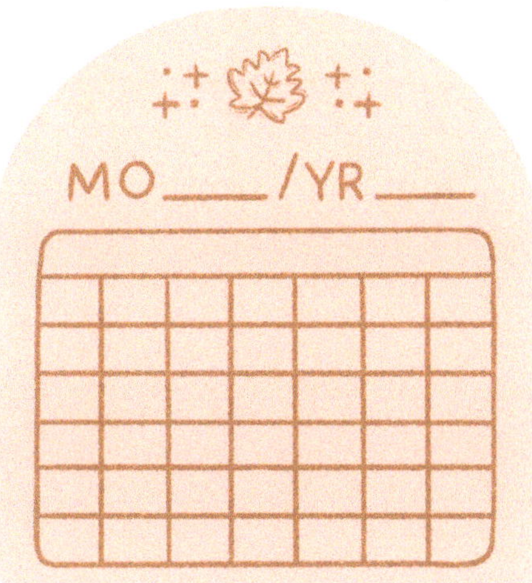

MO____/YR____

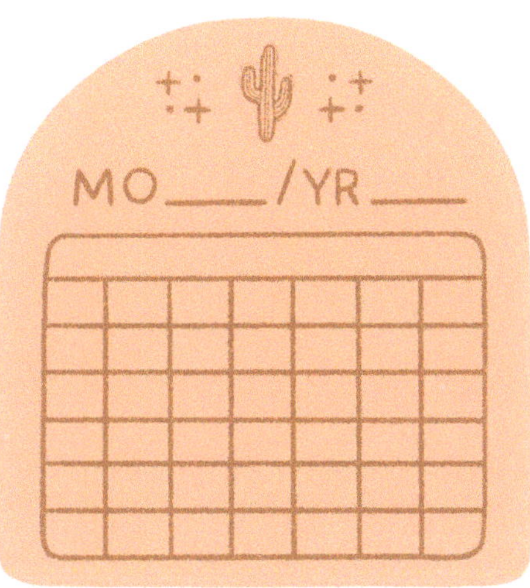

MO____/YR____

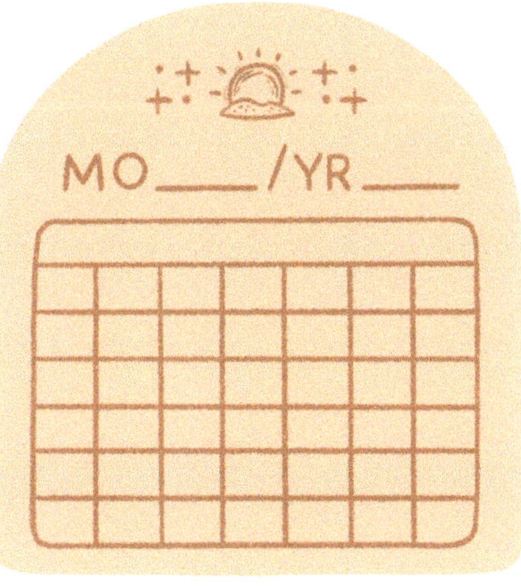

MO____/YR____

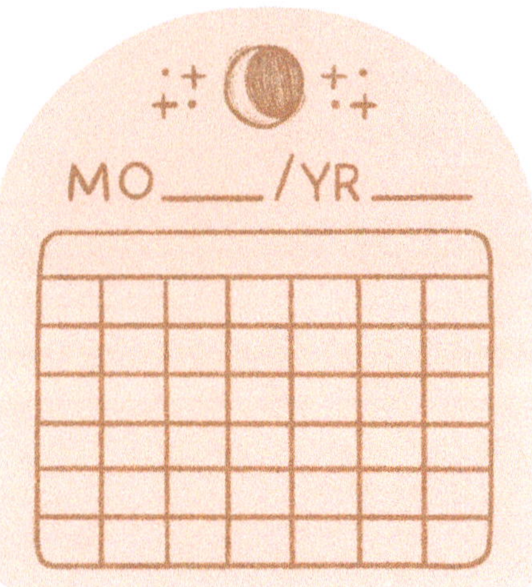
MO____/YR____

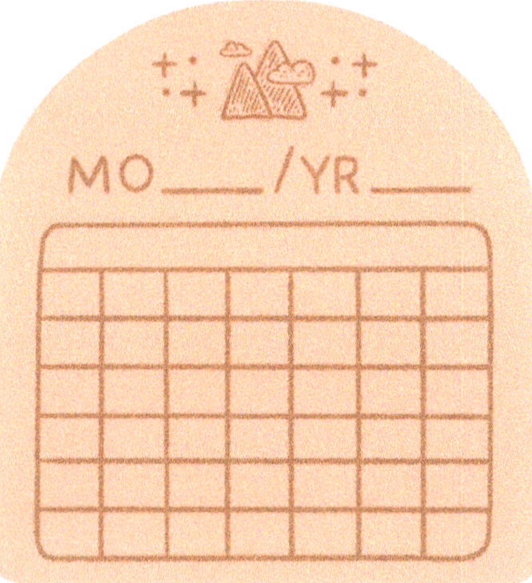
MO____/YR____

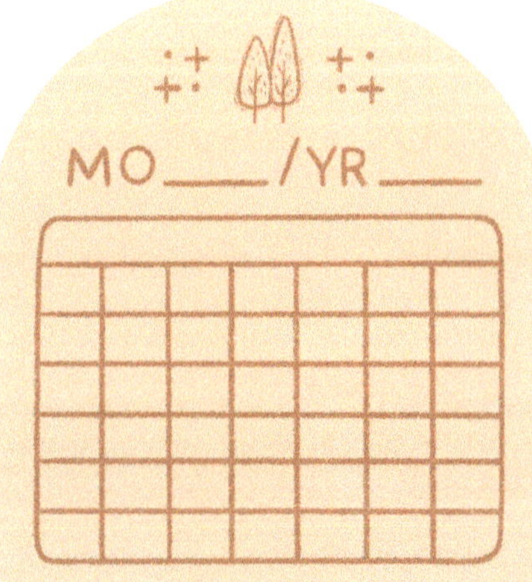
MO____/YR____

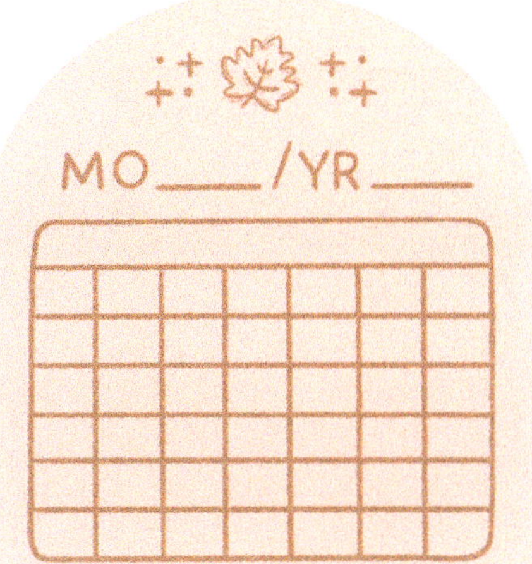
MO____/YR____

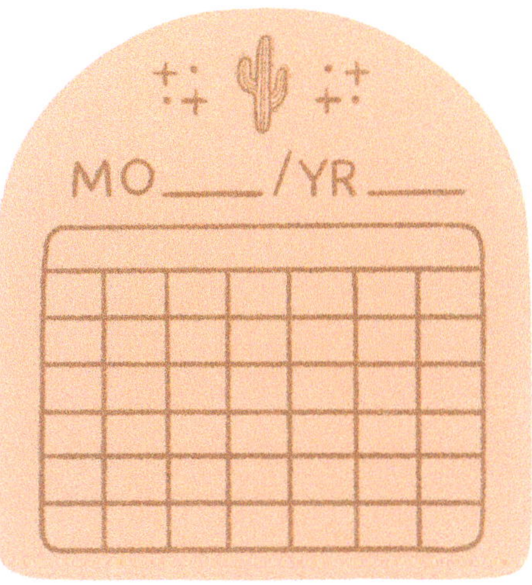
MO____/YR____

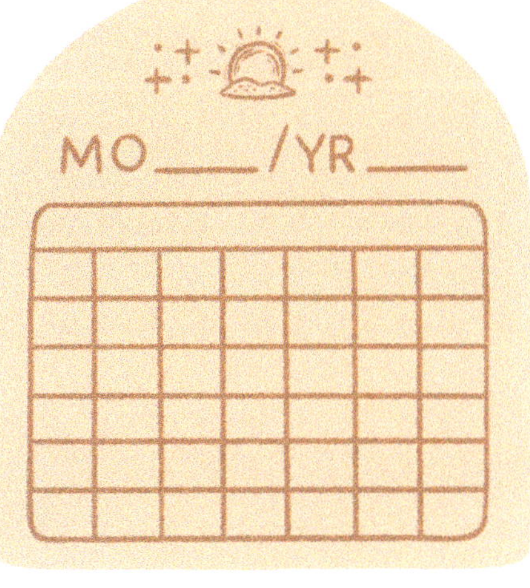
MO____/YR____

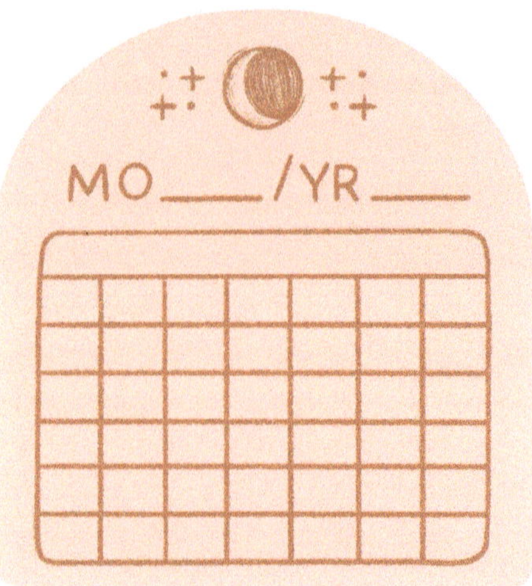

MO____/YR____

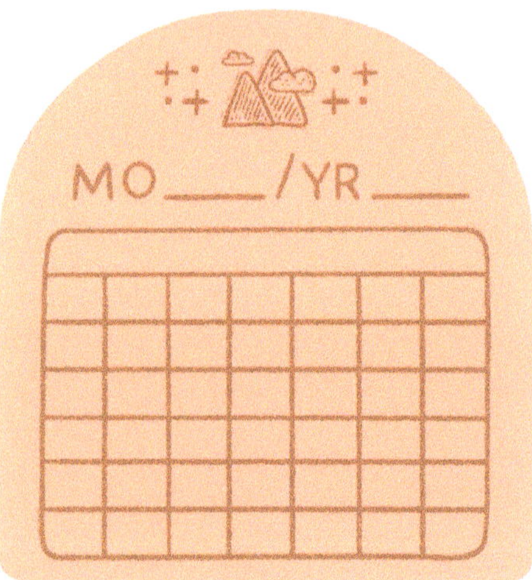

MO____/YR____

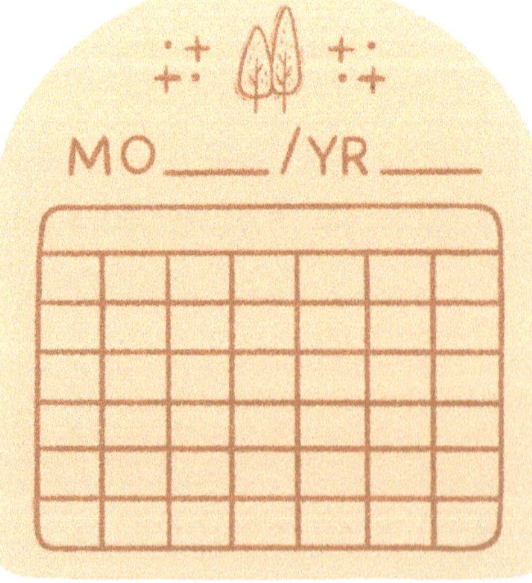

MO____/YR____

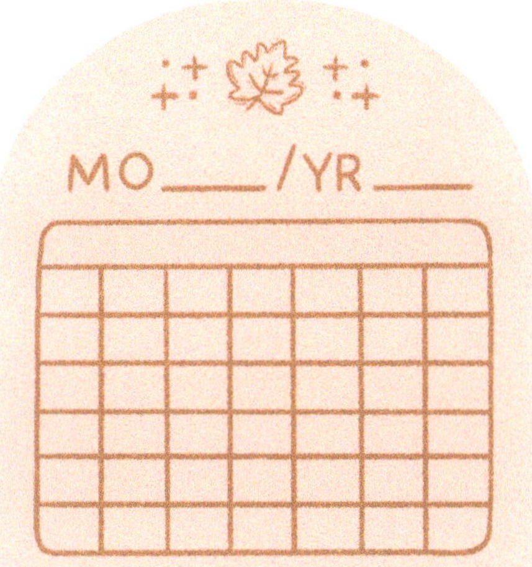
MO____/YR____

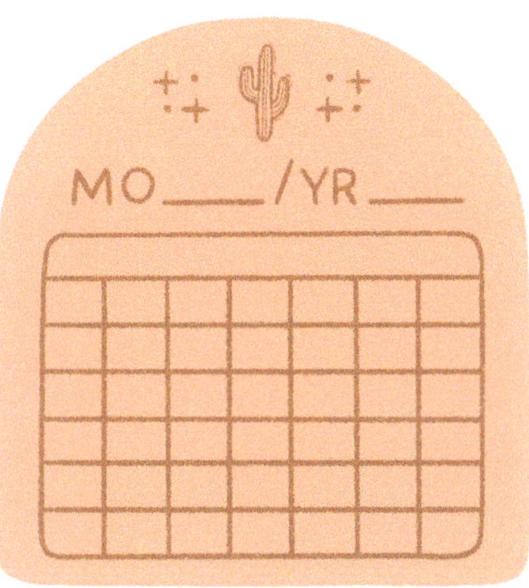
MO____/YR____

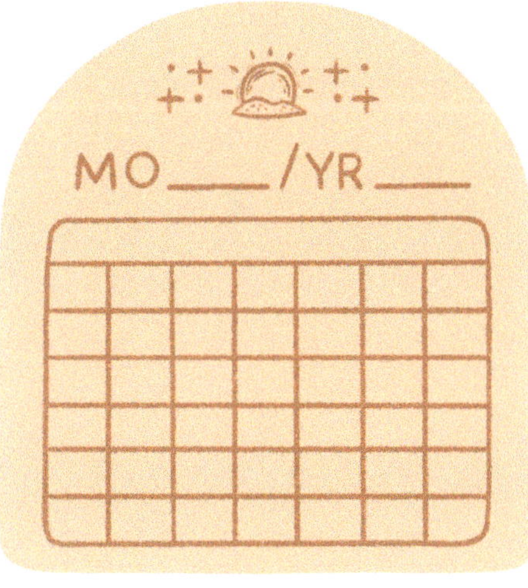
MO____/YR____

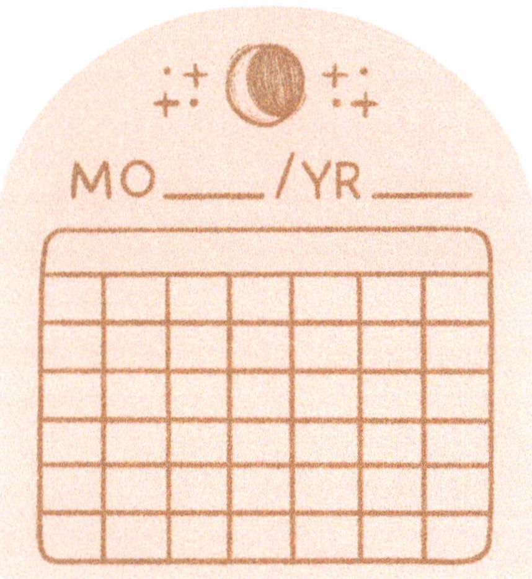
MO____/YR____

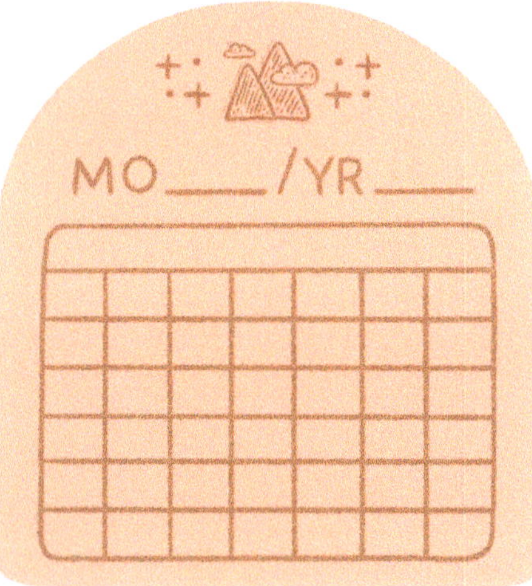
MO____/YR____

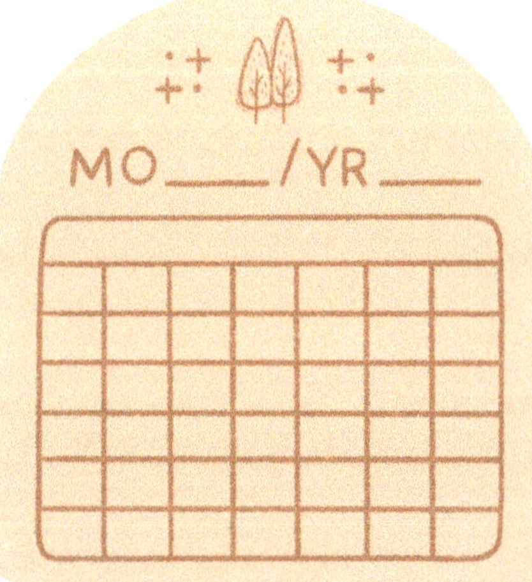
MO____/YR____

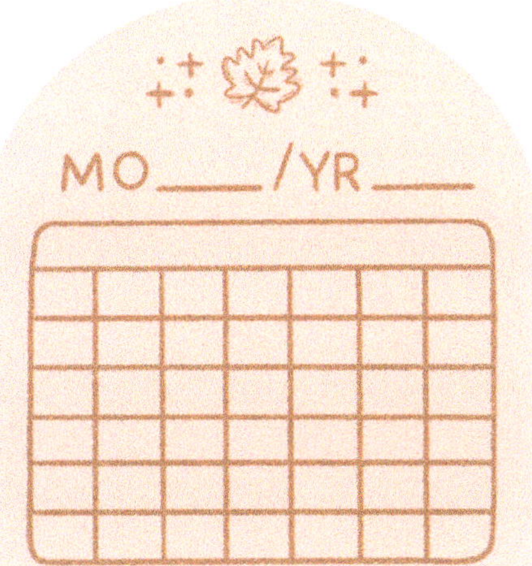

MO____/YR____

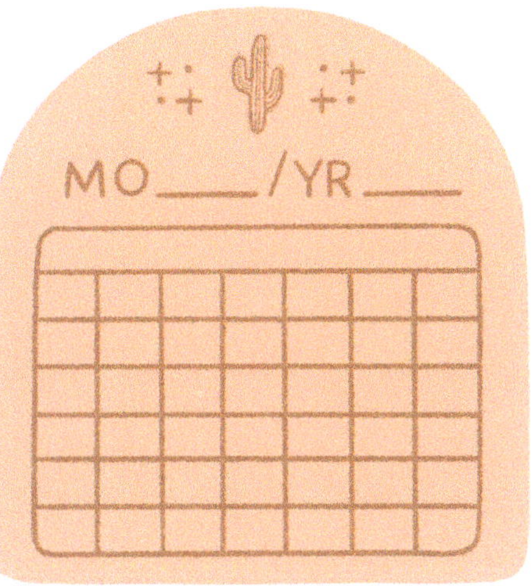

MO____/YR____

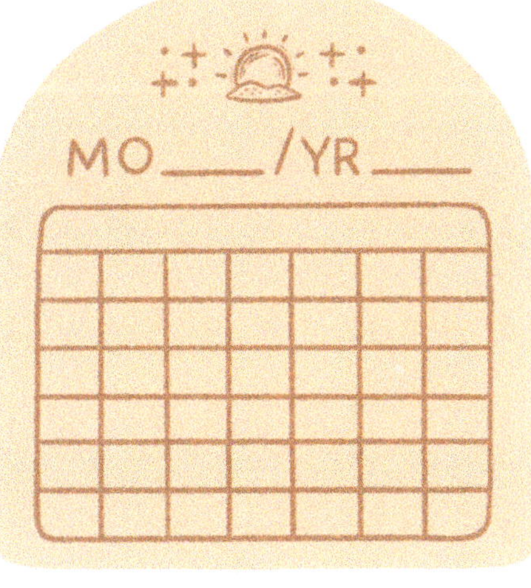

MO____/YR____

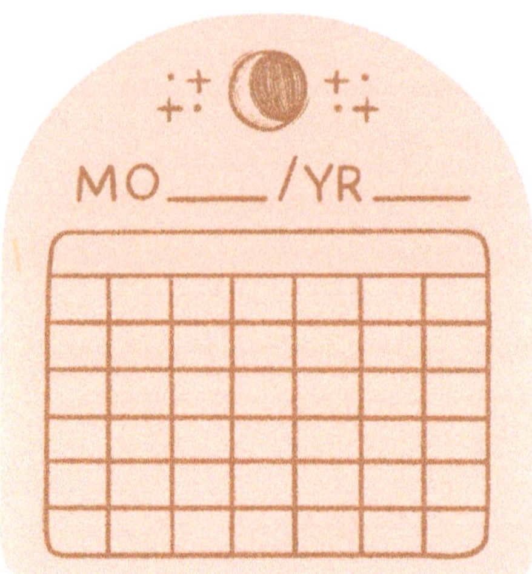
MO____/YR____

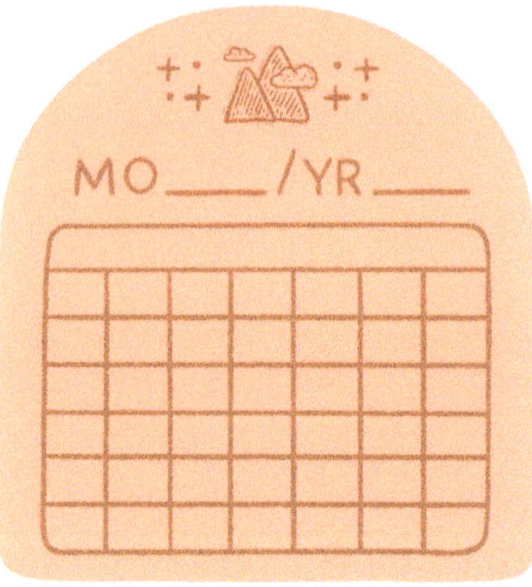
MO____/YR____

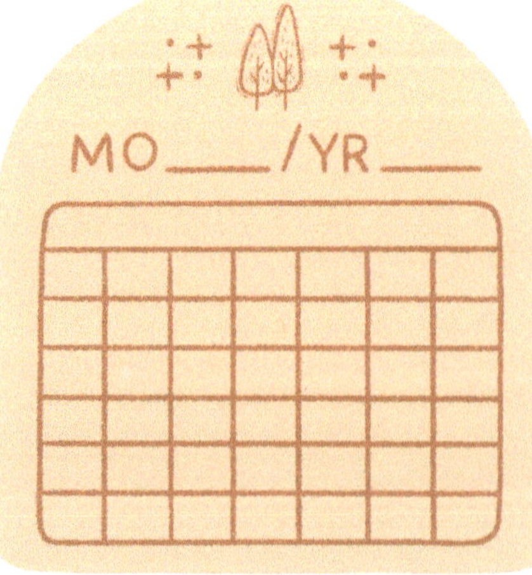
MO____/YR____

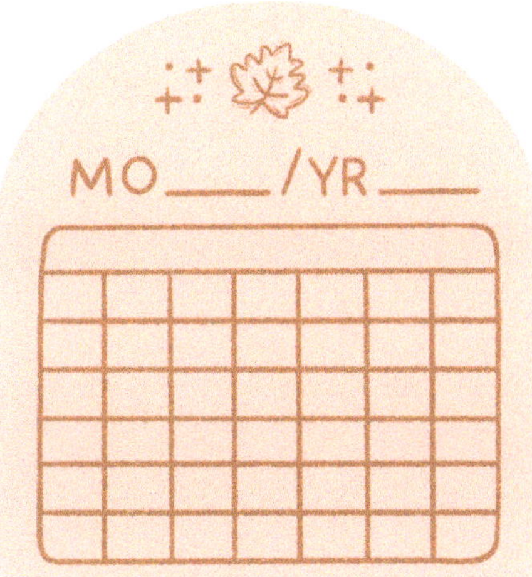
MO____/YR____

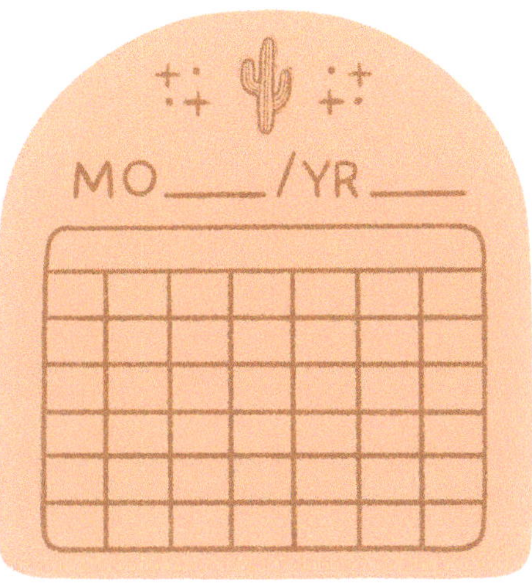
MO____/YR____

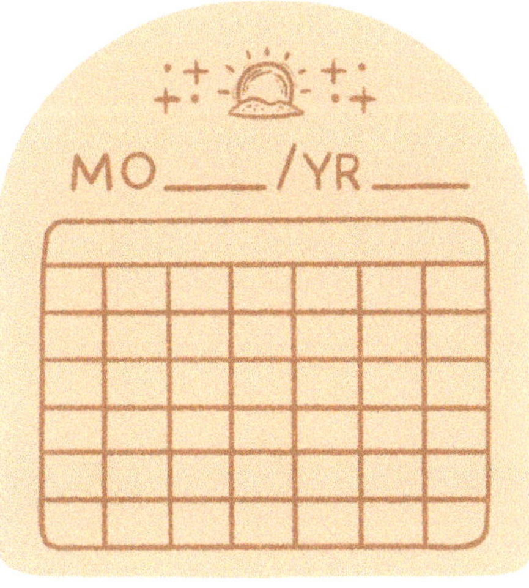
MO____/YR____

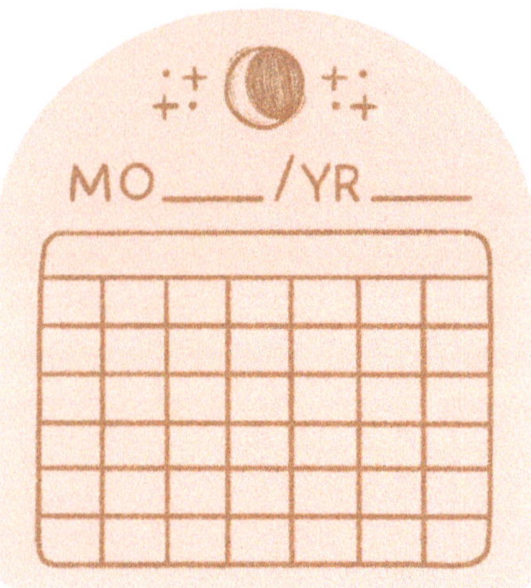
MO___/YR___

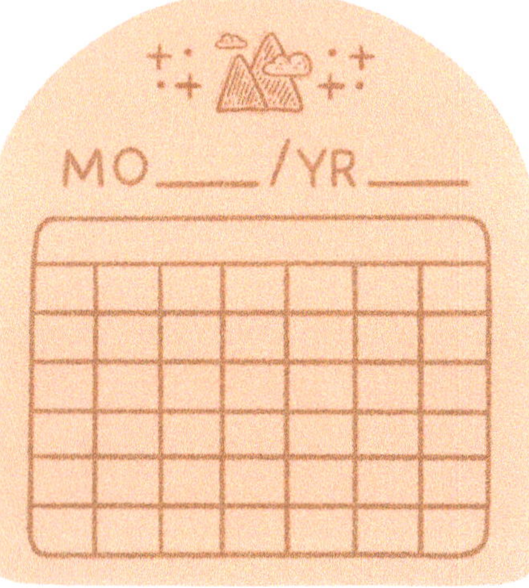
MO___/YR___

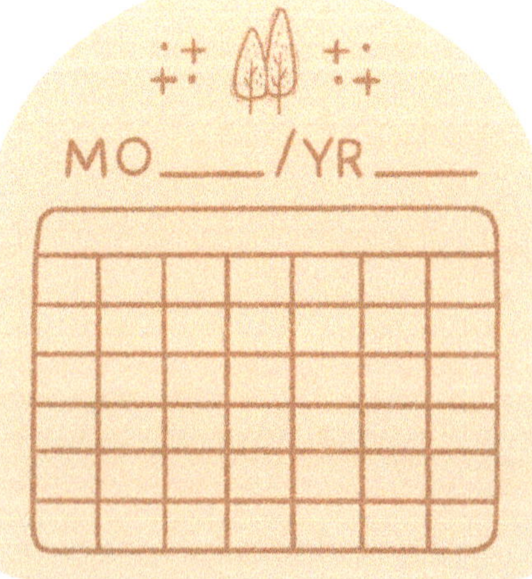
MO___/YR___

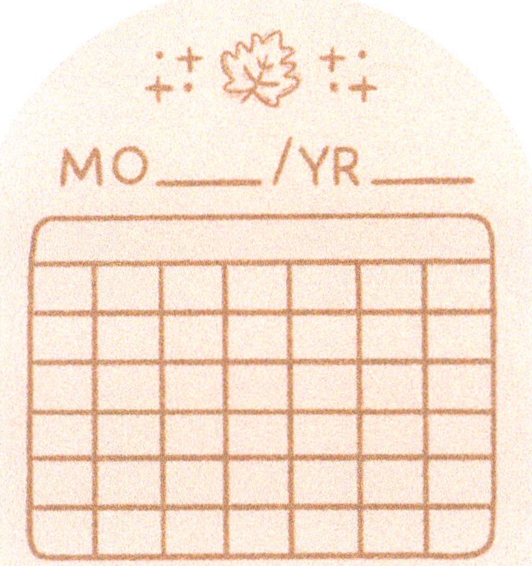
MO____/YR____

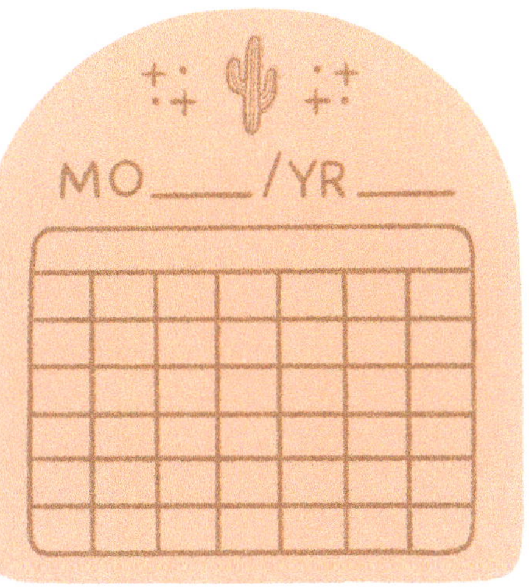
MO____/YR____

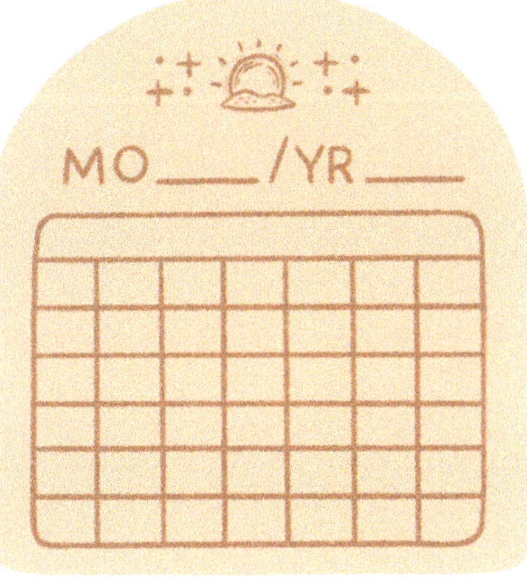
MO____/YR____

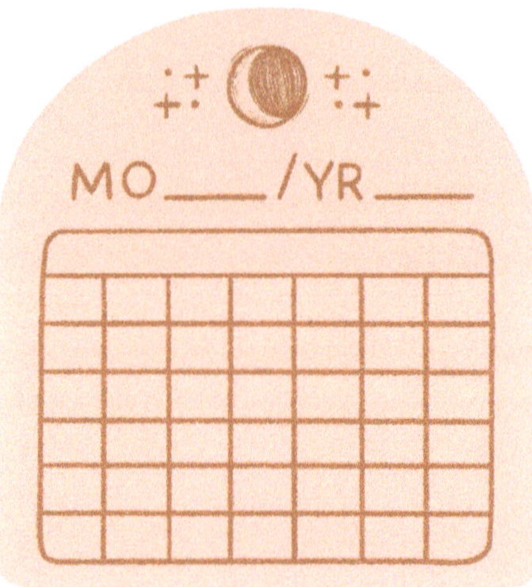
MO____/YR____

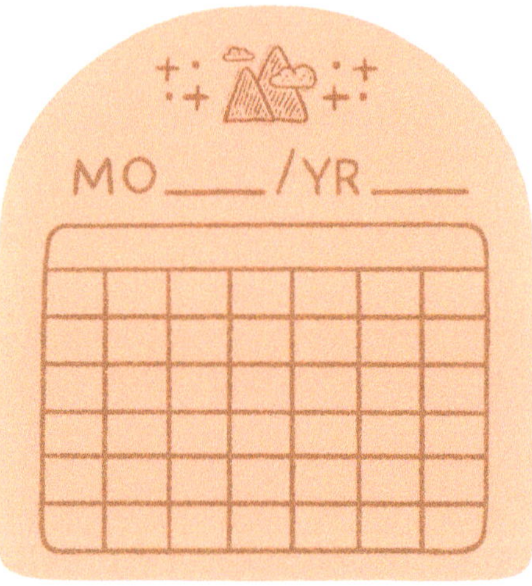
MO____/YR____

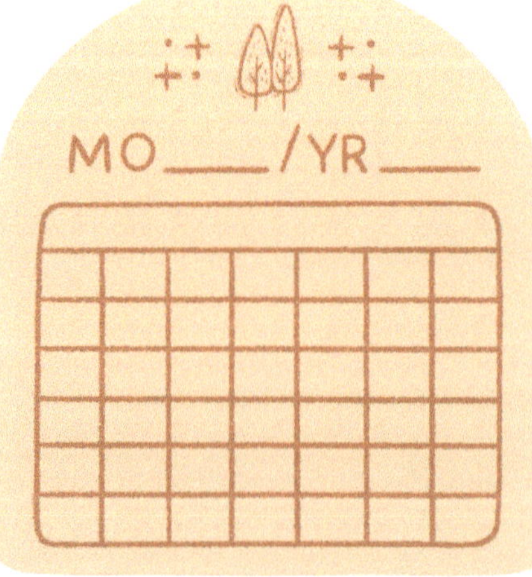
MO____/YR____

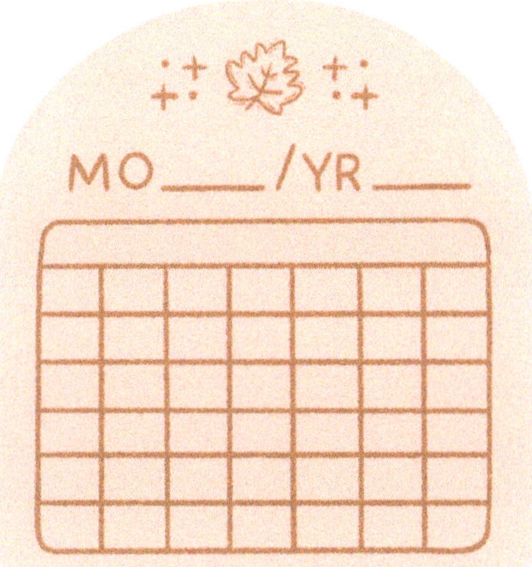
MO____/YR____

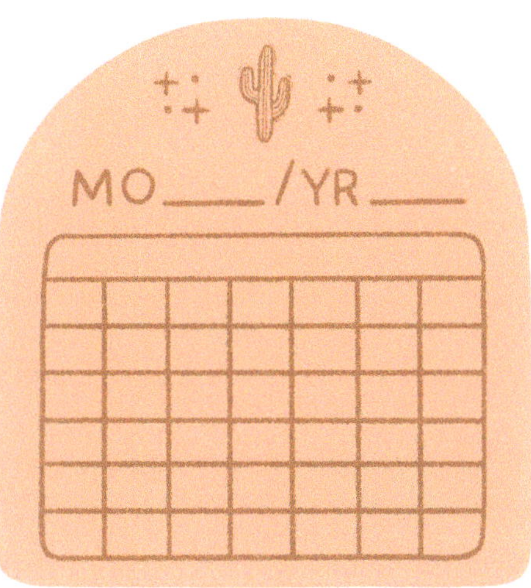
MO____/YR____

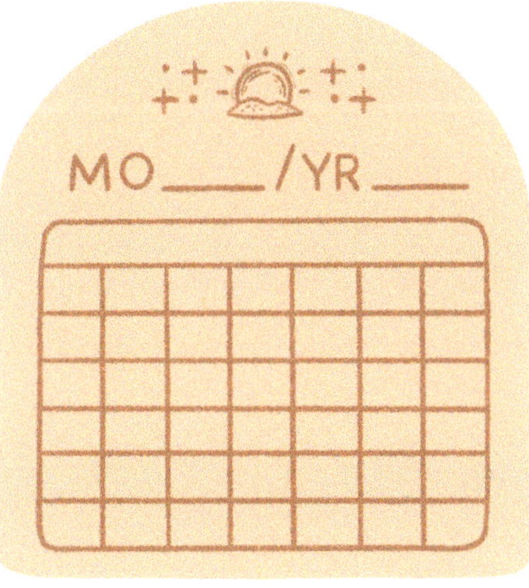
MO____/YR____

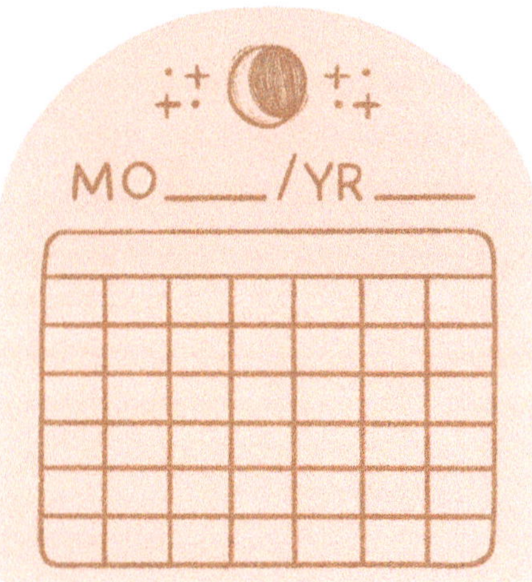

MO_____/YR_____

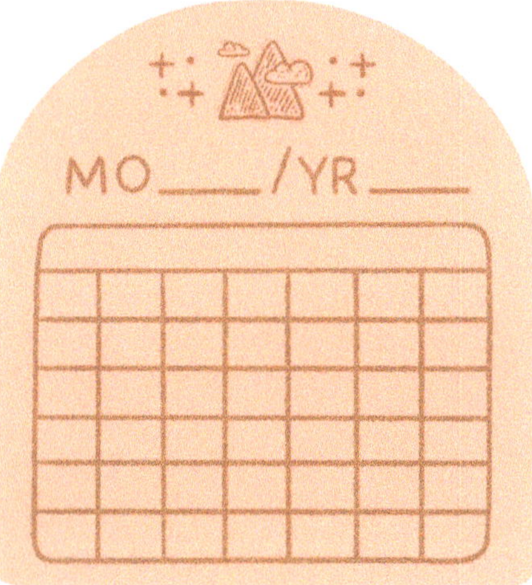

MO_____/YR_____

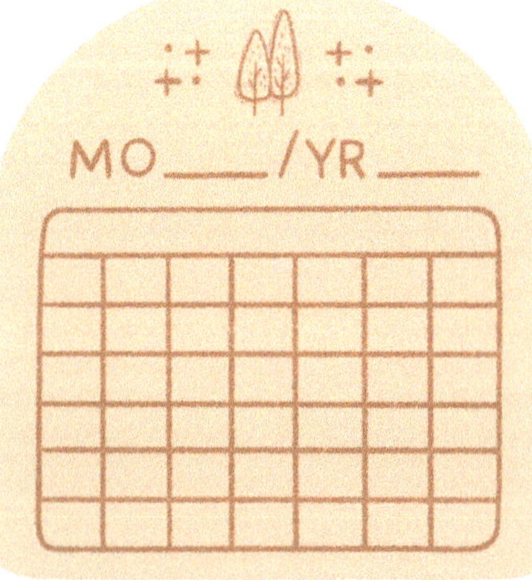

MO_____/YR_____

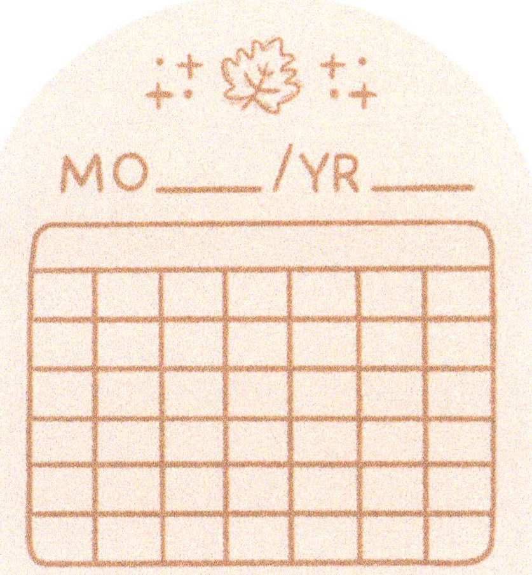
MO_____/YR_____

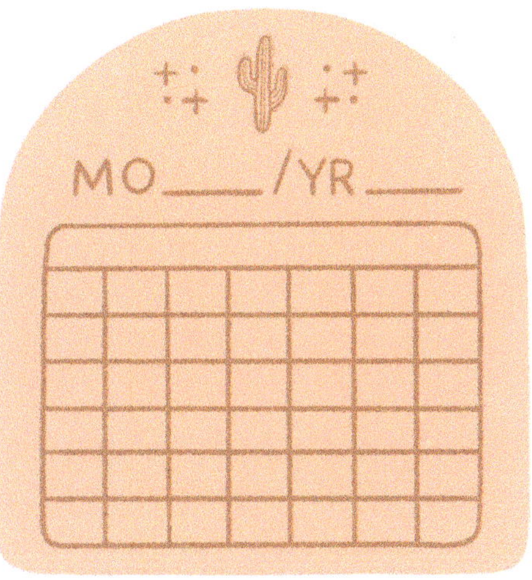
MO_____/YR_____

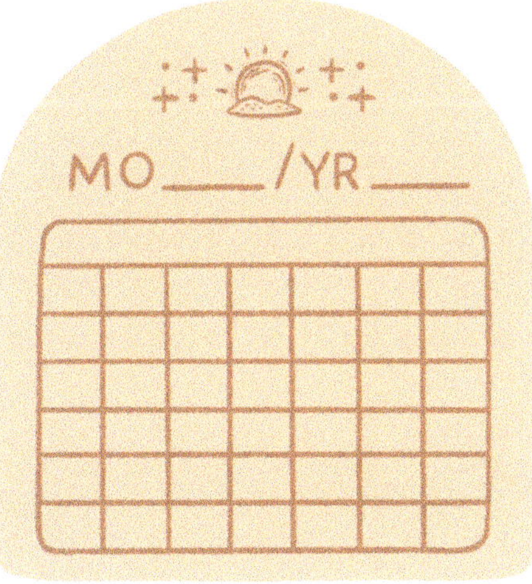
MO_____/YR_____

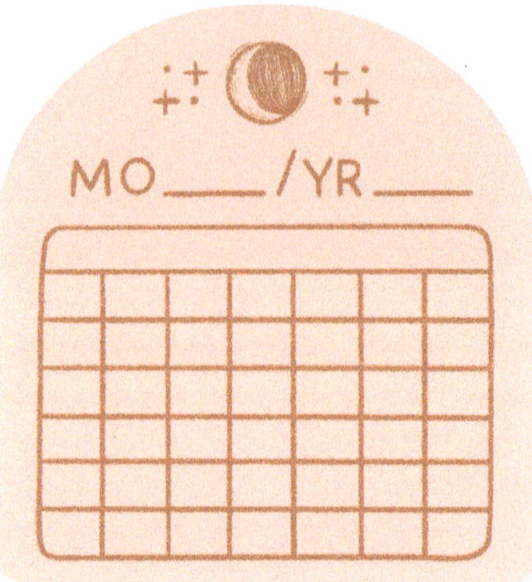
MO____/YR____

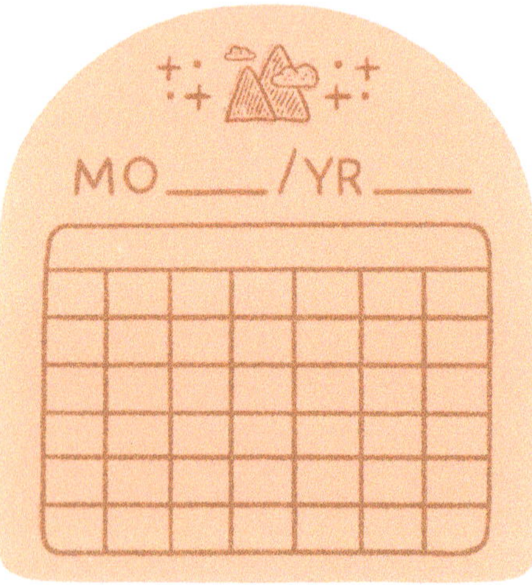
MO____/YR____

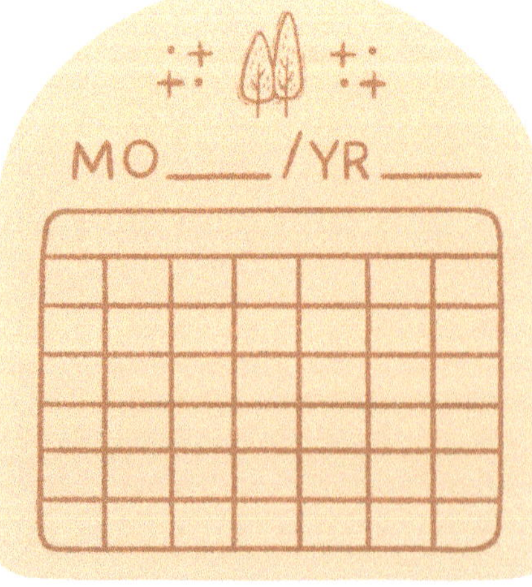
MO____/YR____

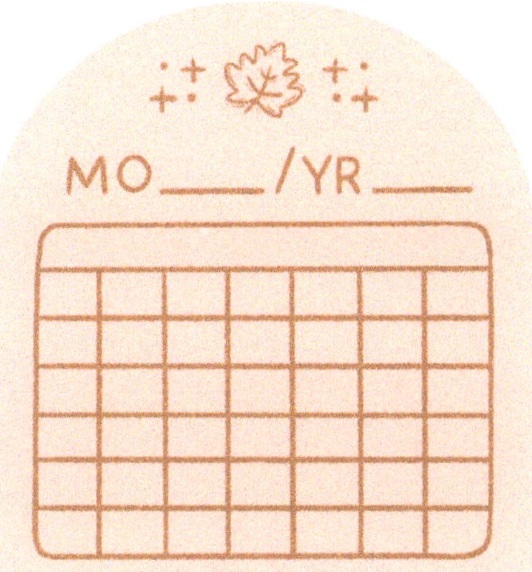
MO____/YR____

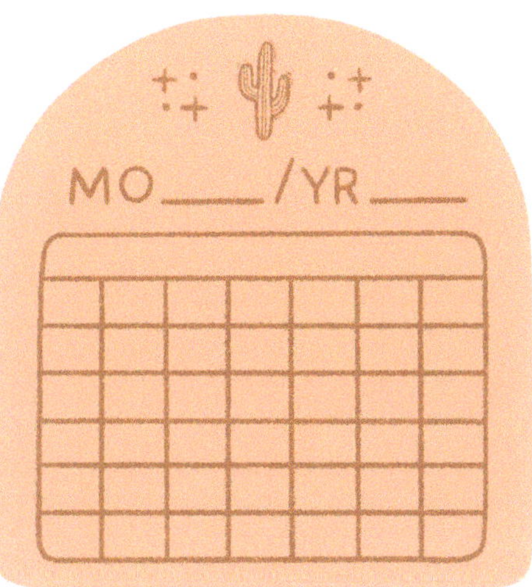
MO____/YR____

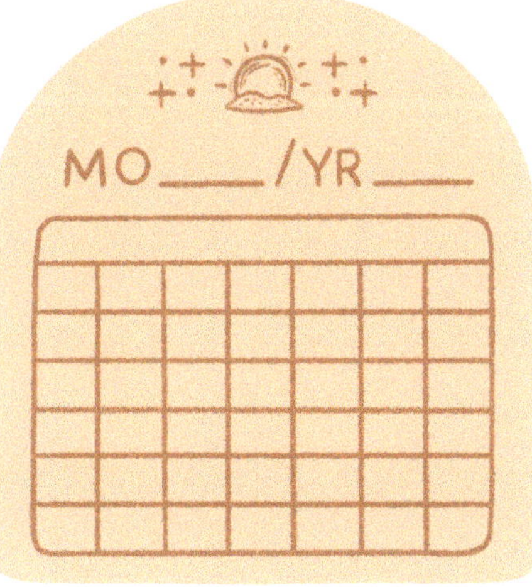
MO____/YR____

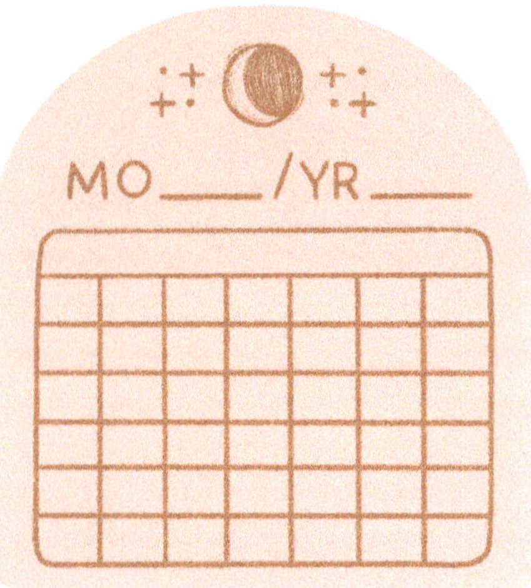
MO____/YR____

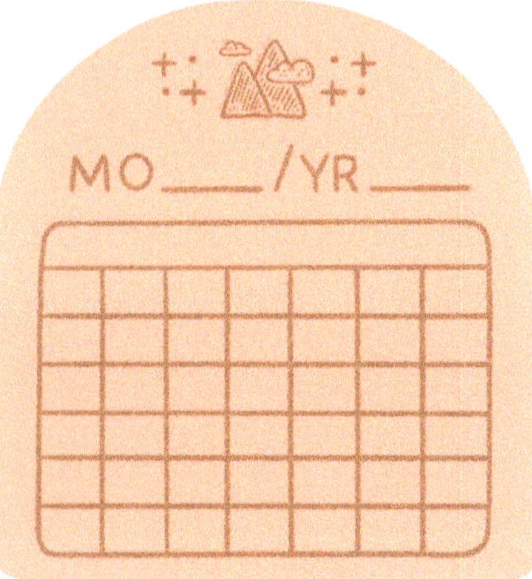
MO____/YR____

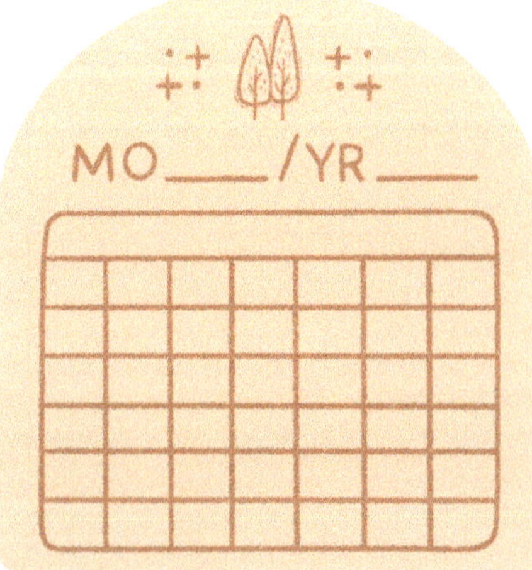
MO____/YR____

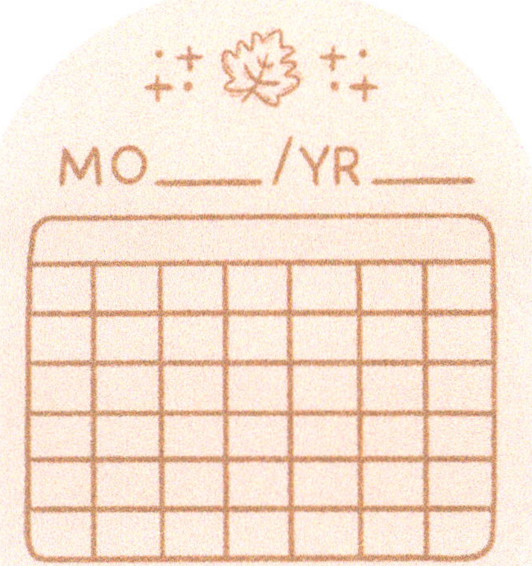
MO____/YR____

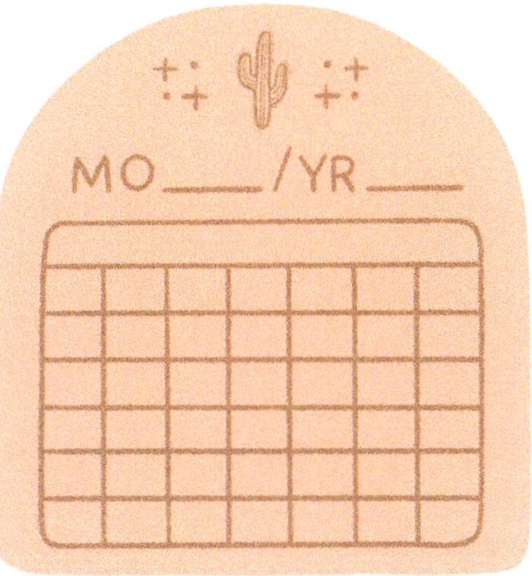
MO____/YR____

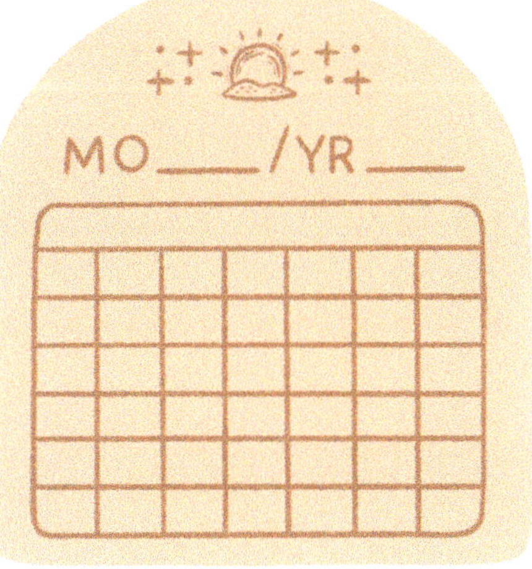
MO____/YR____

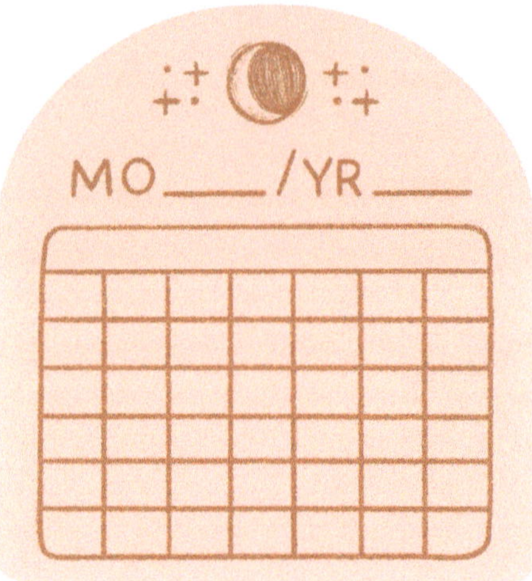

MO____/YR____

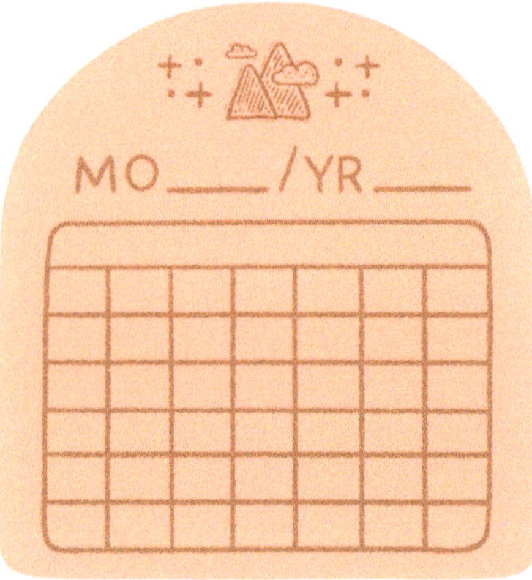

MO____/YR____

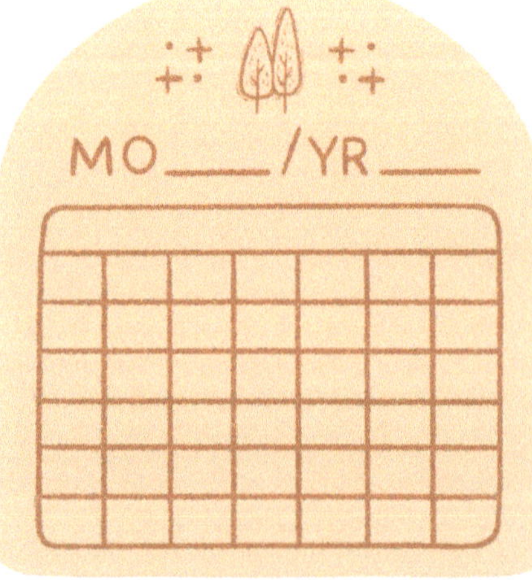

MO____/YR____

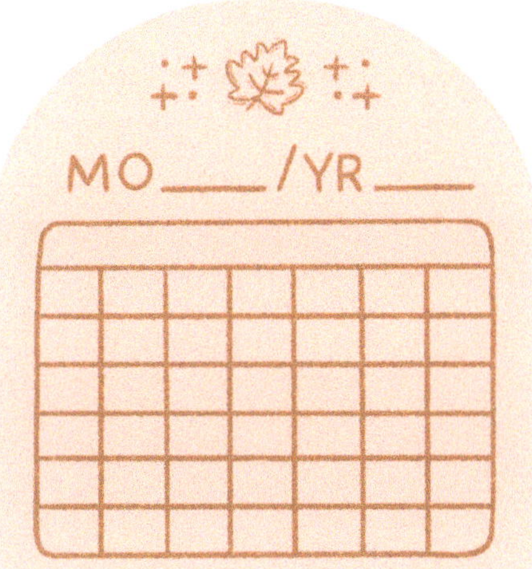
MO____/YR____

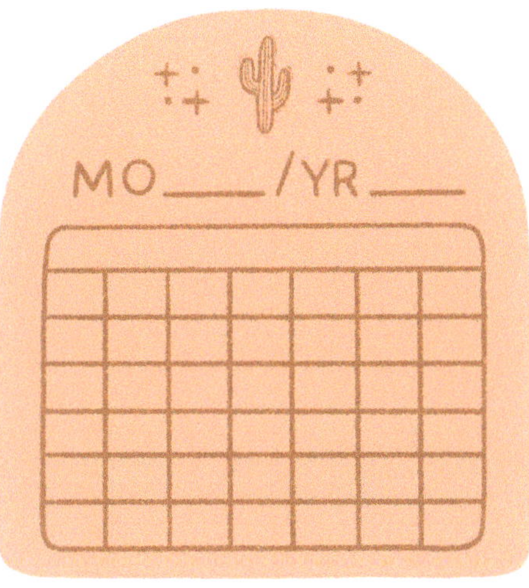
MO____/YR____

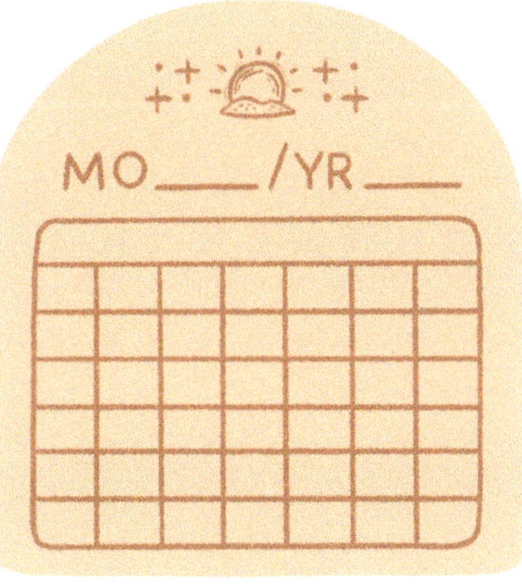
MO____/YR____

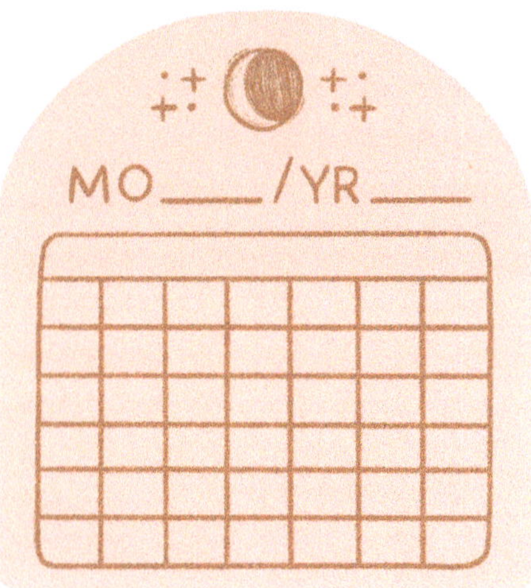
MO____/YR____

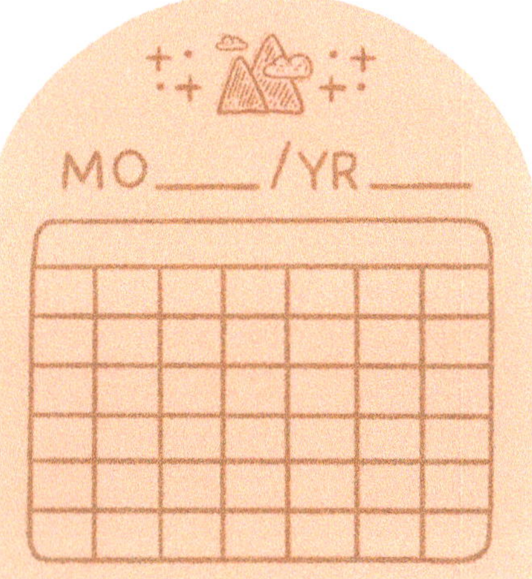
MO____/YR____

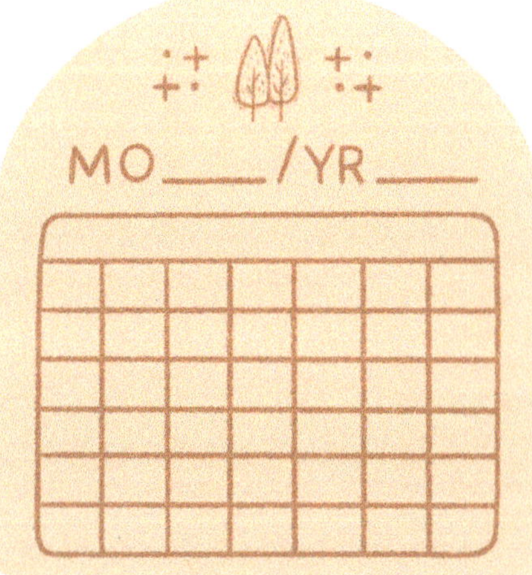
MO____/YR____

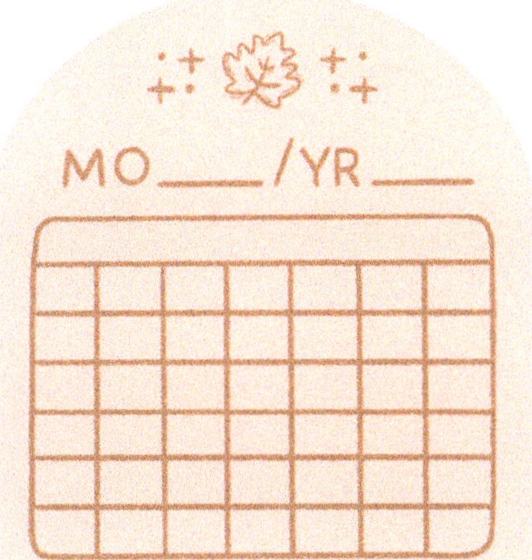

MO____/YR____

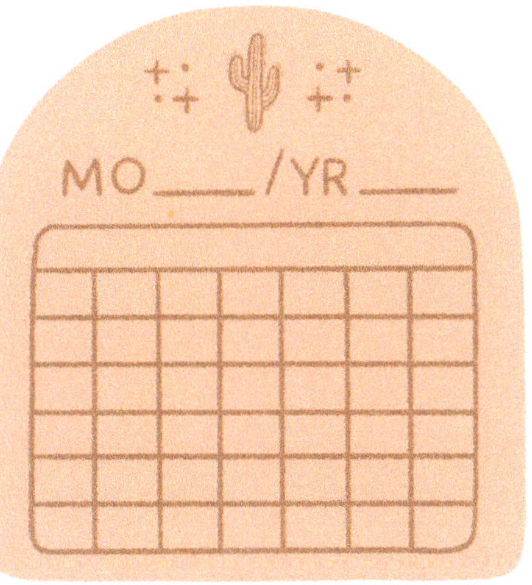

MO____/YR____

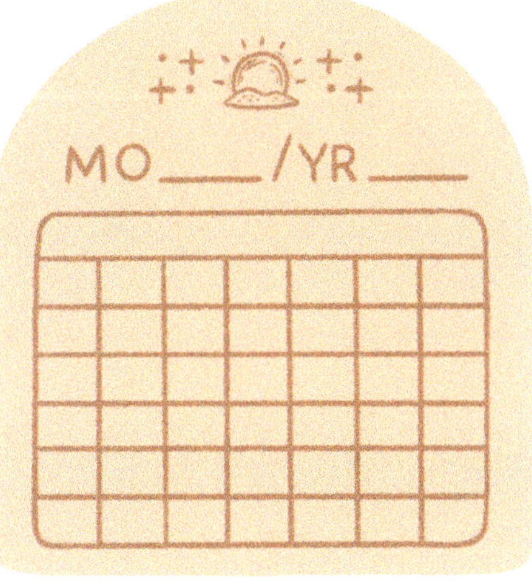

MO____/YR____

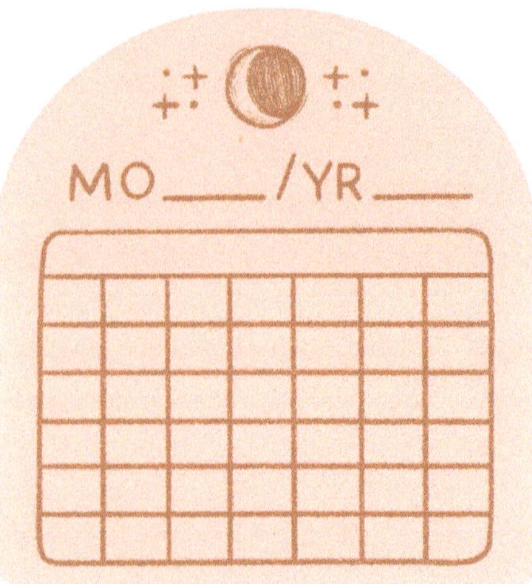
MO____/YR____

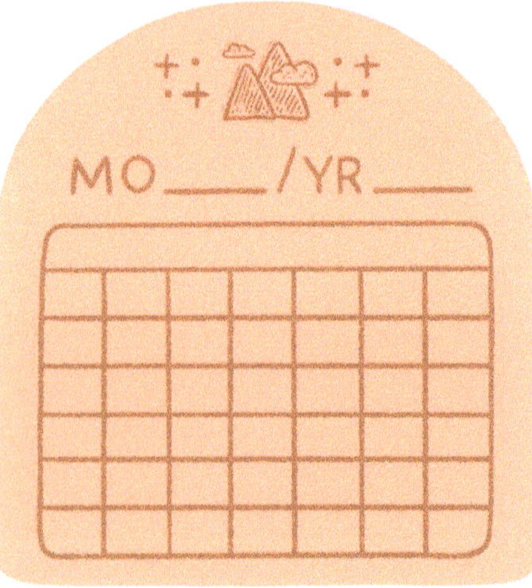
MO____/YR____

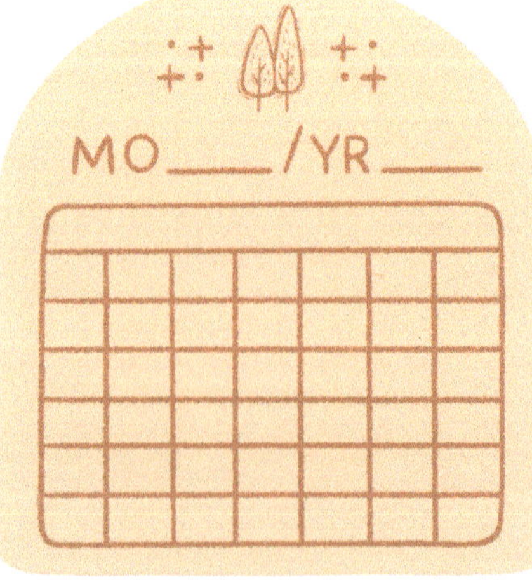
MO____/YR____

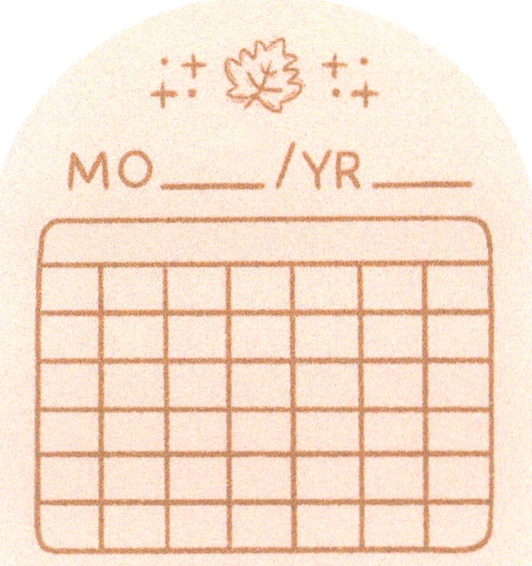
MO____/YR____

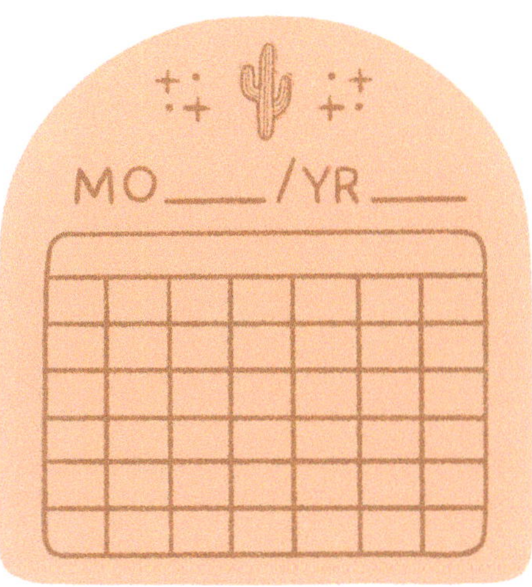
MO____/YR____

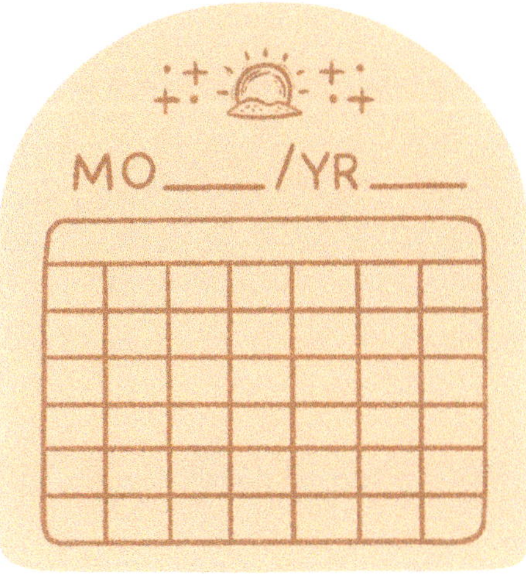
MO____/YR____

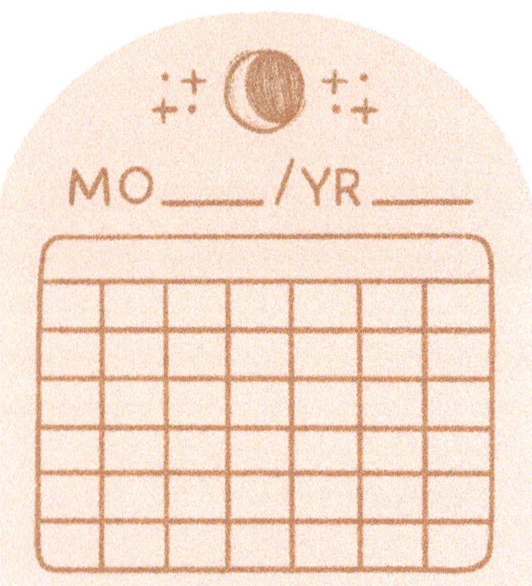

MO____/YR____

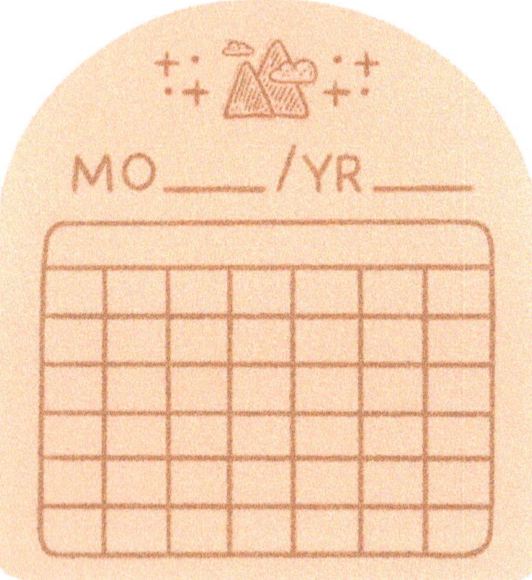

MO____/YR____

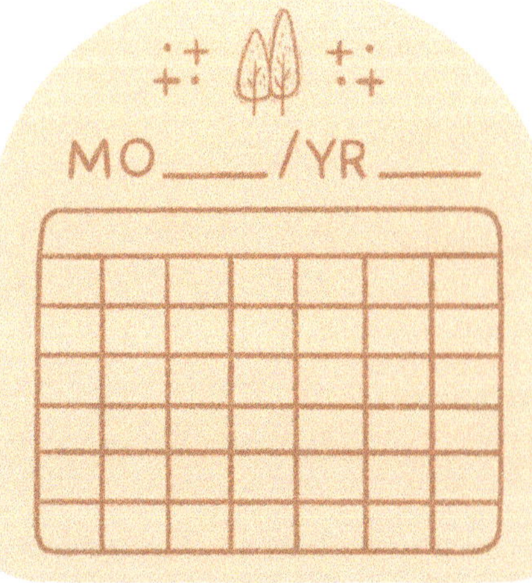

MO____/YR____

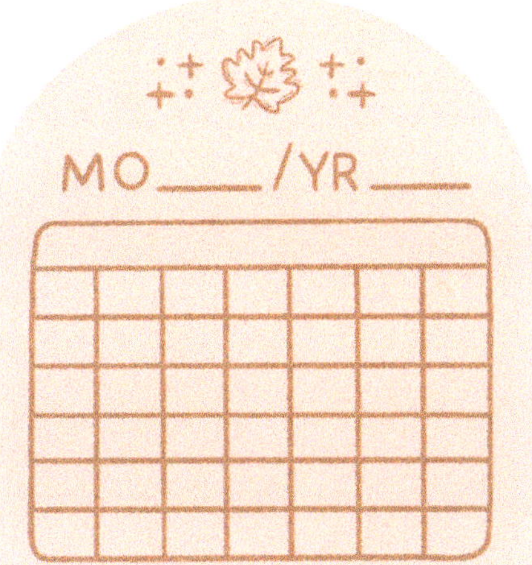

MO_____/YR_____

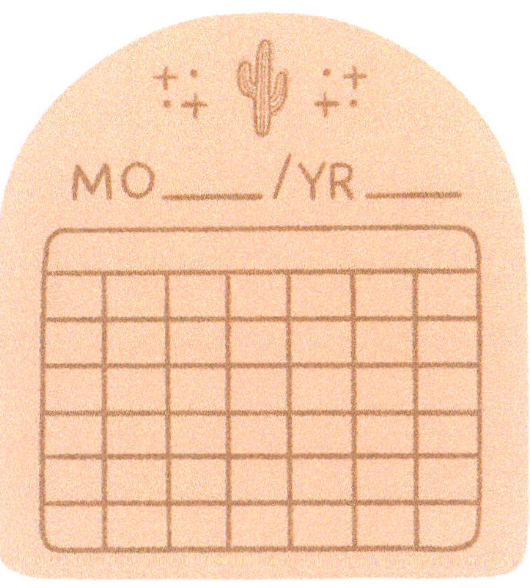

MO_____/YR_____

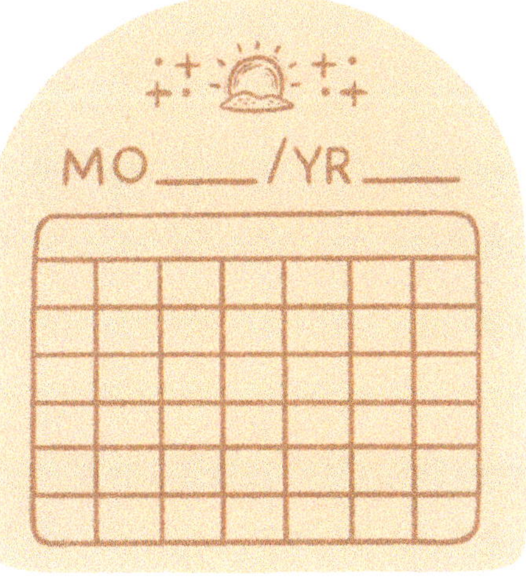

MO_____/YR_____

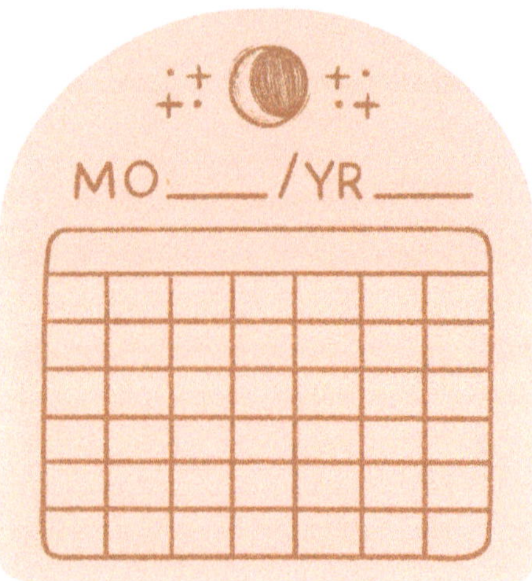
MO____/YR____

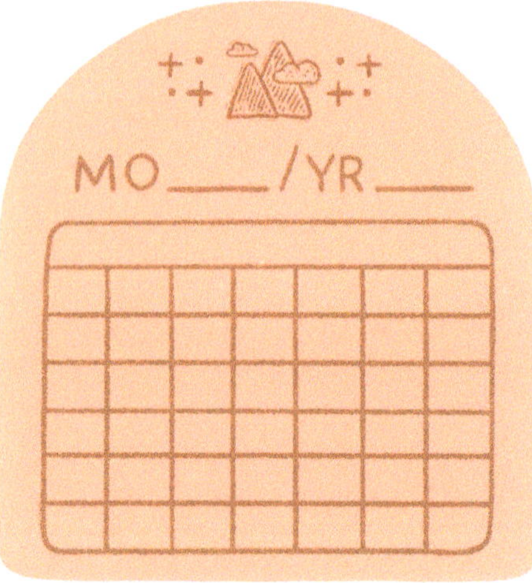
MO____/YR____

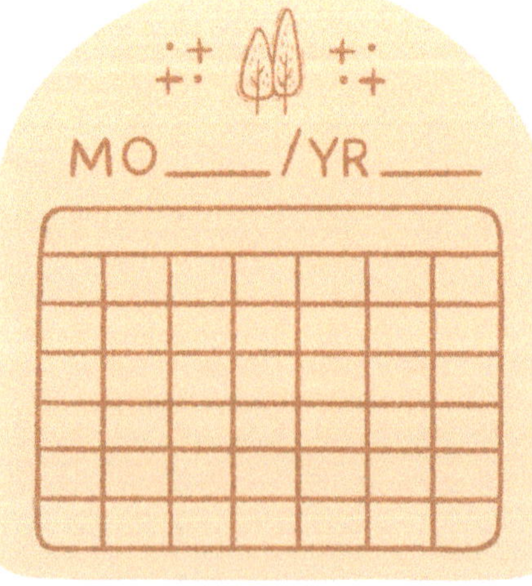
MO____/YR____

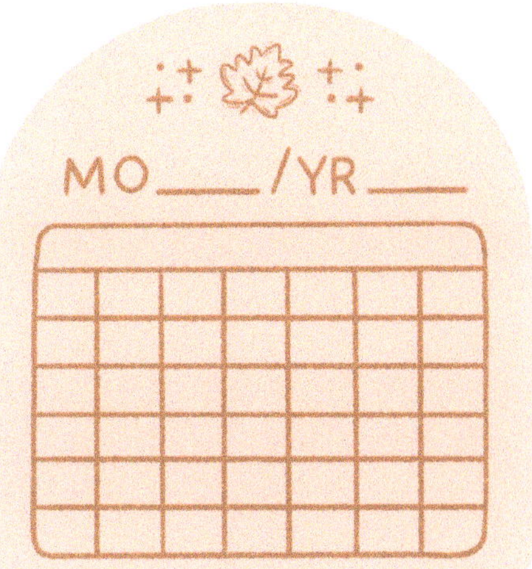
MO____/YR____

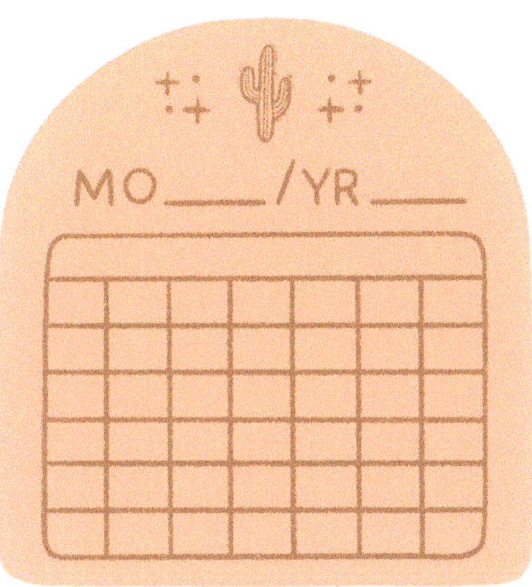
MO____/YR____

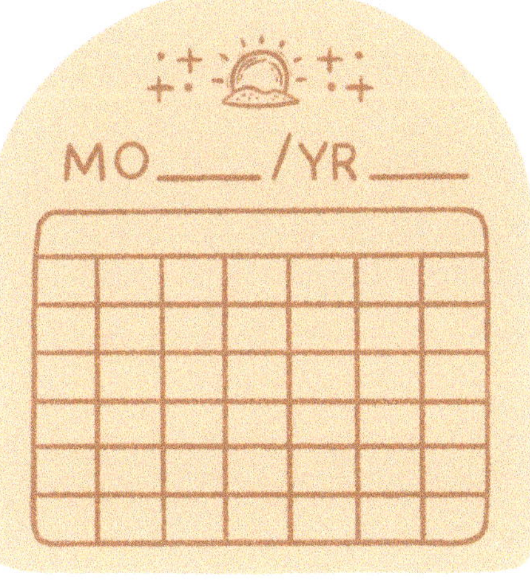
MO____/YR____

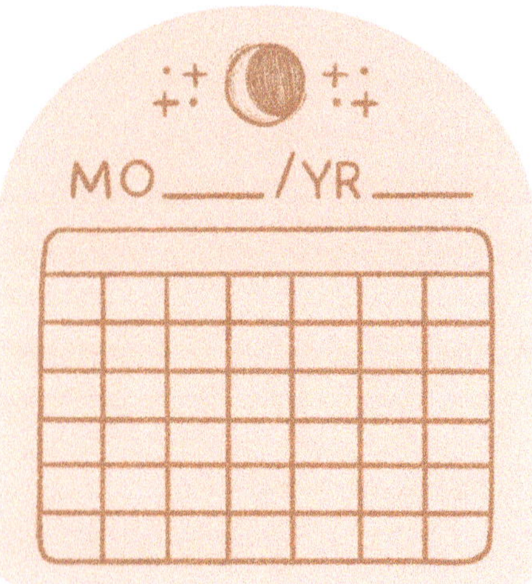
MO____/YR____

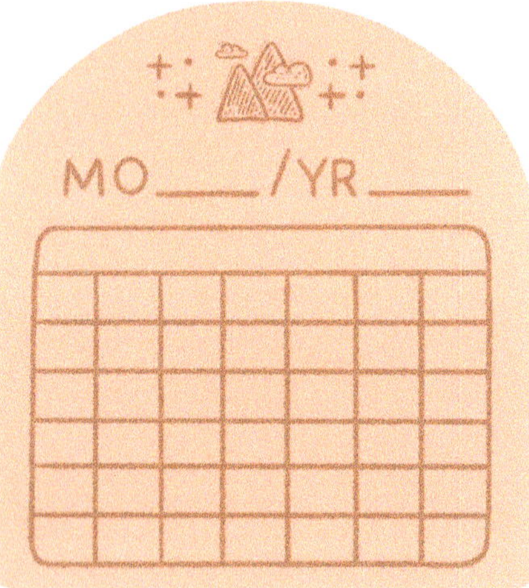
MO____/YR____

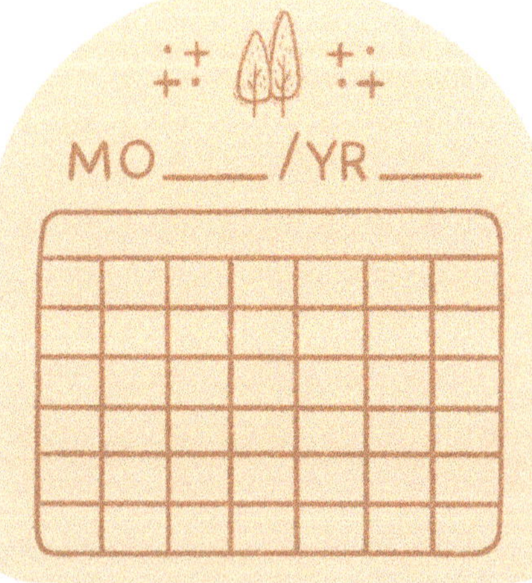
MO____/YR____

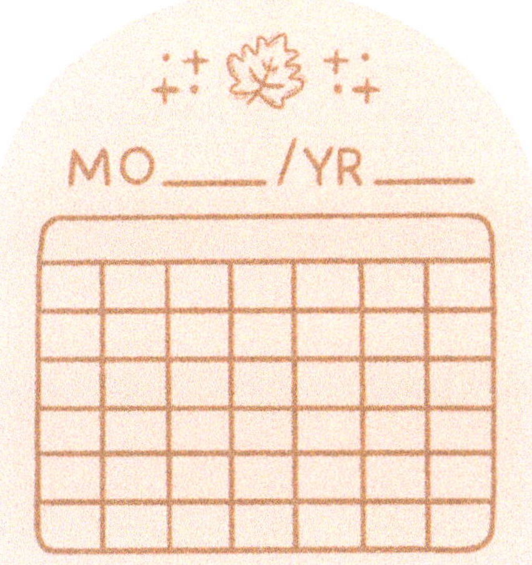
MO_____/YR_____

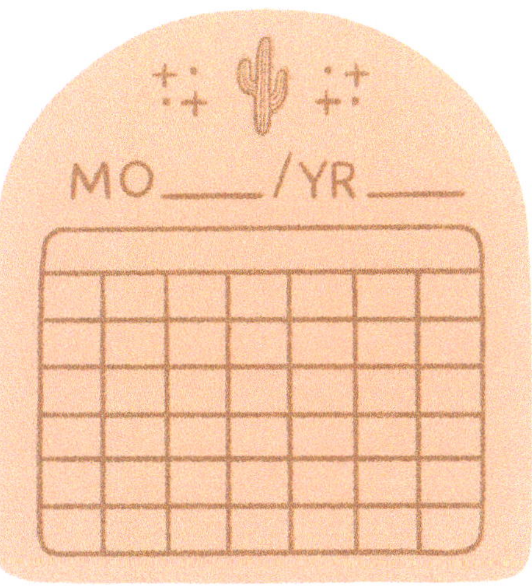
MO_____/YR_____

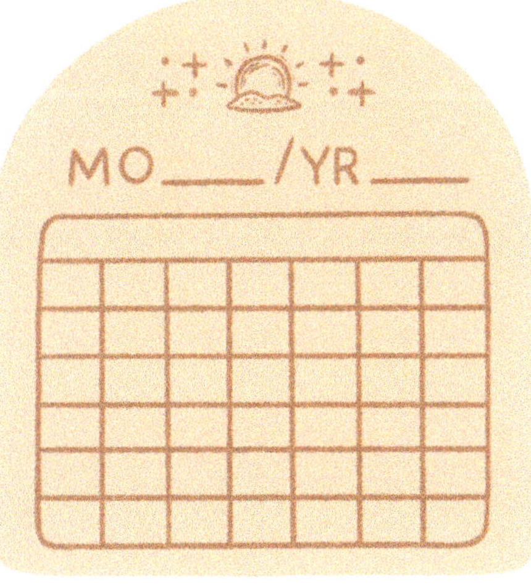
MO_____/YR_____

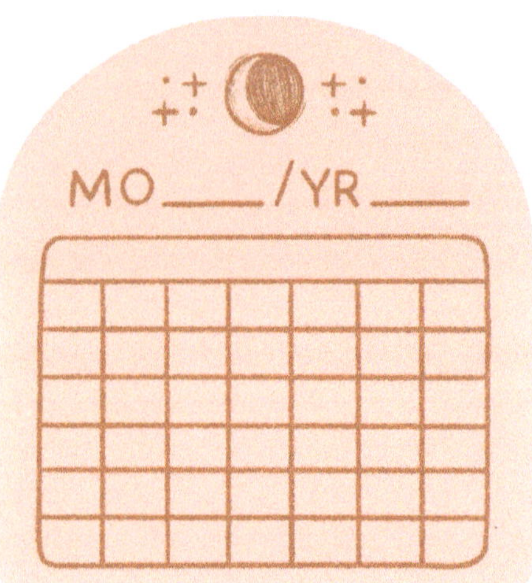

MO_____/YR_____

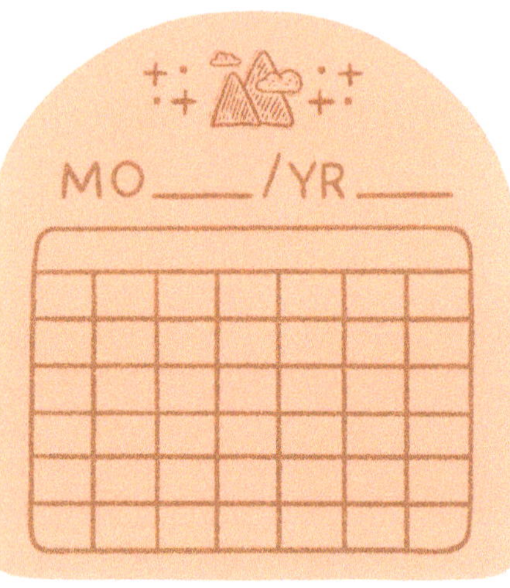

MO_____/YR_____

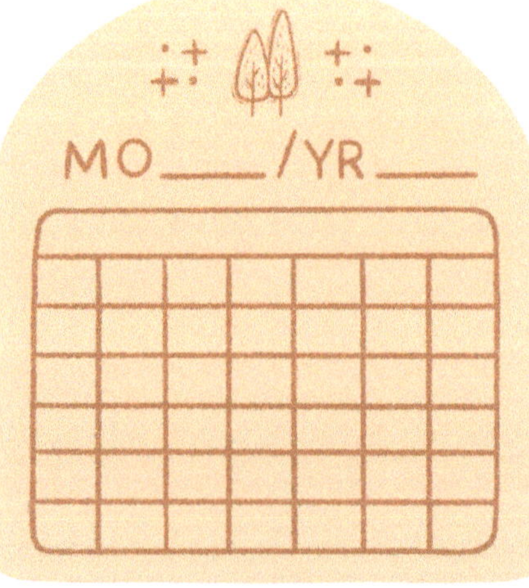

MO_____/YR_____

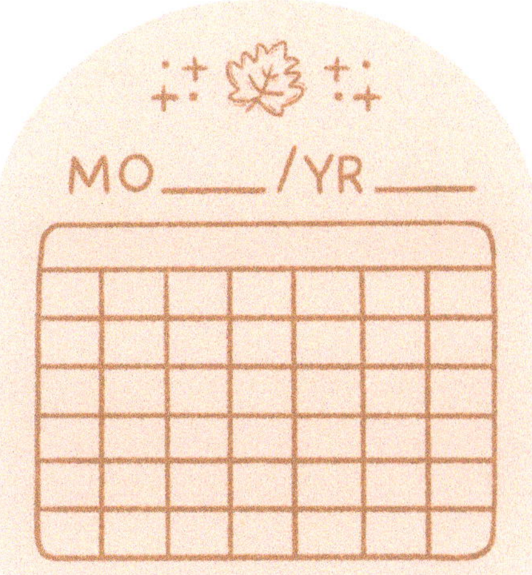

MO____/YR____

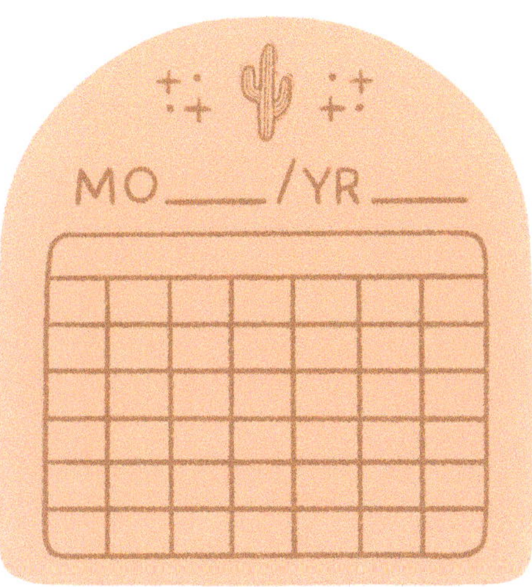

MO____/YR____

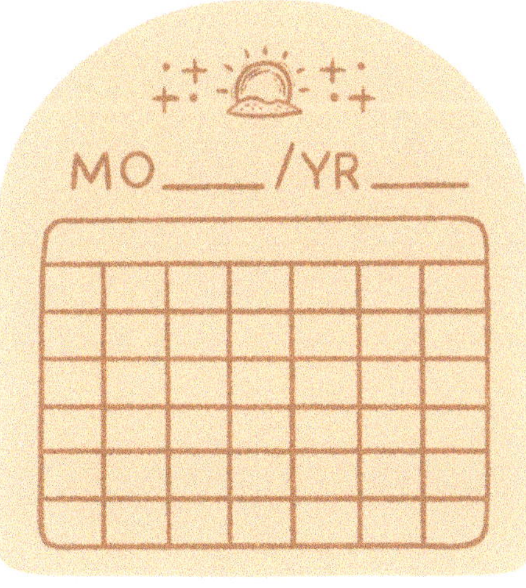

MO____/YR____

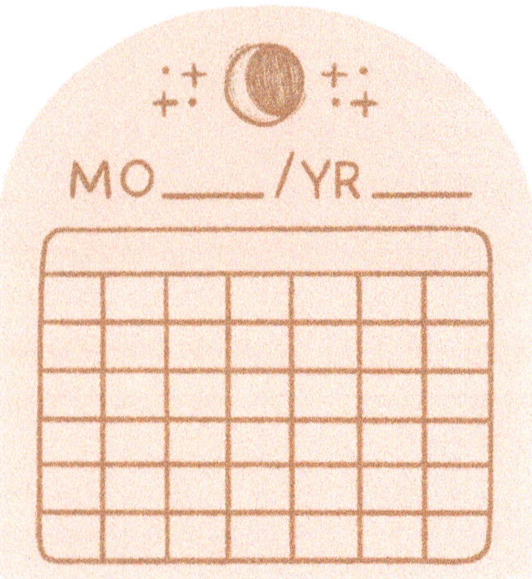
MO_____/YR_____

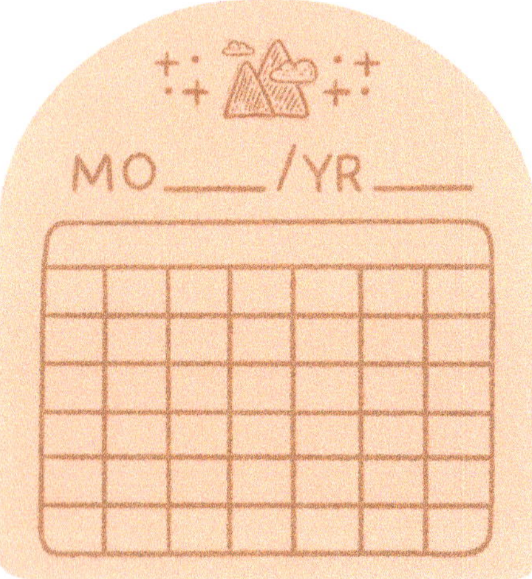
MO_____/YR_____

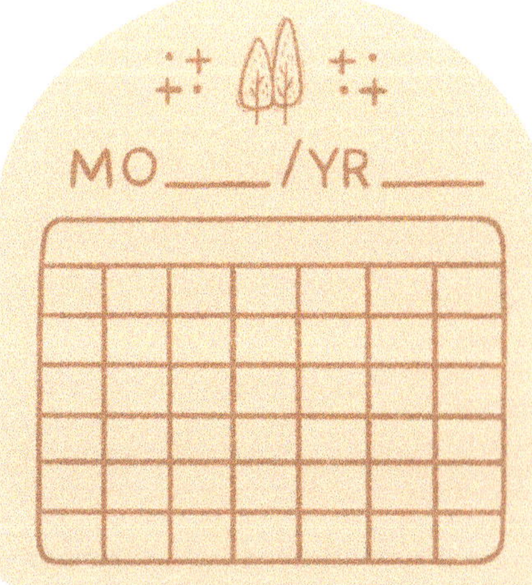
MO_____/YR_____

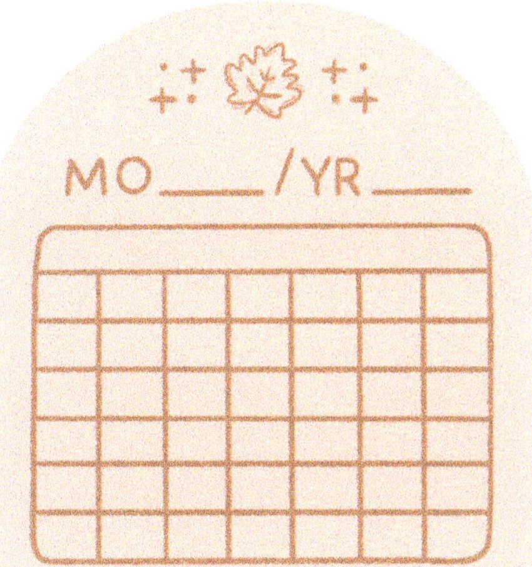

MO____/YR____

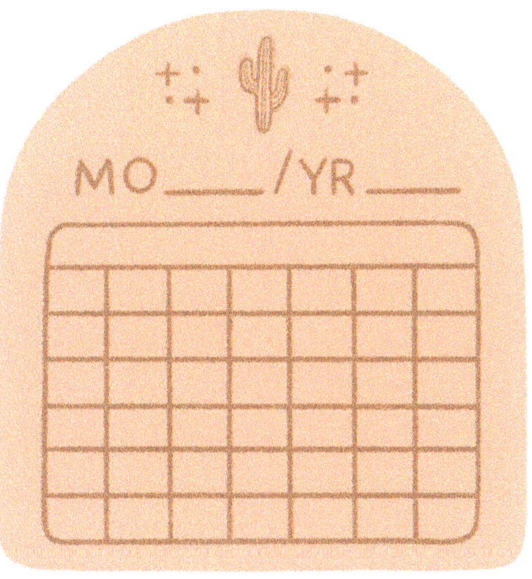

MO____/YR____

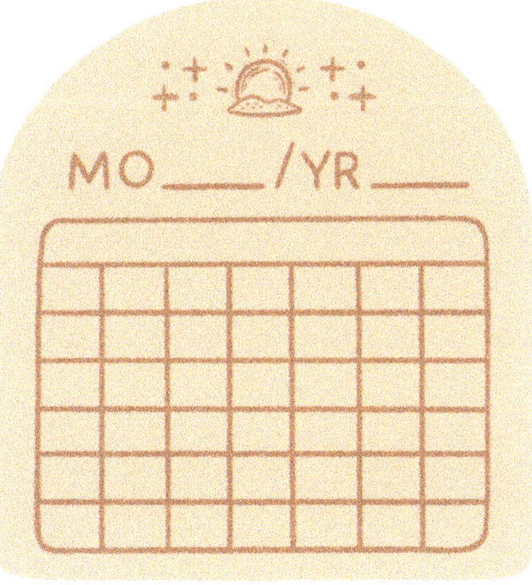

MO____/YR____

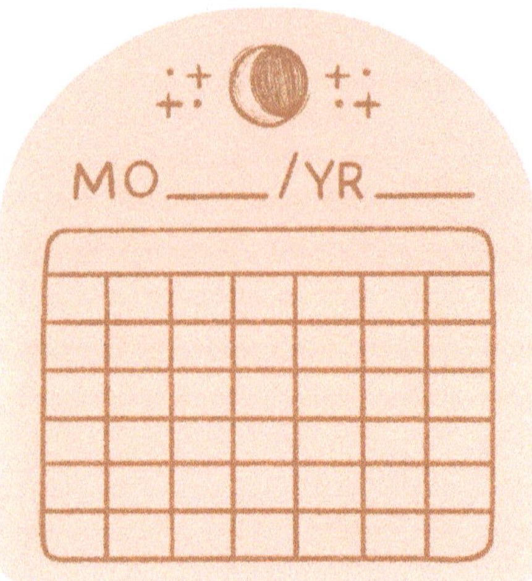
MO____/YR____

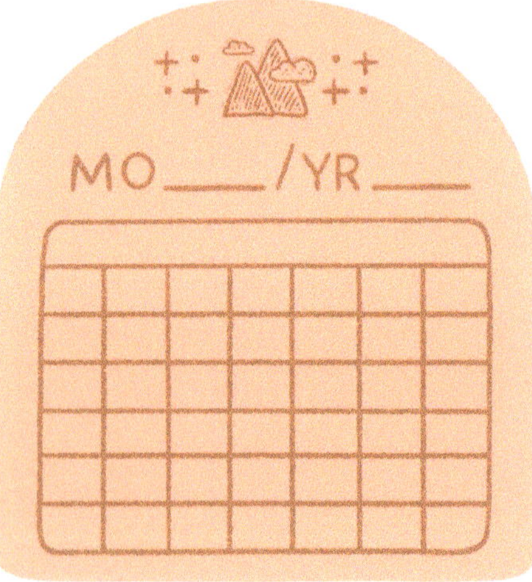
MO____/YR____

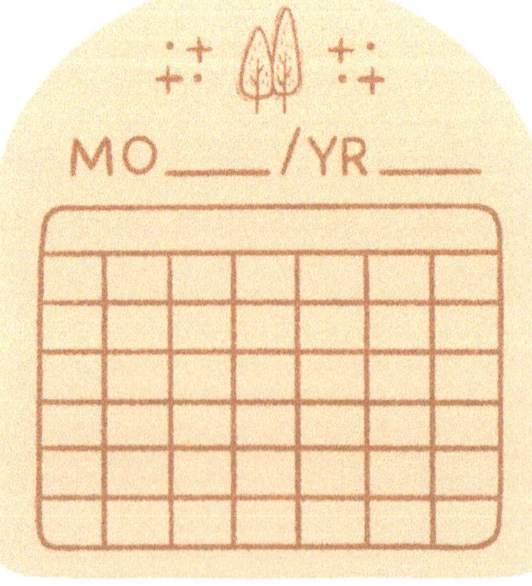
MO____/YR____

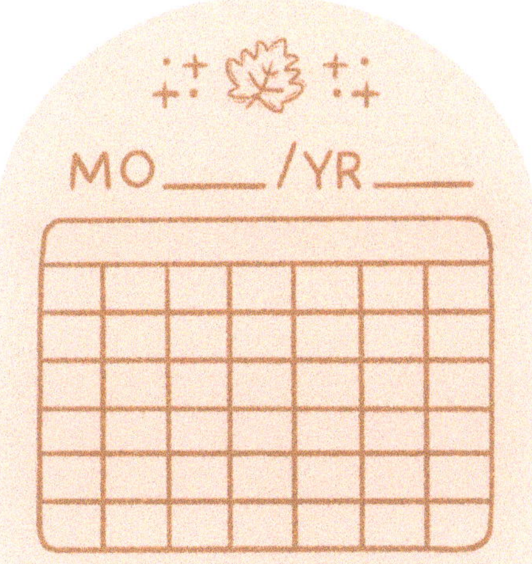
MO____/YR____

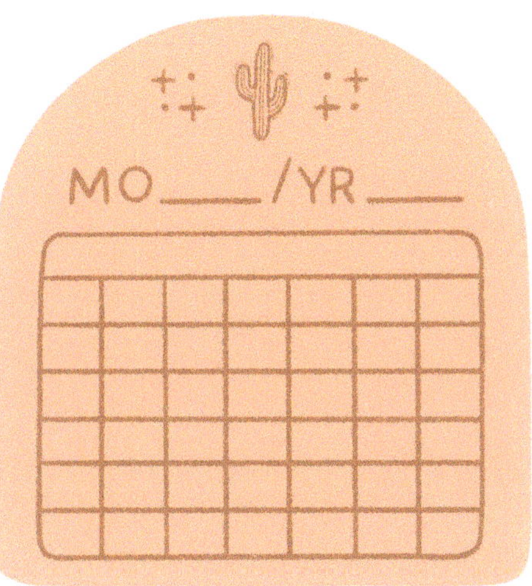
MO____/YR____

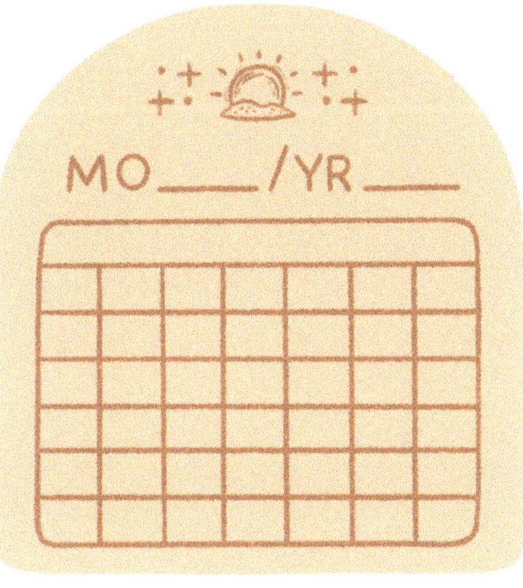
MO____/YR____

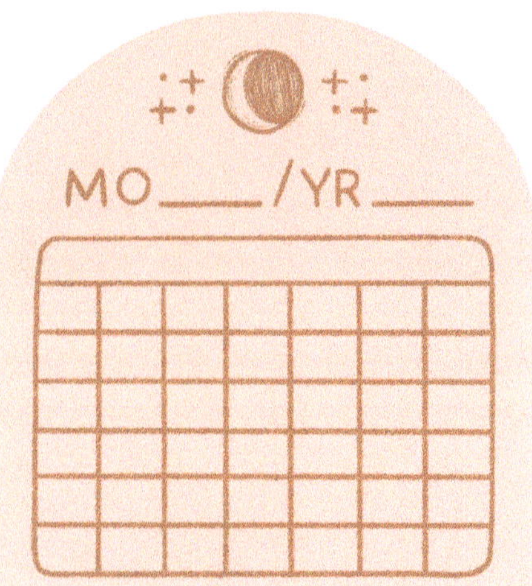
MO____ /YR____

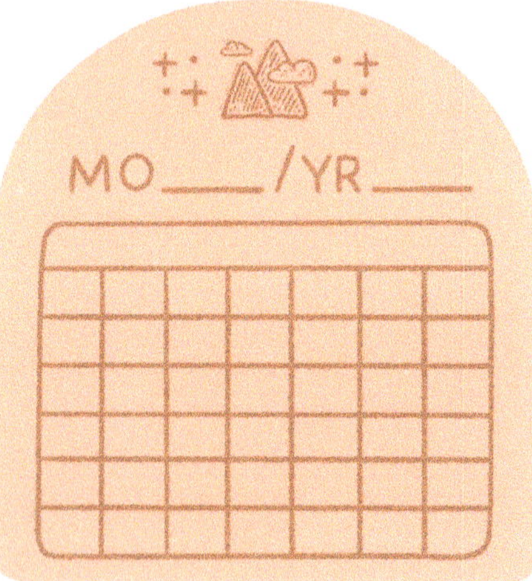
MO____ /YR____

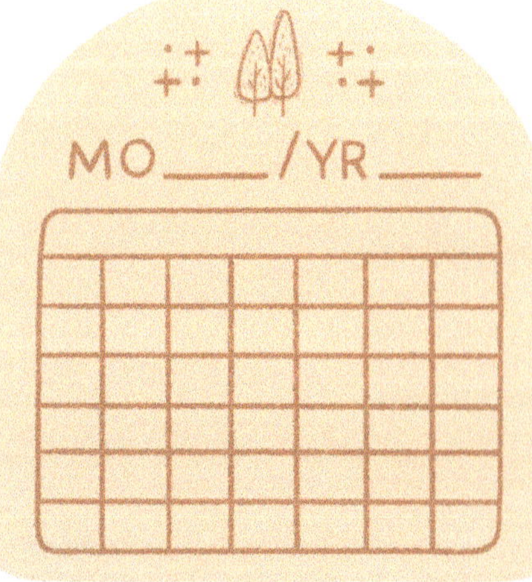
MO____ /YR____

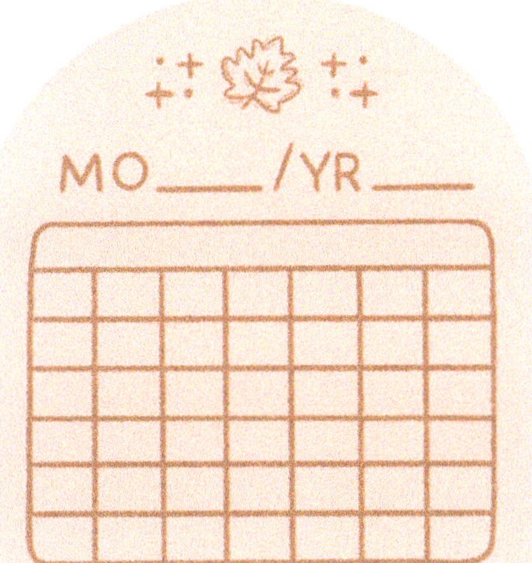

MO____/YR____

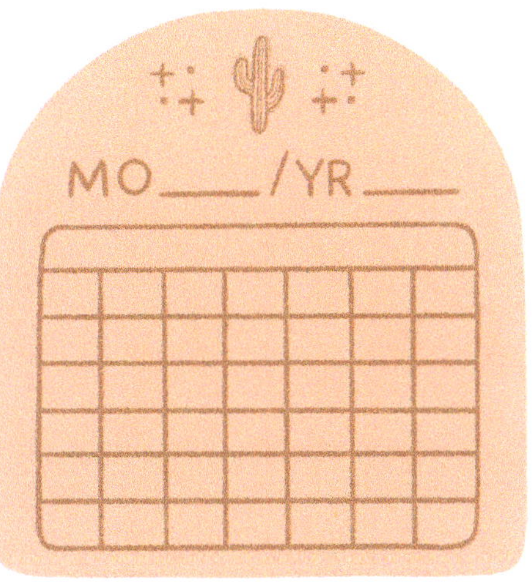

MO____/YR____

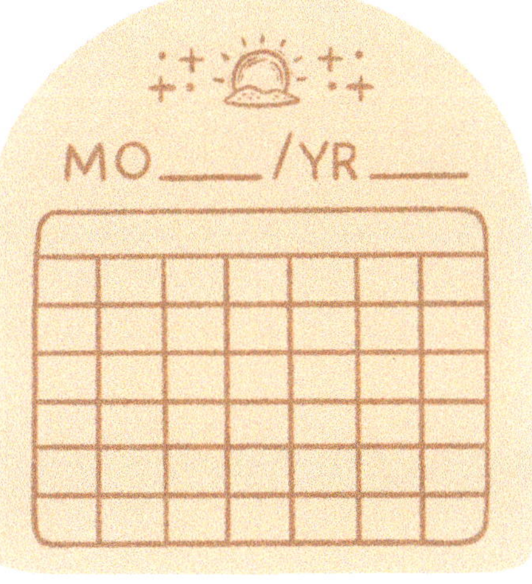

MO____/YR____

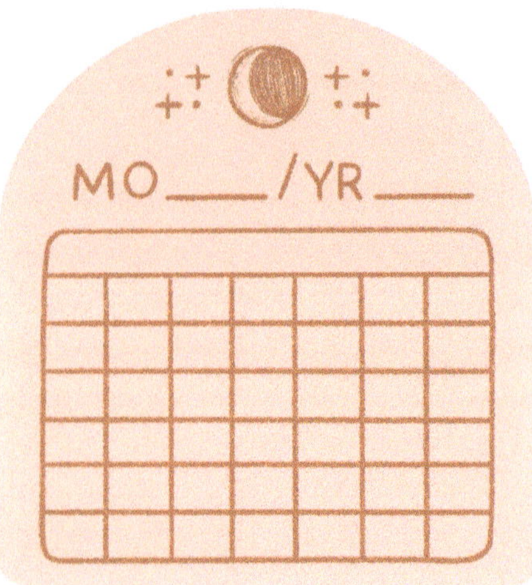

MO____/YR____

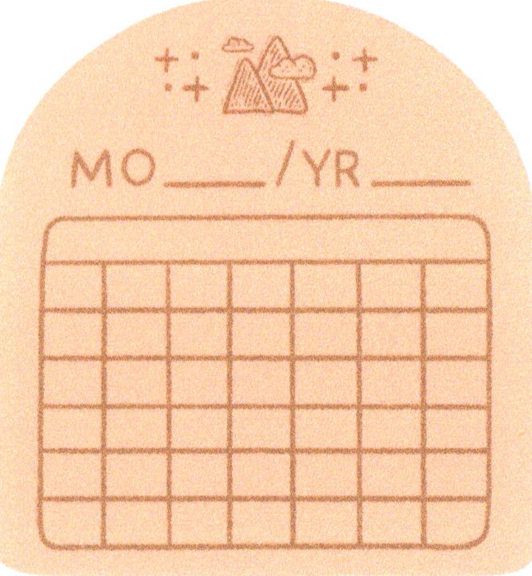

MO____/YR____

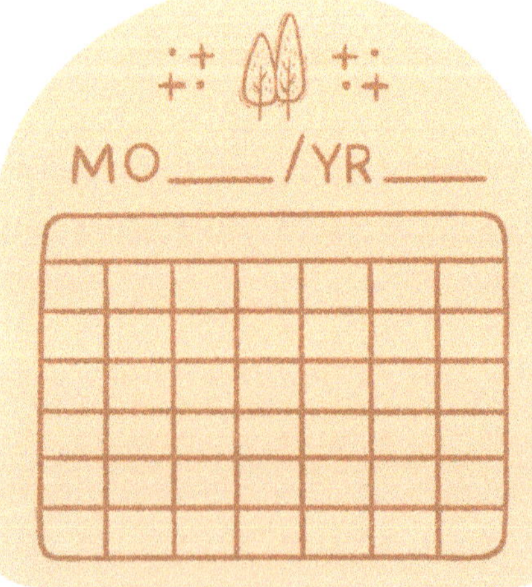

MO____/YR____

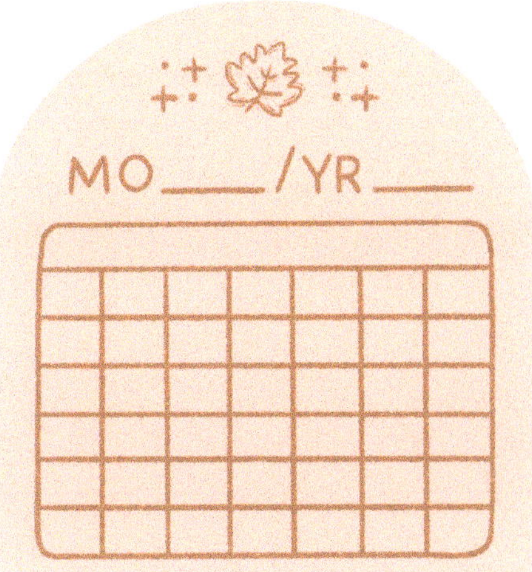
MO____/YR____

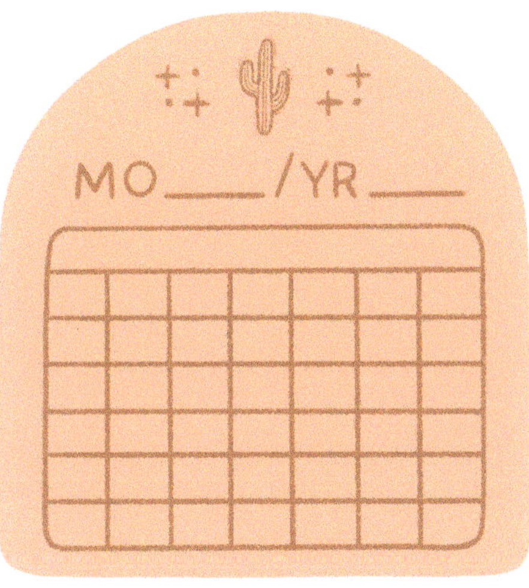
MO____/YR____

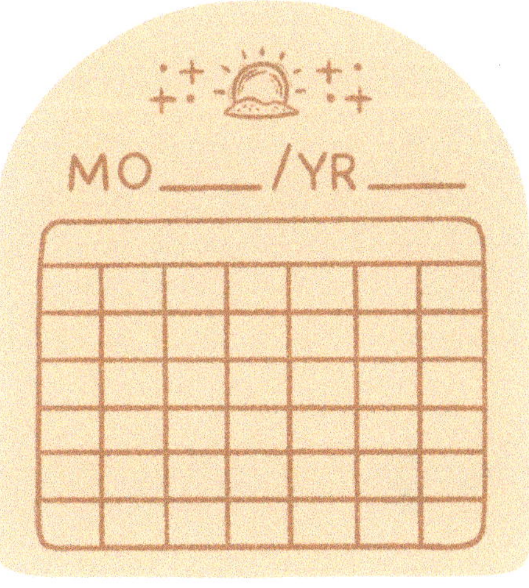
MO____/YR____

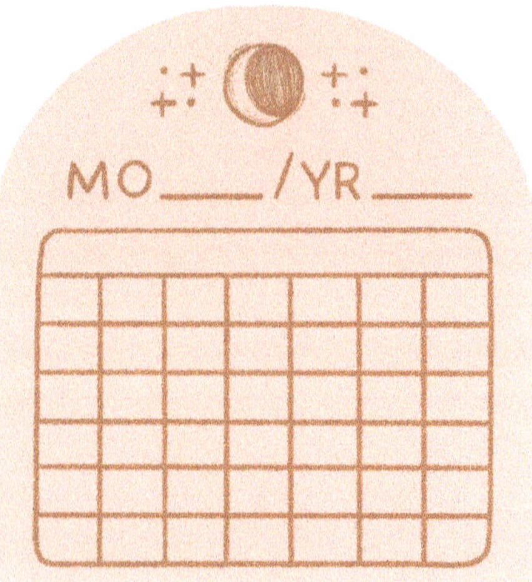
MO____/YR____

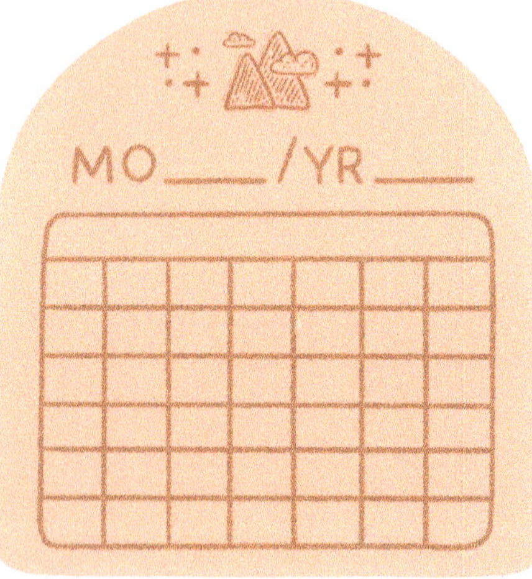
MO____/YR____

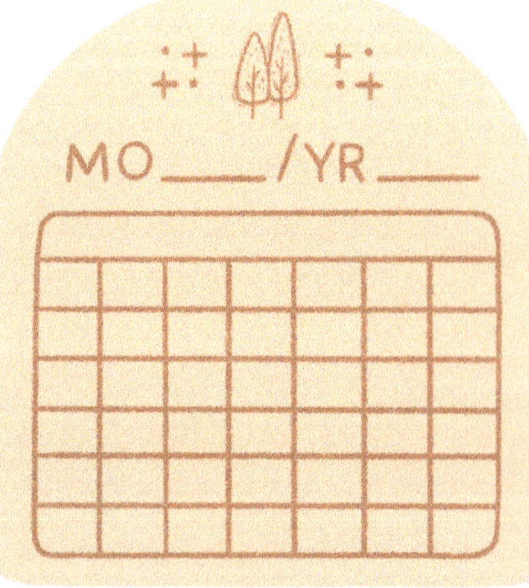
MO____/YR____

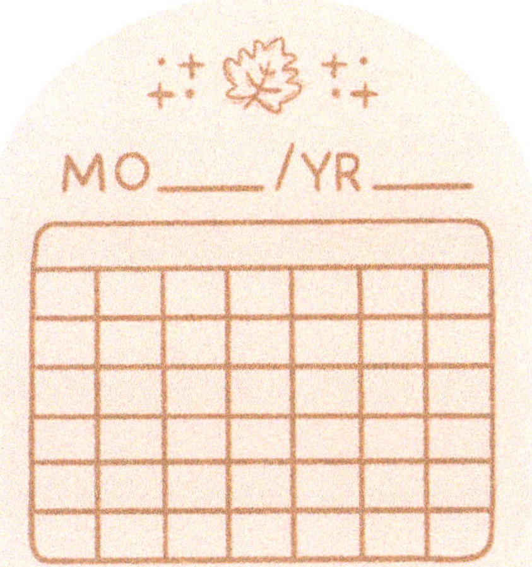

MO____/YR____

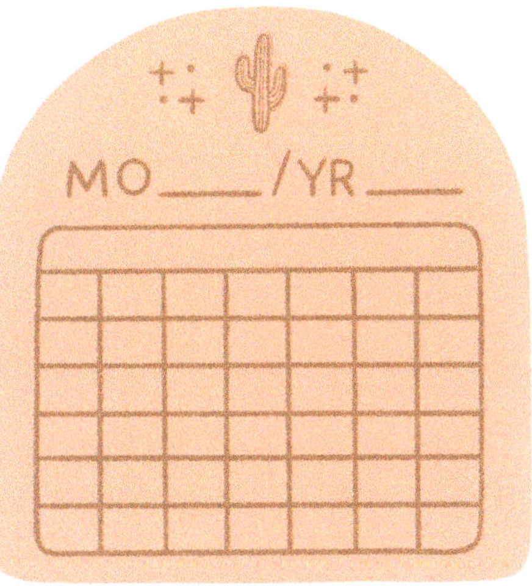

MO____/YR____

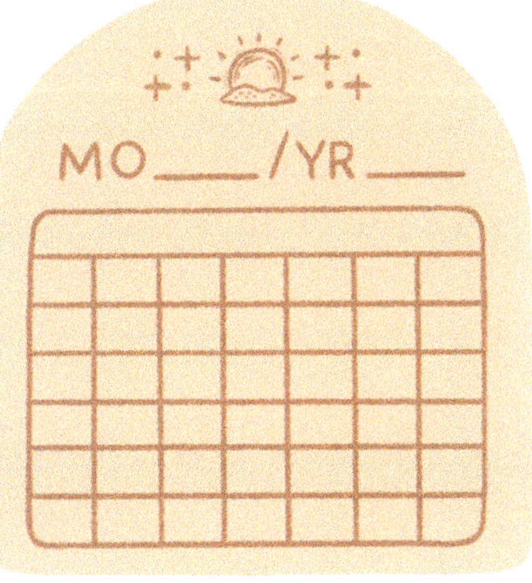

MO____/YR____

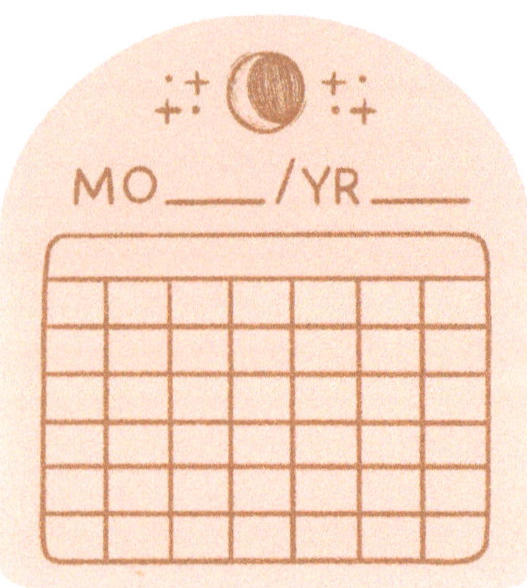
MO____/YR____

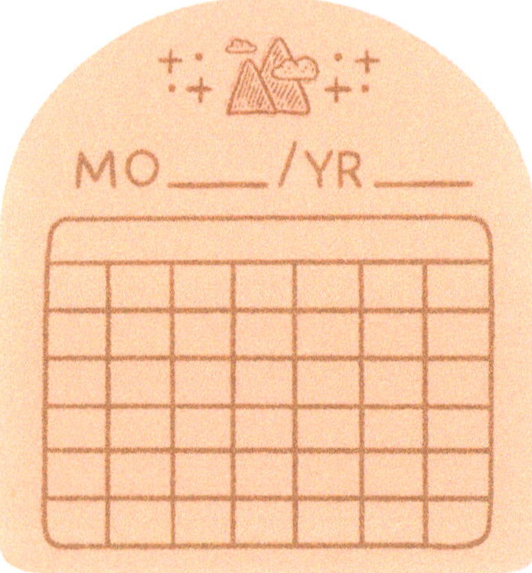
MO____/YR____

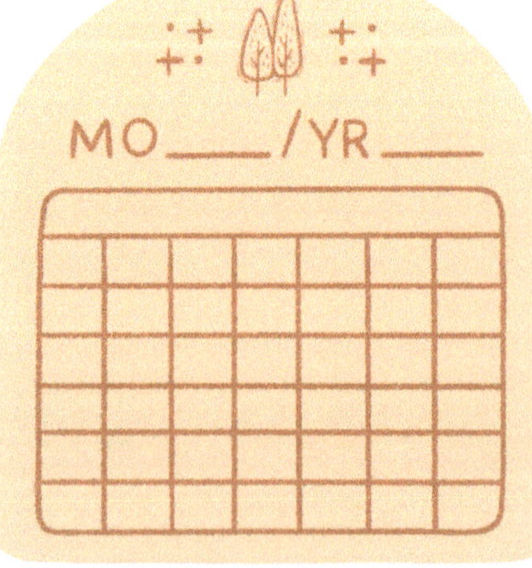
MO____/YR____

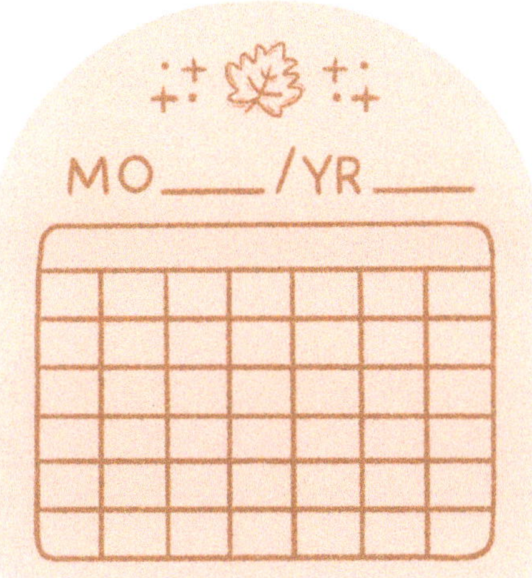
MO____/YR____

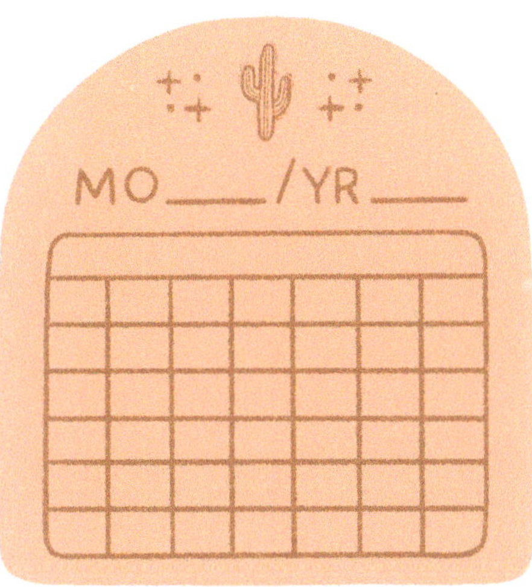
MO____/YR____

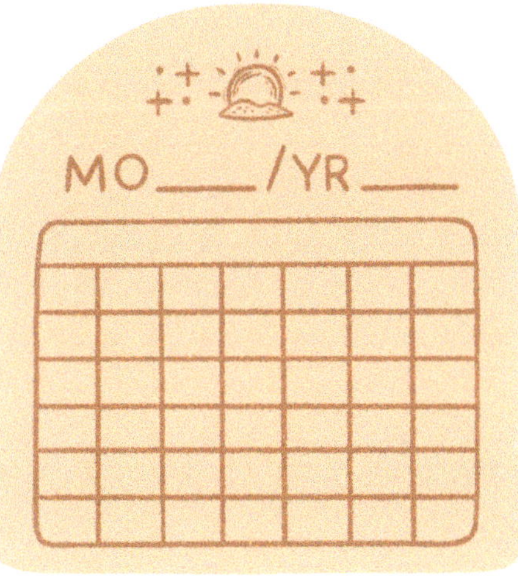
MO____/YR____

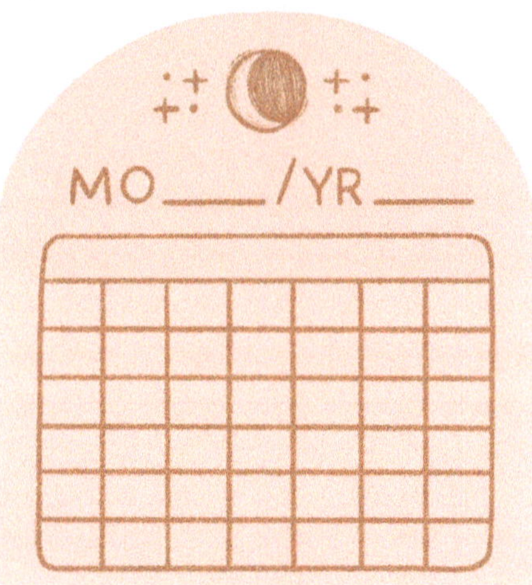

MO_____/YR_____

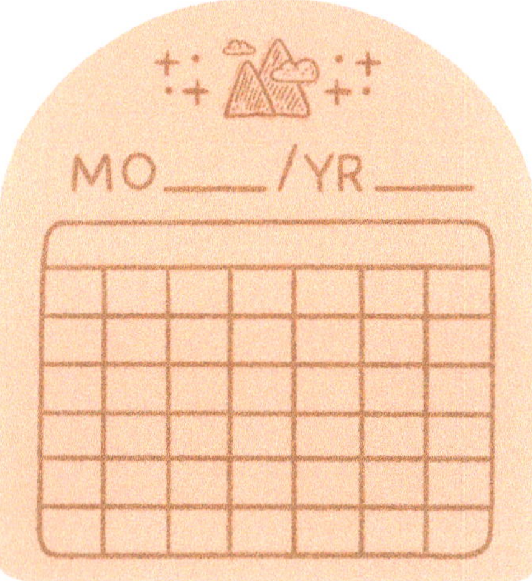

MO_____/YR_____

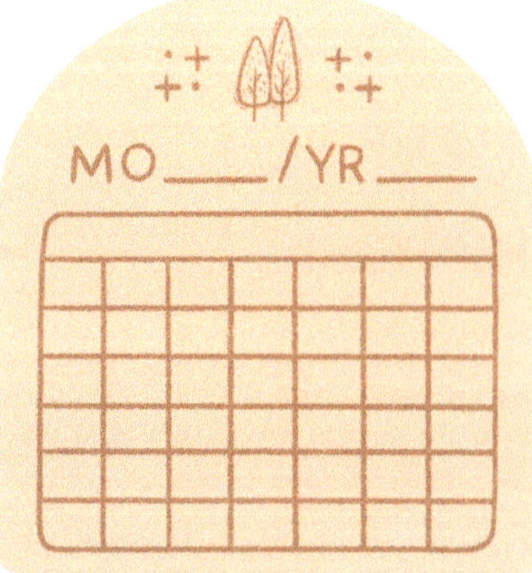

MO_____/YR_____

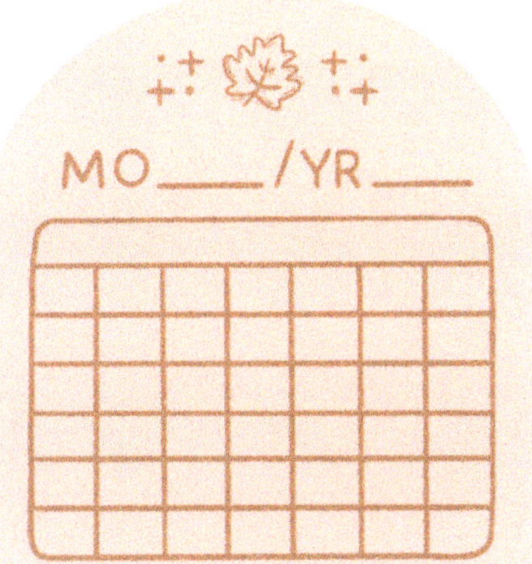

MO____/YR____

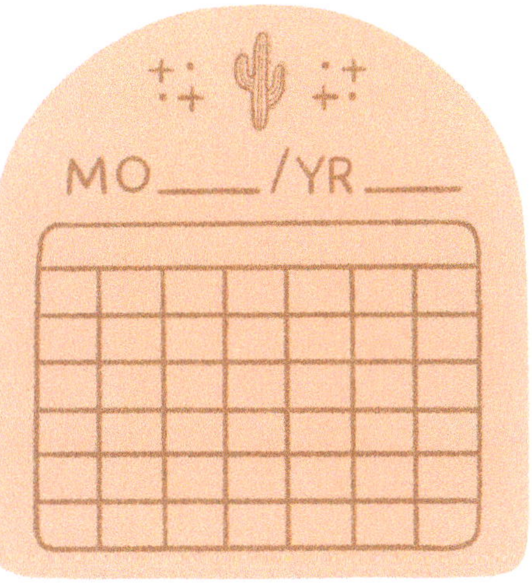

MO____/YR____

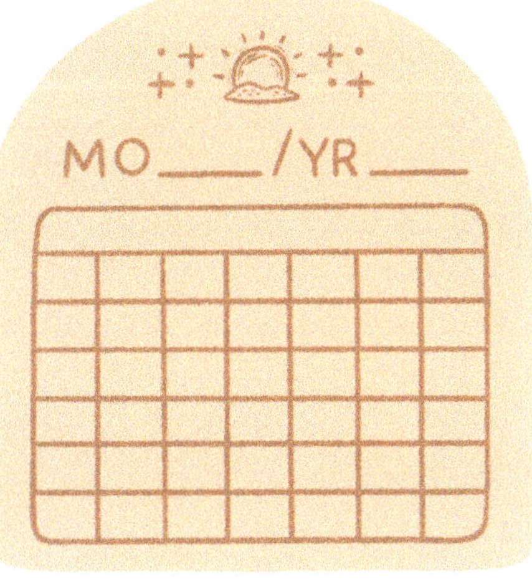

MO____/YR____

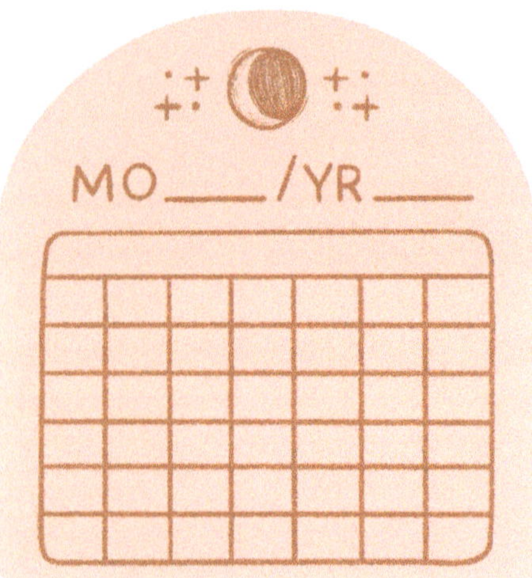

MO____/YR____

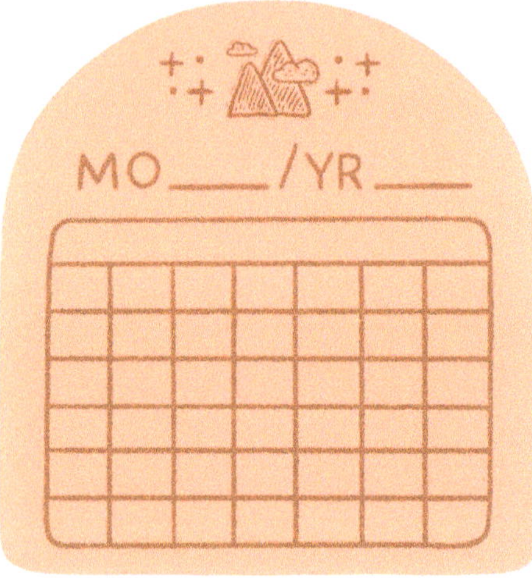

MO____/YR____

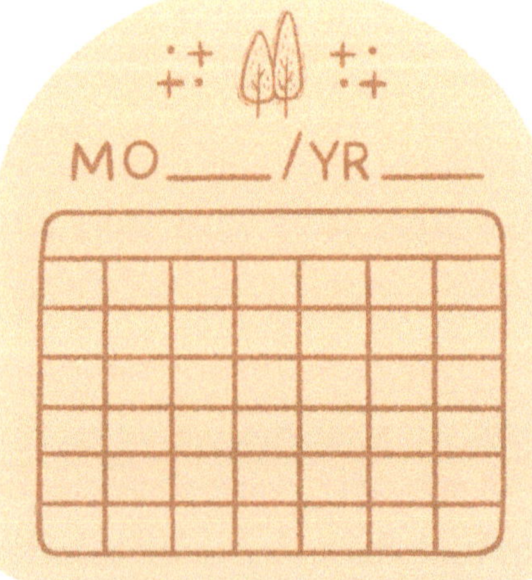

MO____/YR____

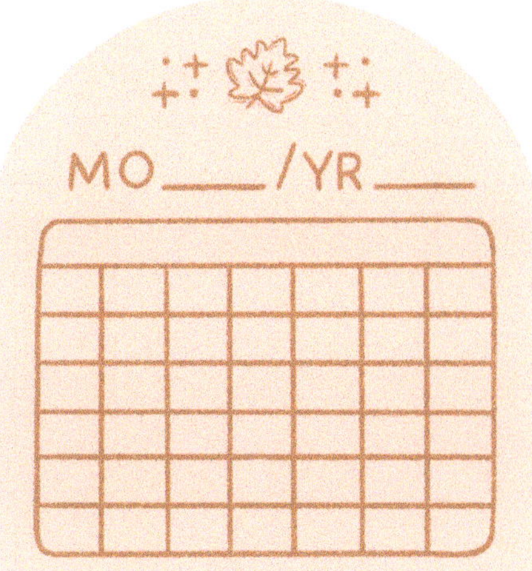
MO____/YR____
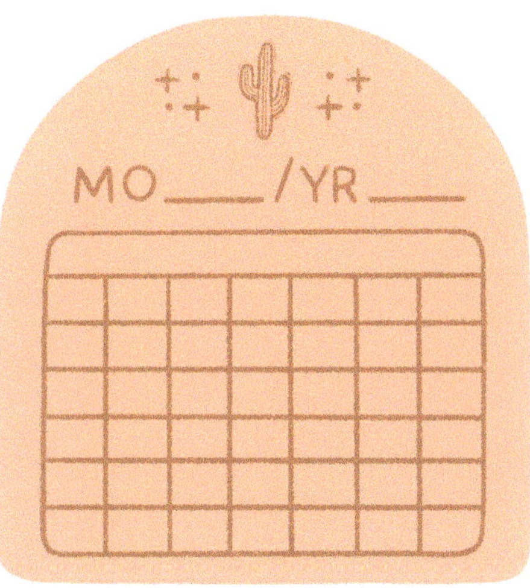
MO____/YR____
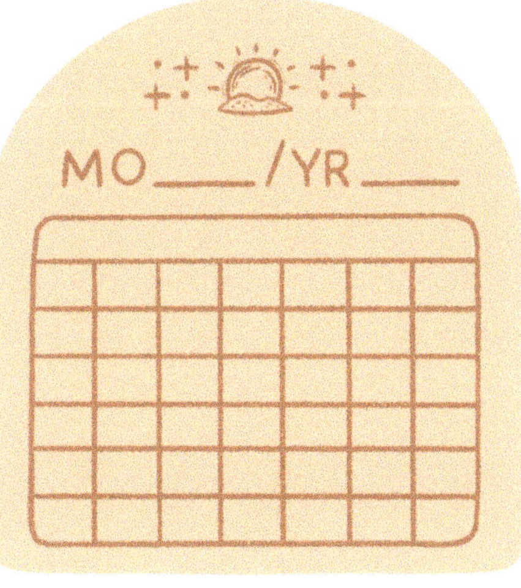
MO____/YR____

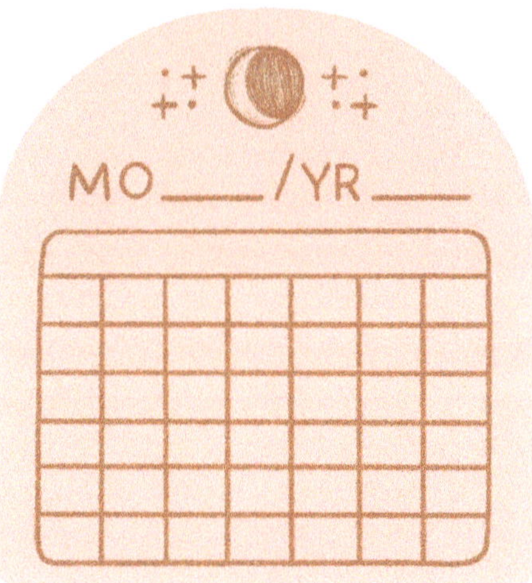

MO____/YR____

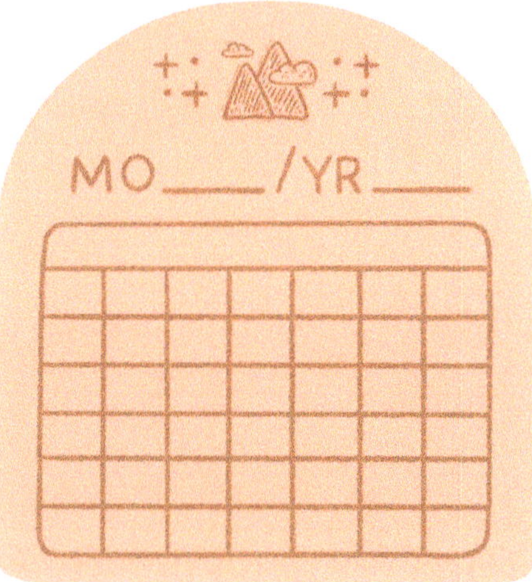

MO____/YR____

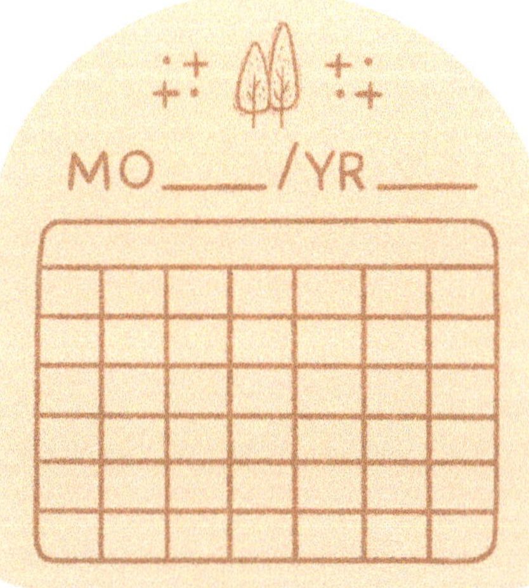

MO____/YR____

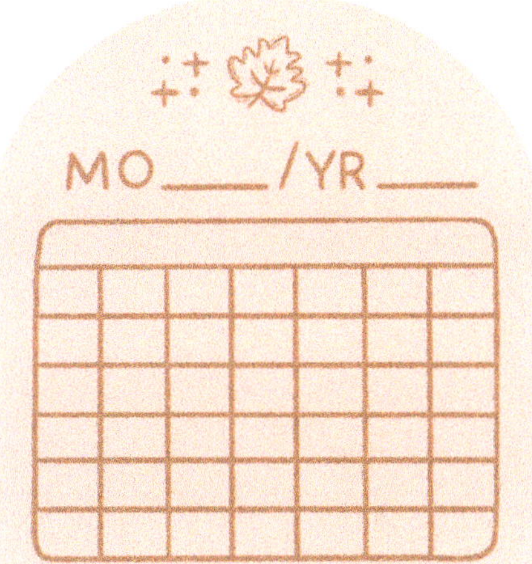

MO ____ /YR ____

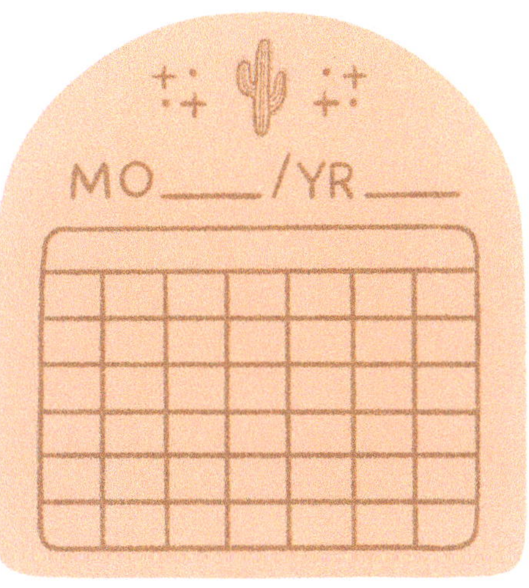

MO ____ /YR ____

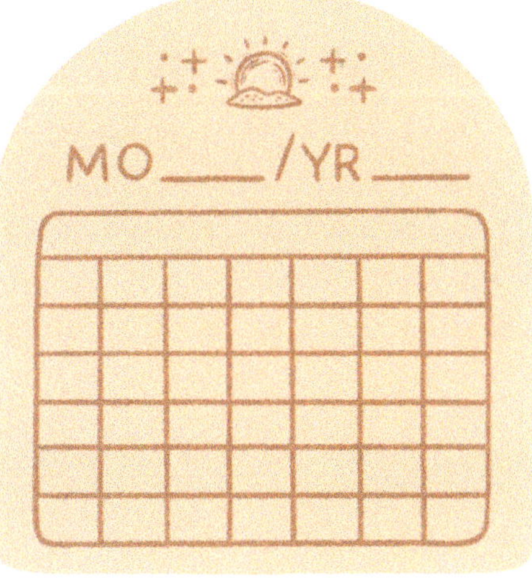

MO ____ /YR ____

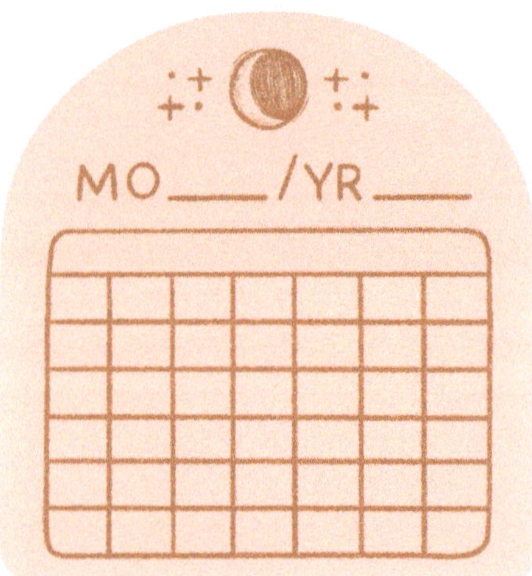

MO____/YR____

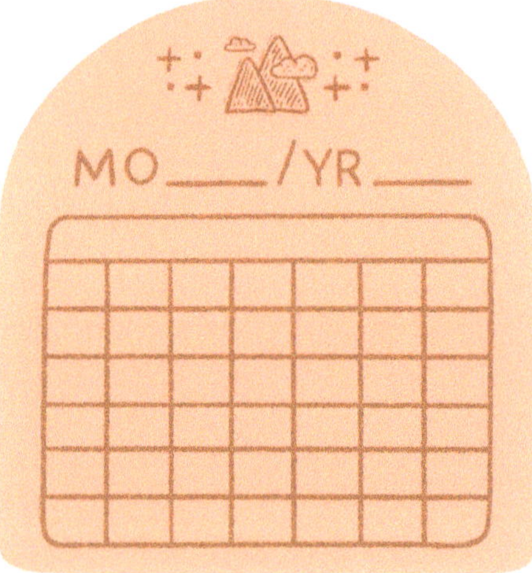

MO____/YR____

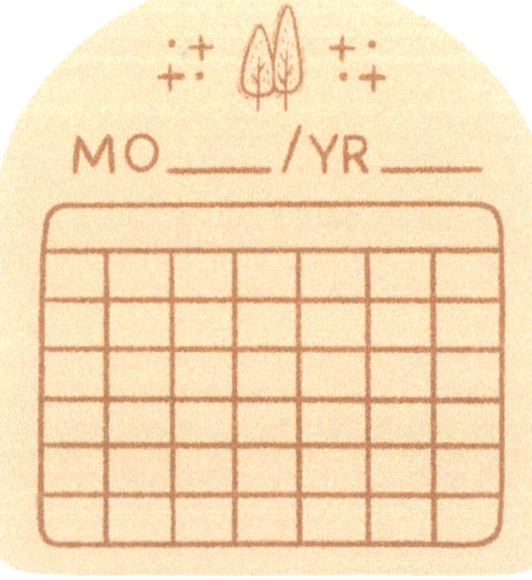

MO____/YR____

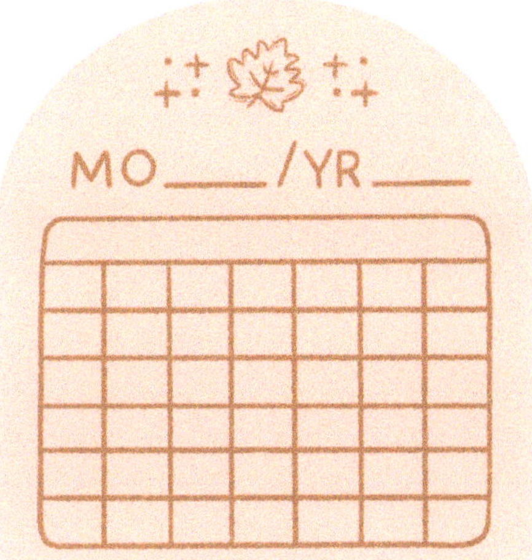

MO____/YR____

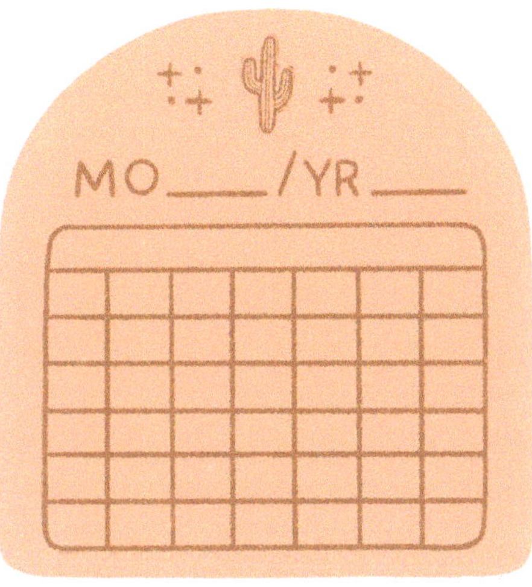

MO____/YR____

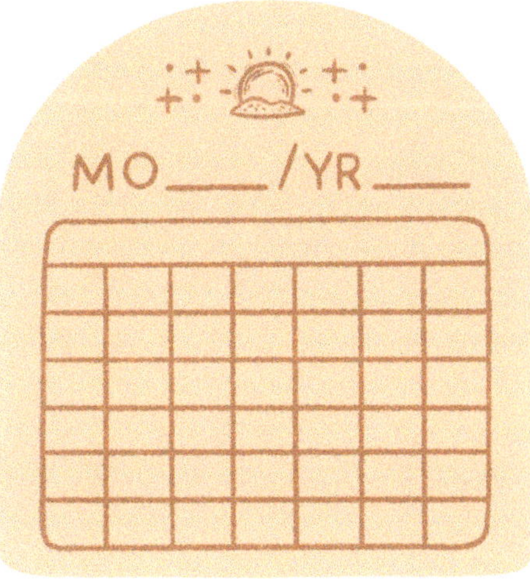

MO____/YR____

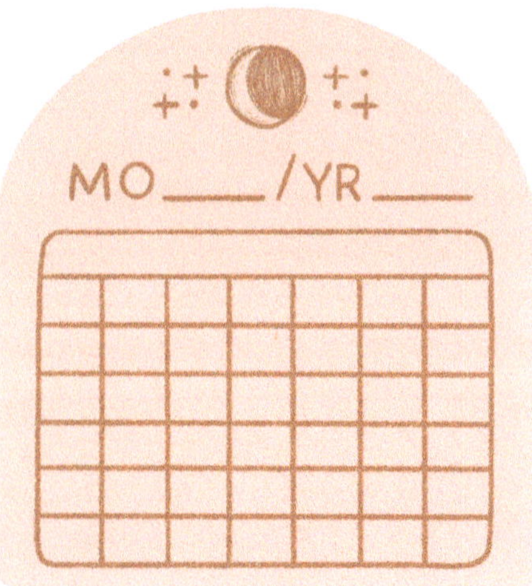

MO____/YR____

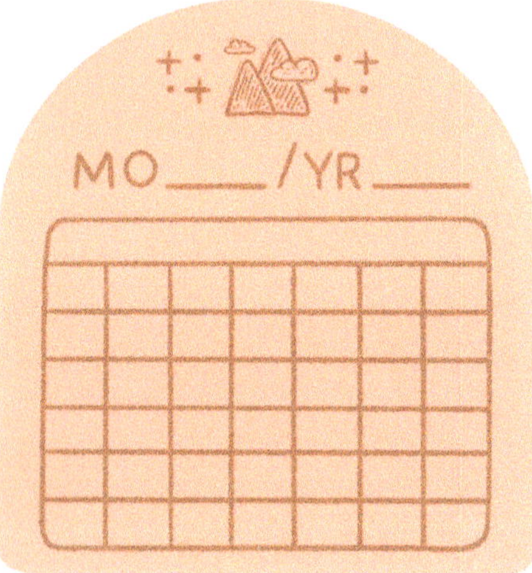

MO____/YR____

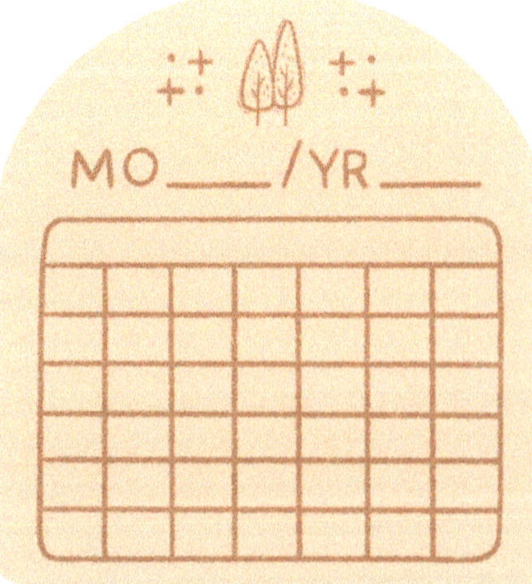

MO____/YR____

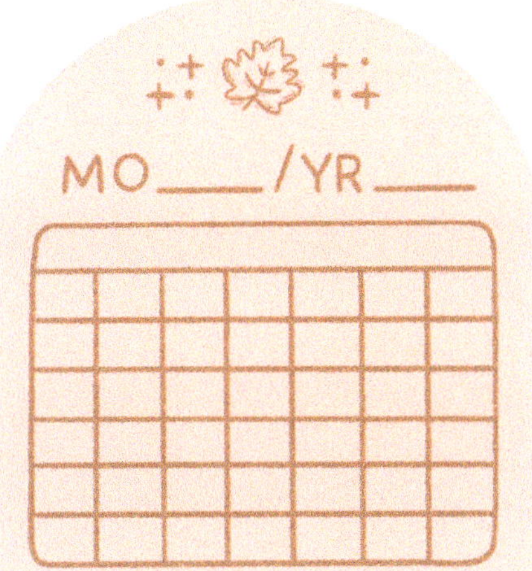
MO____/YR____

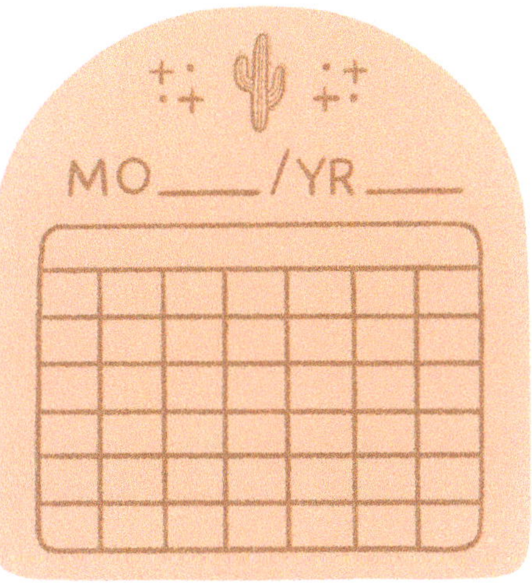
MO____/YR____

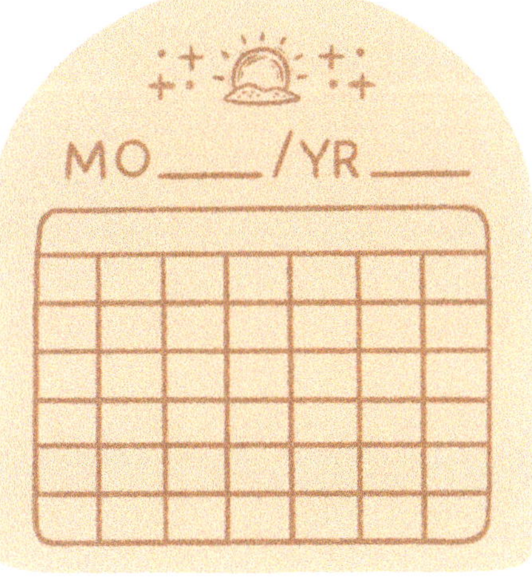
MO____/YR____

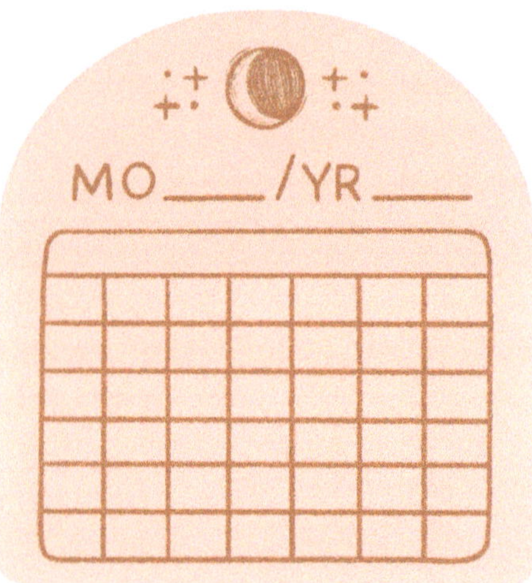

MO____/YR____

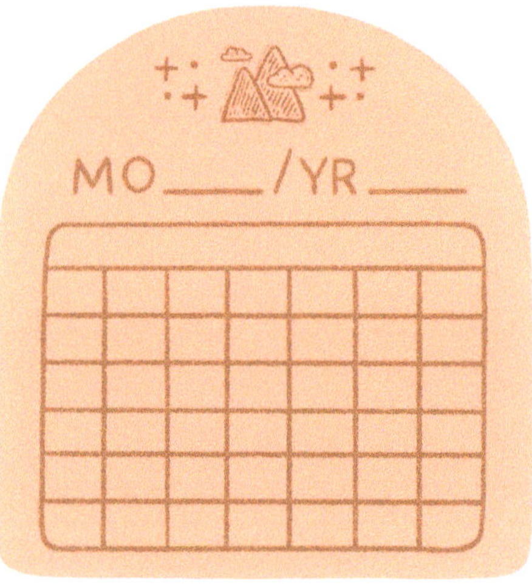

MO____/YR____

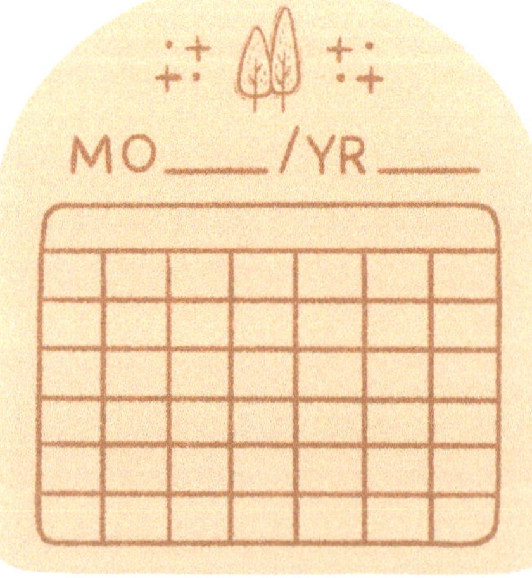

MO____/YR____

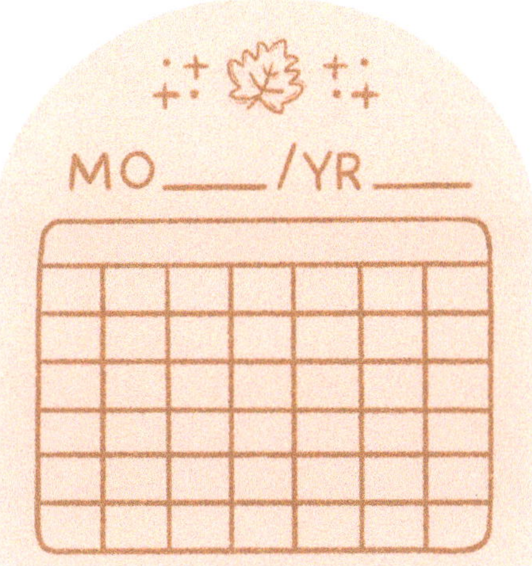

MO____/YR____

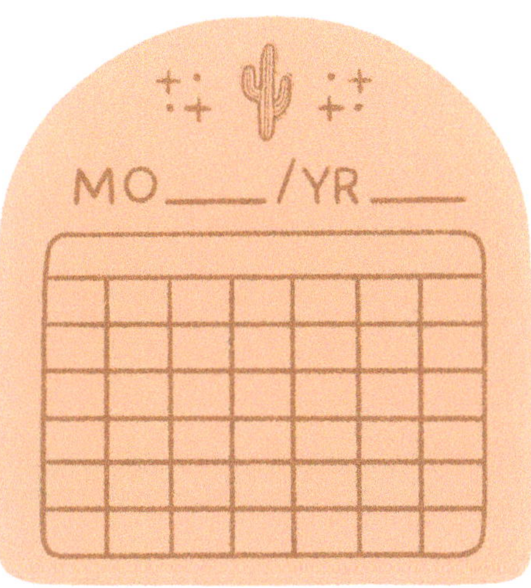

MO____/YR____

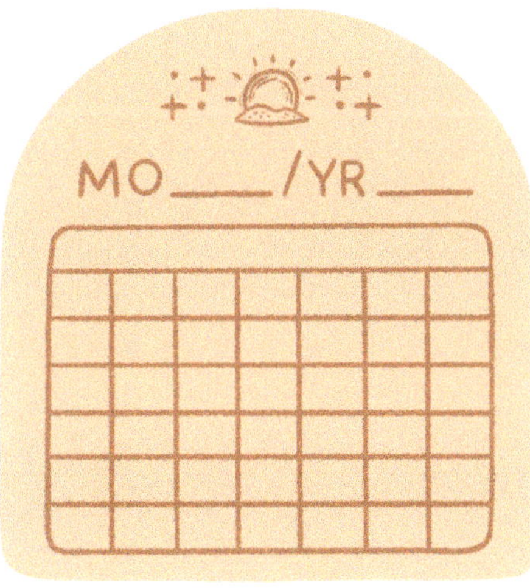

MO____/YR____

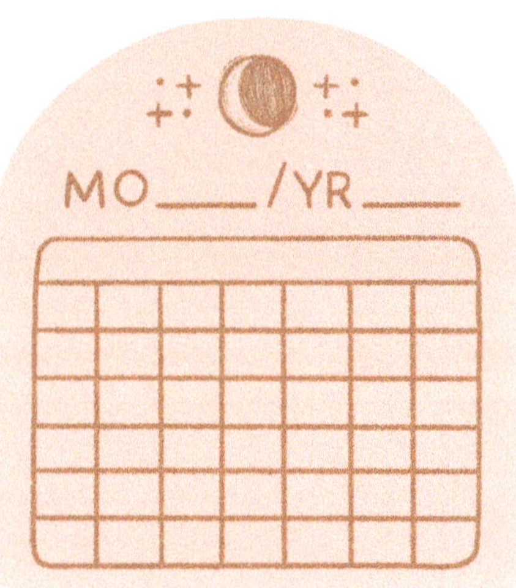

MO_____/YR_____

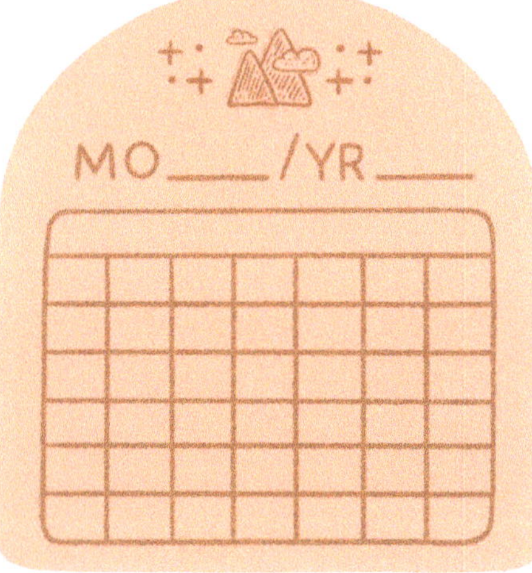

MO_____/YR_____

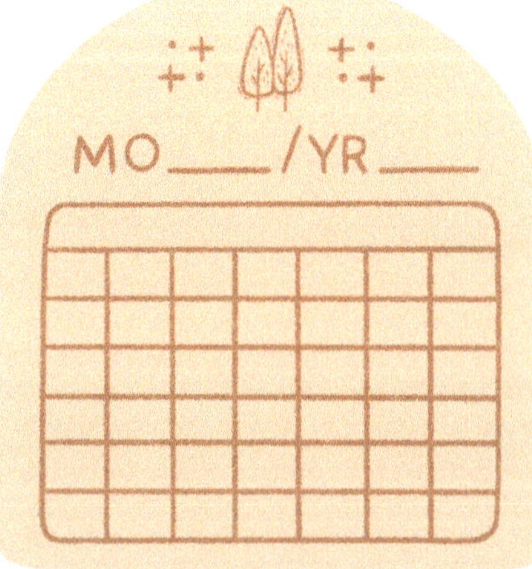

MO_____/YR_____

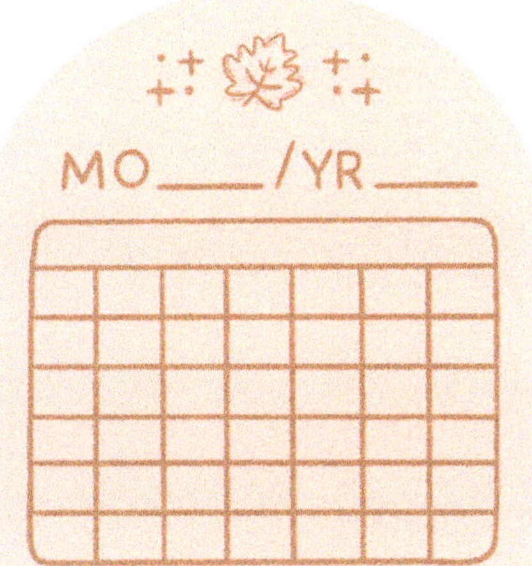

MO____/YR____

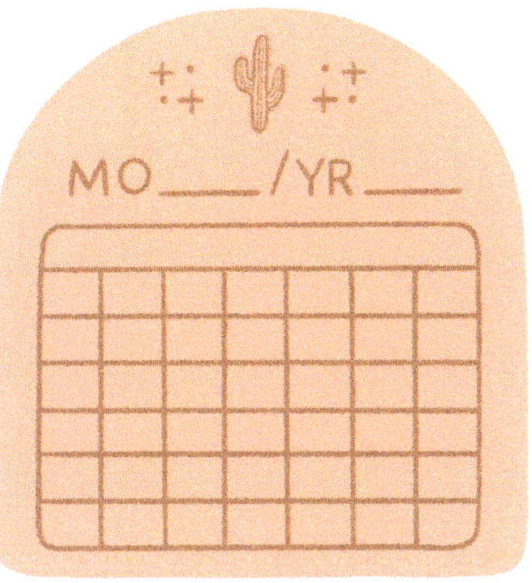

MO____/YR____

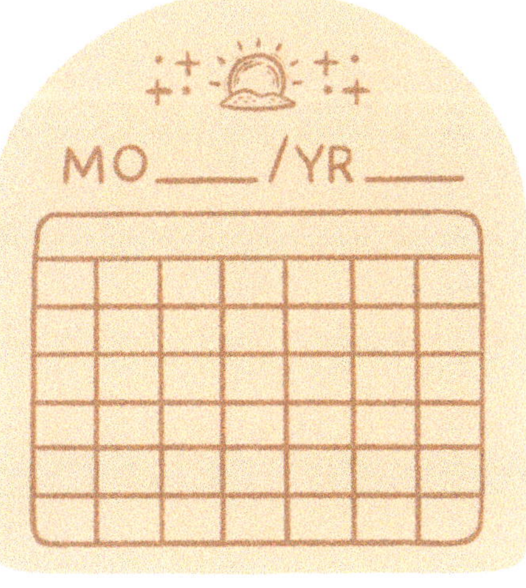

MO____/YR____

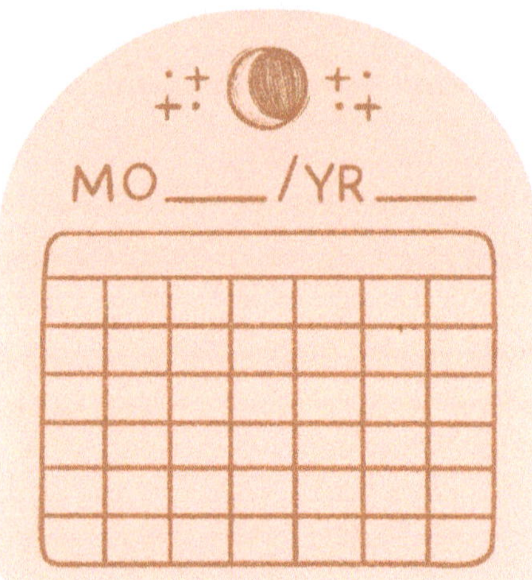

MO____/YR____

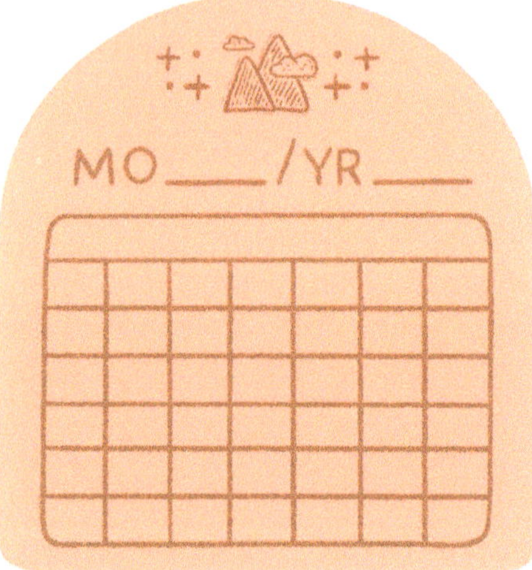

MO____/YR____

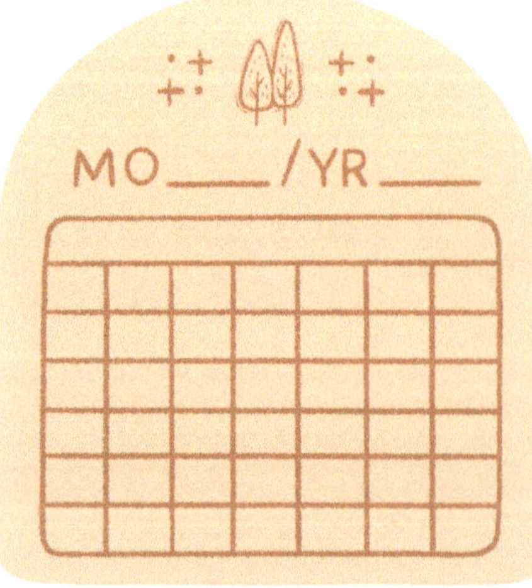

MO____/YR____

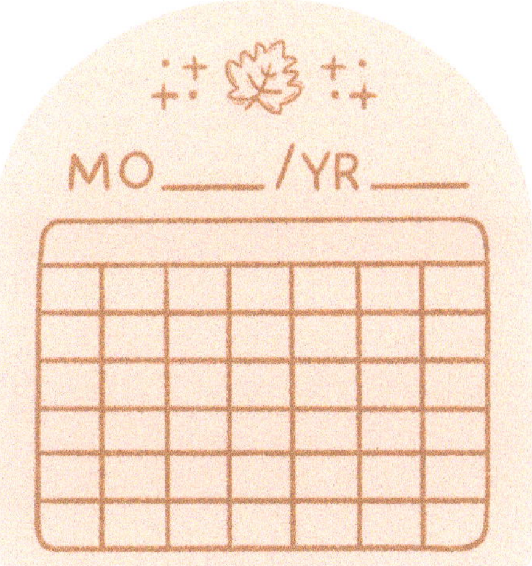
MO____/YR____

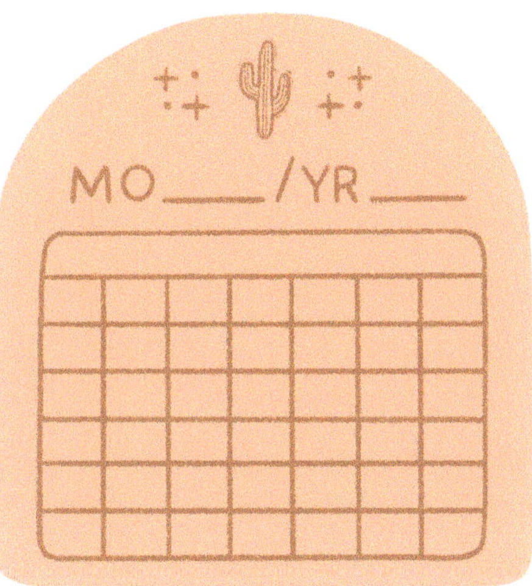
MO____/YR____

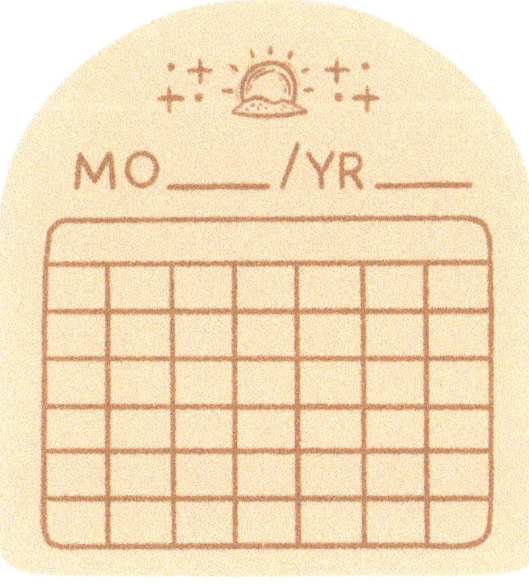
MO____/YR____

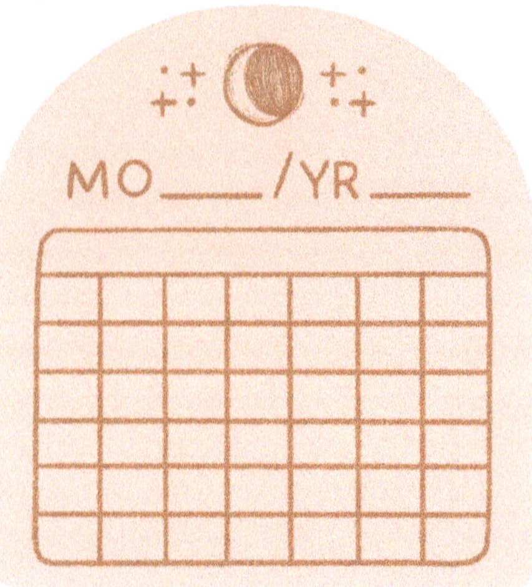

MO____/YR____

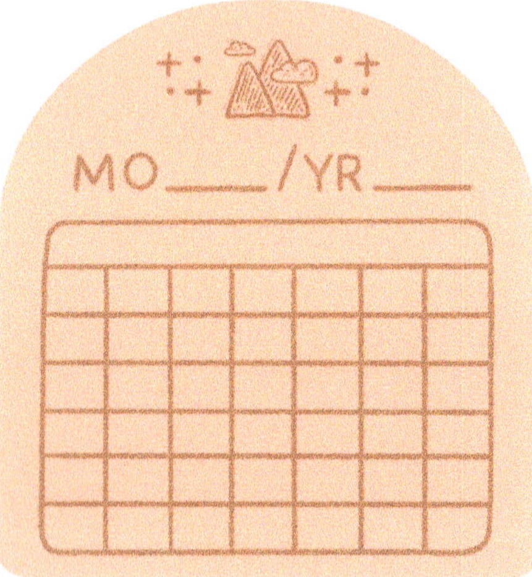

MO____/YR____

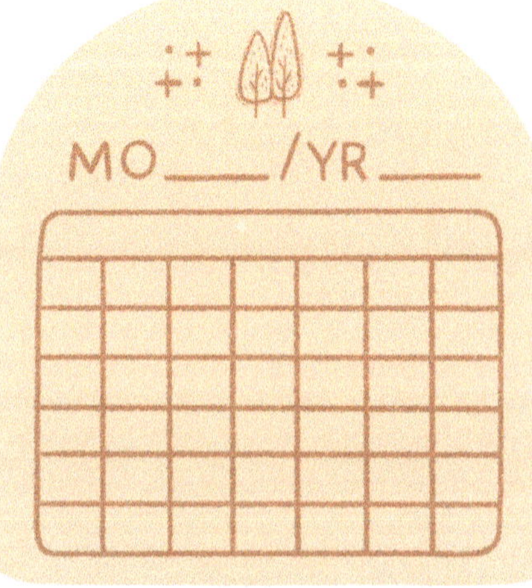

MO____/YR____

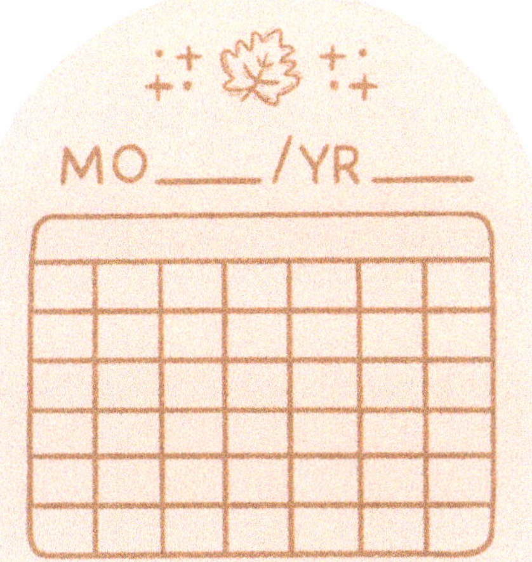

MO____/YR____

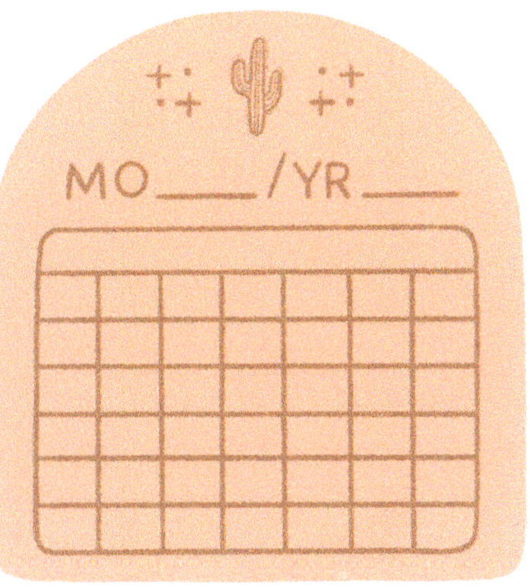

MO____/YR____

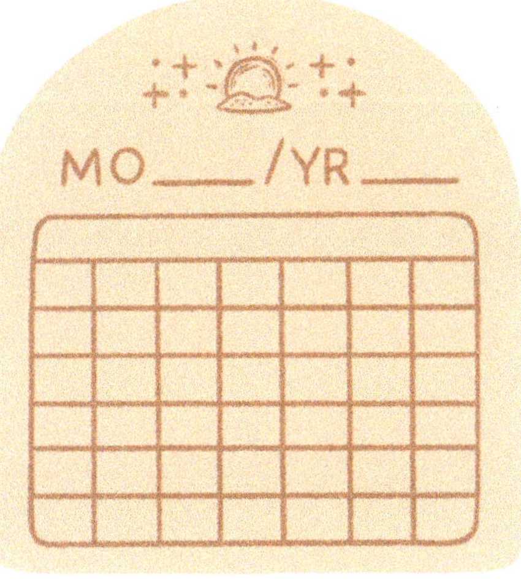

MO____/YR____

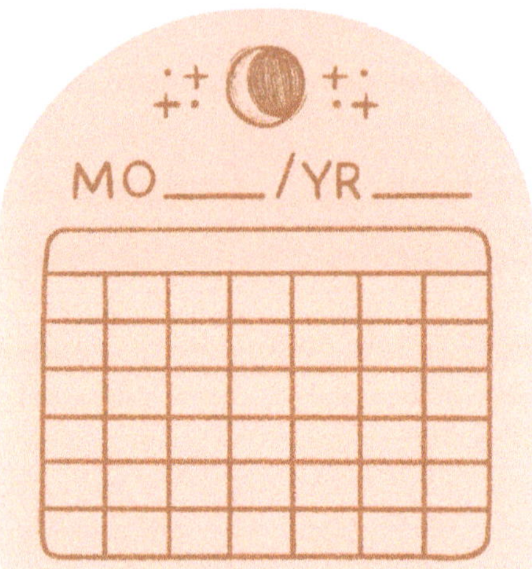
MO____/YR____

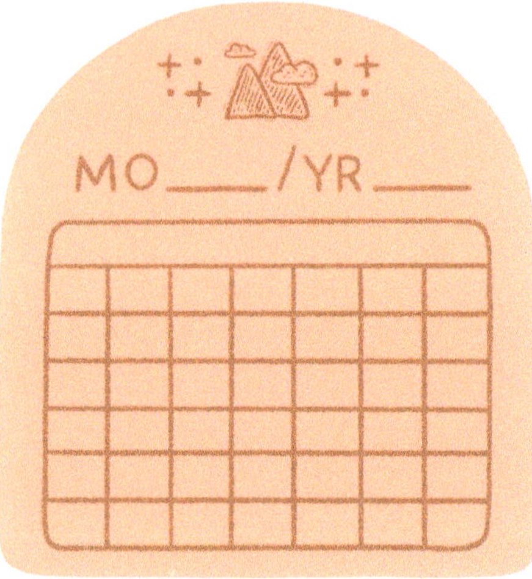
MO____/YR____

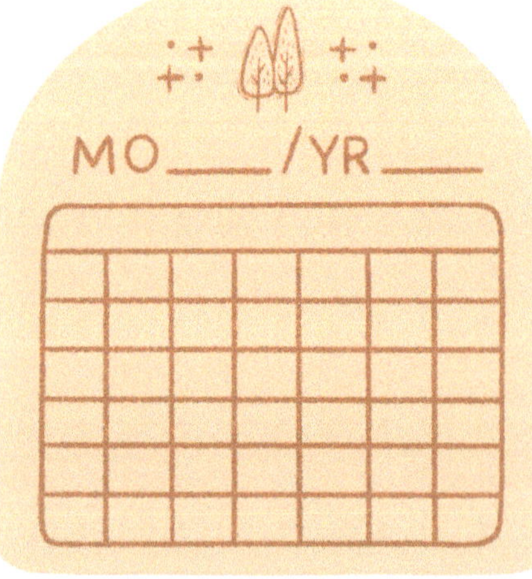
MO____/YR____

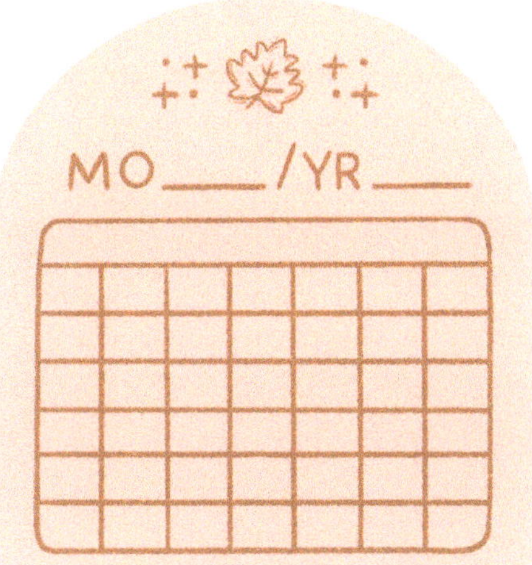

MO____/YR____

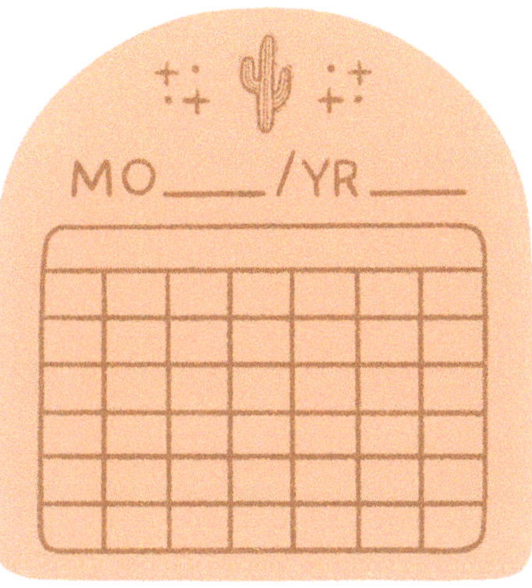

MO____/YR____

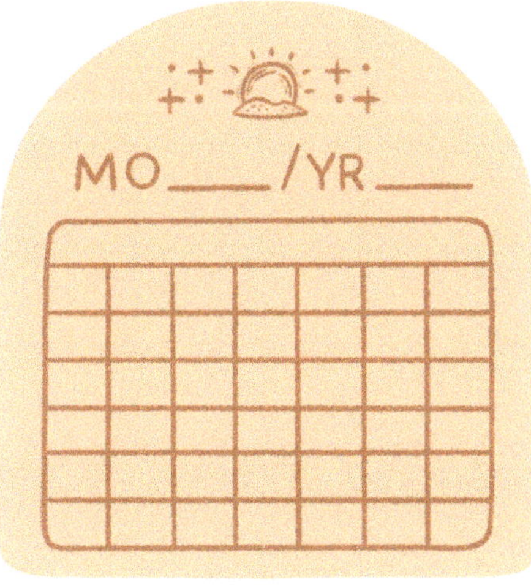

MO____/YR____

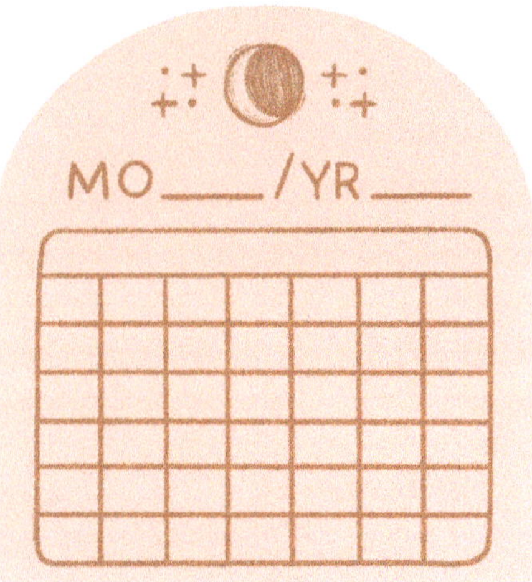
MO____/YR____

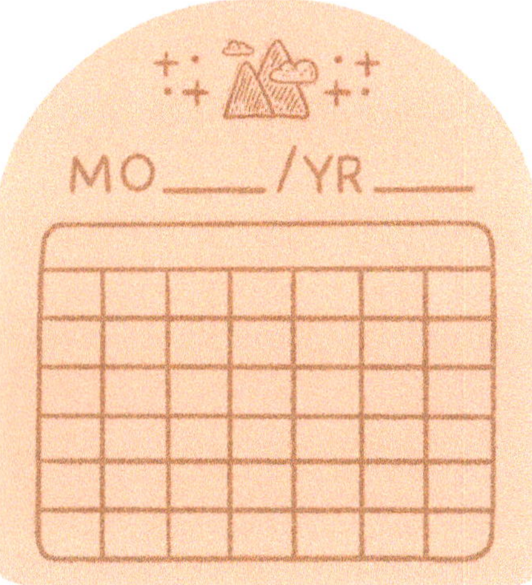
MO____/YR____

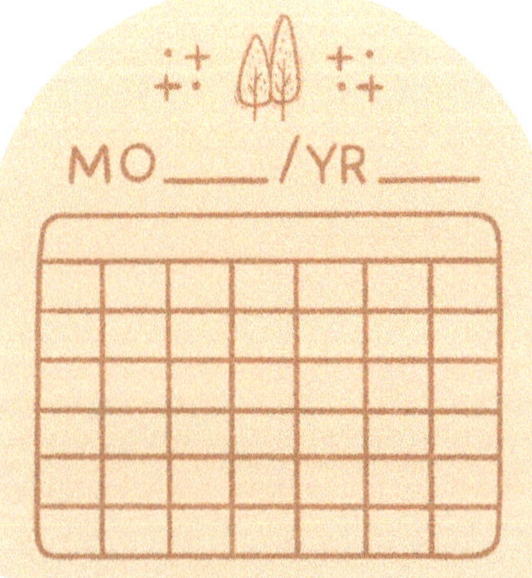
MO____/YR____

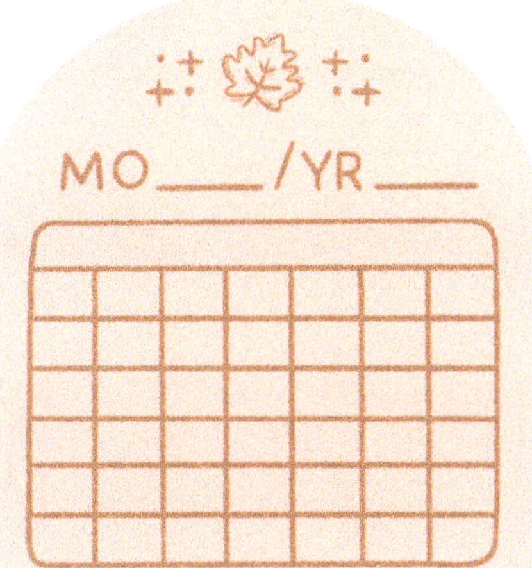
MO____ /YR____

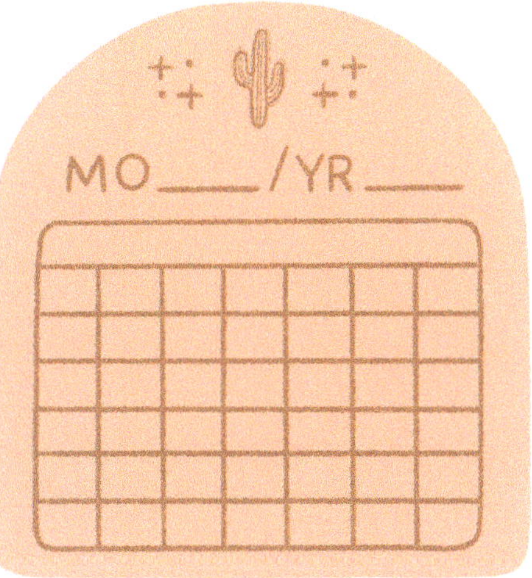
MO____ /YR____

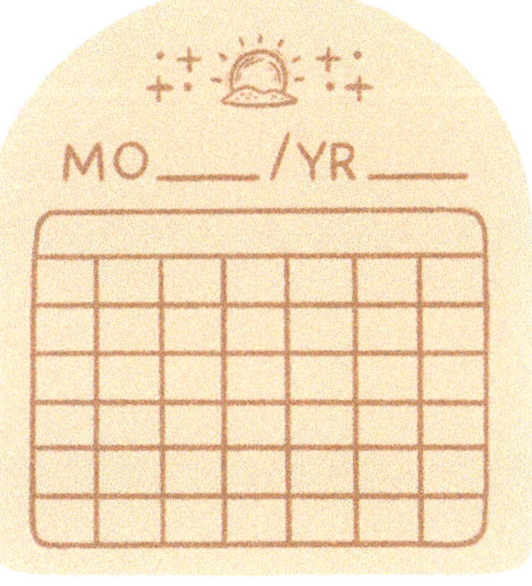
MO____ /YR____

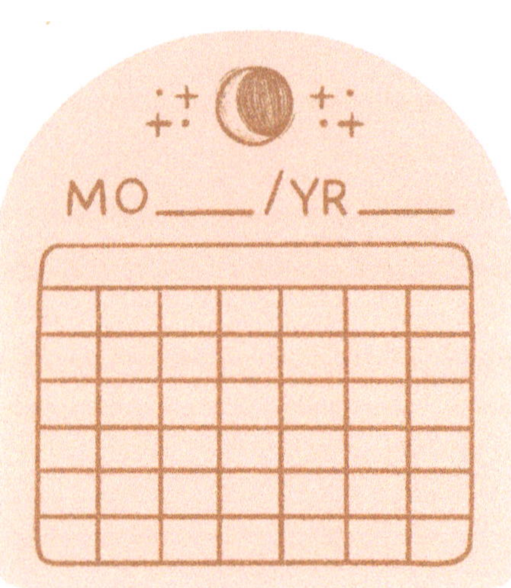

MO____/YR____

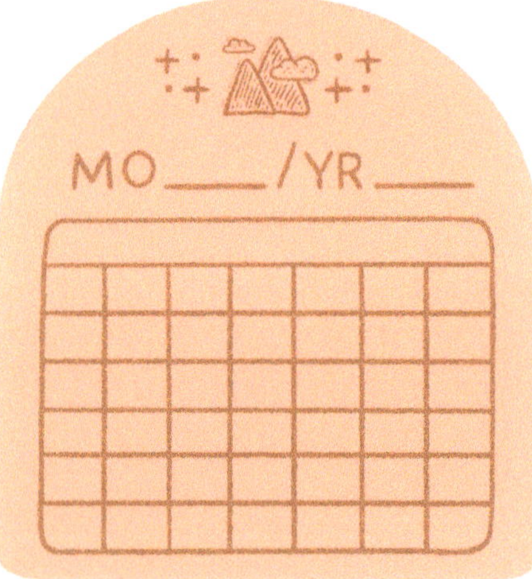

MO____/YR____

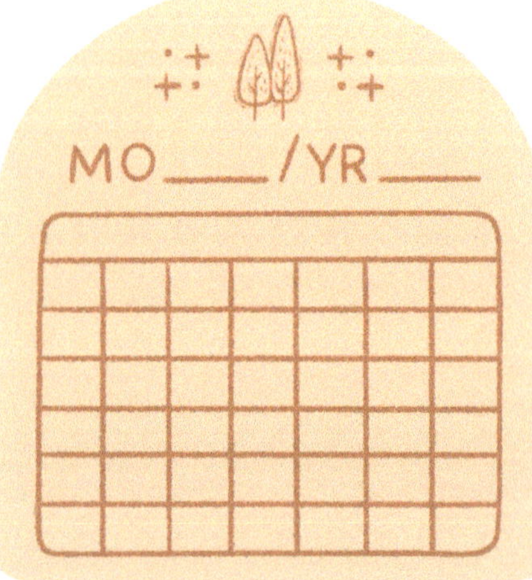

MO____/YR____

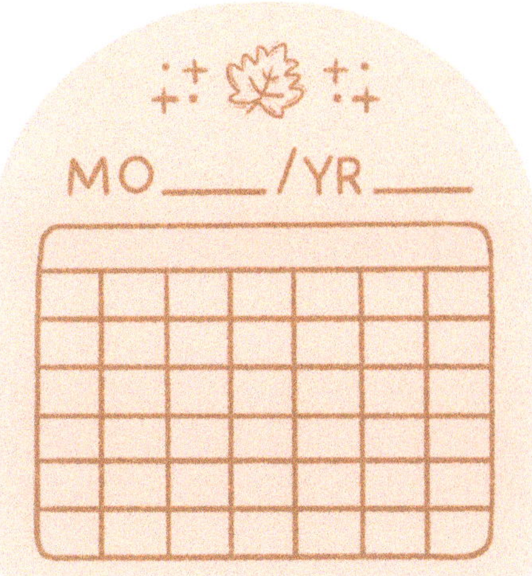

MO_____/YR_____

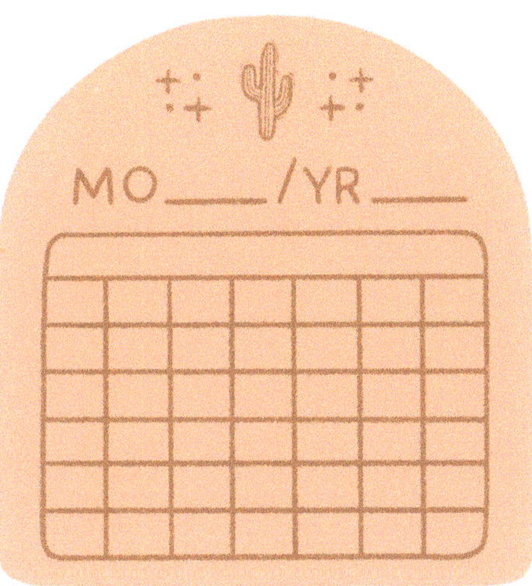

MO_____/YR_____

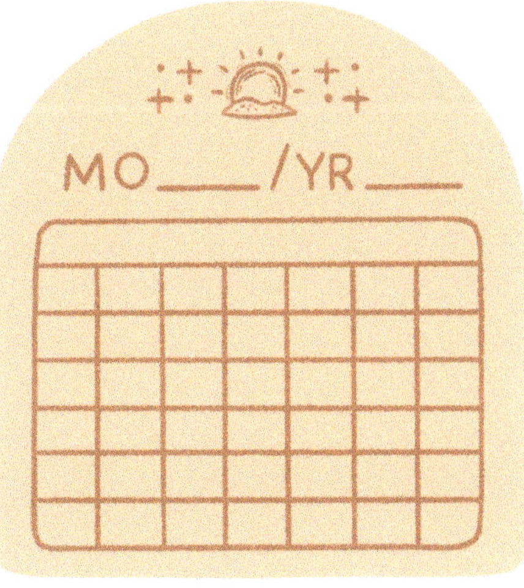

MO_____/YR_____

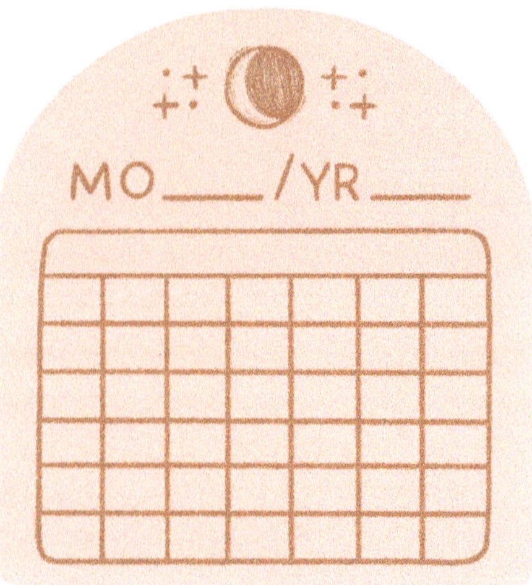
MO____/YR____

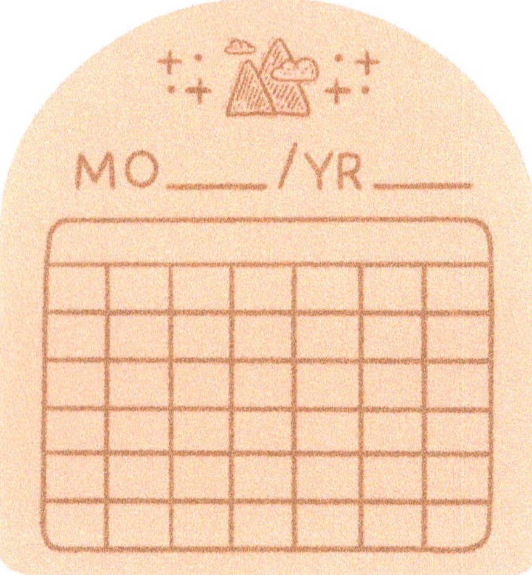
MO____/YR____

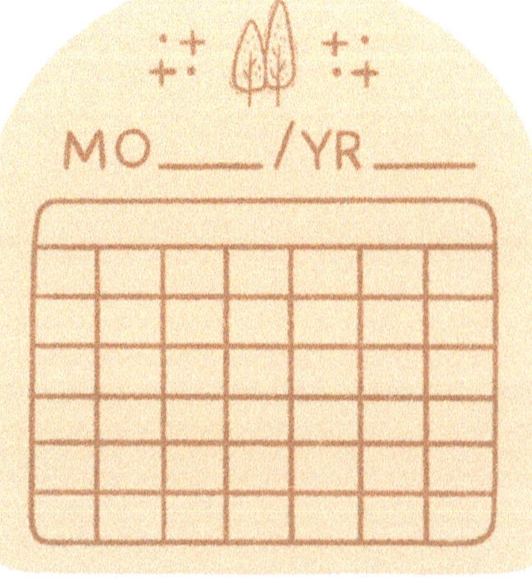
MO____/YR____

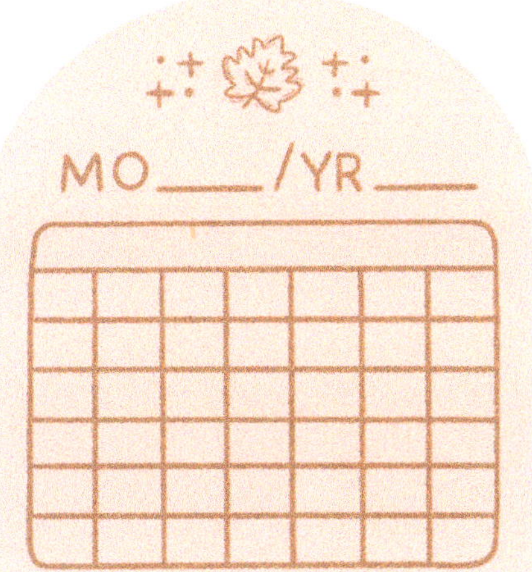
MO____ /YR ____

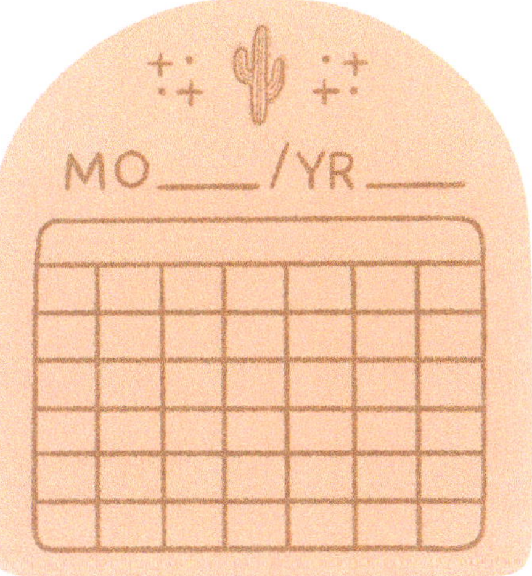
MO____ /YR ____

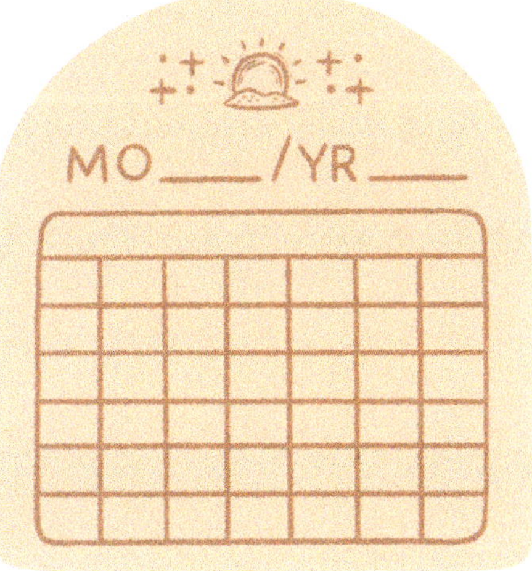
MO____ /YR ____

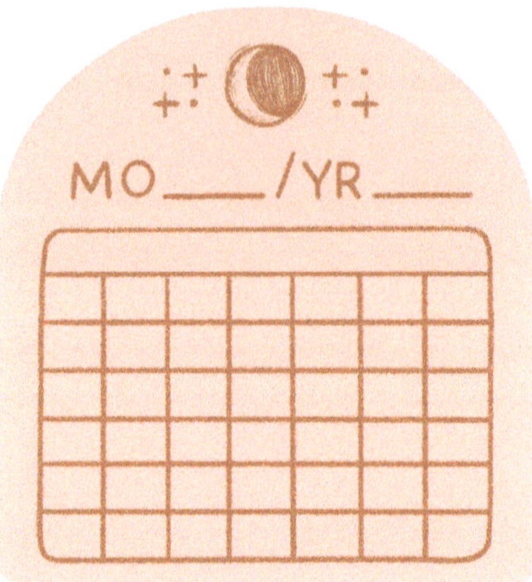

MO____/YR____

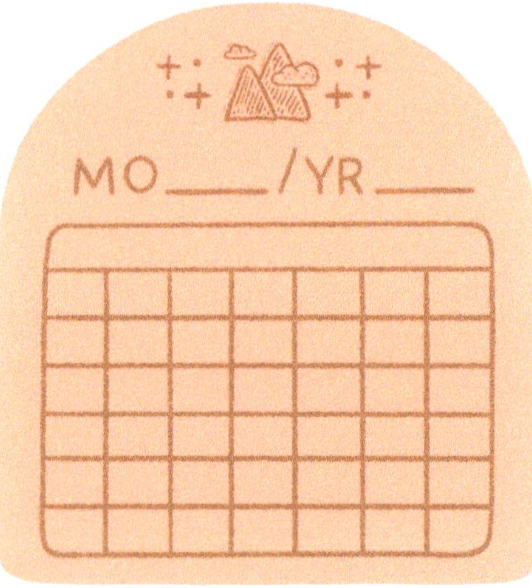

MO____/YR____

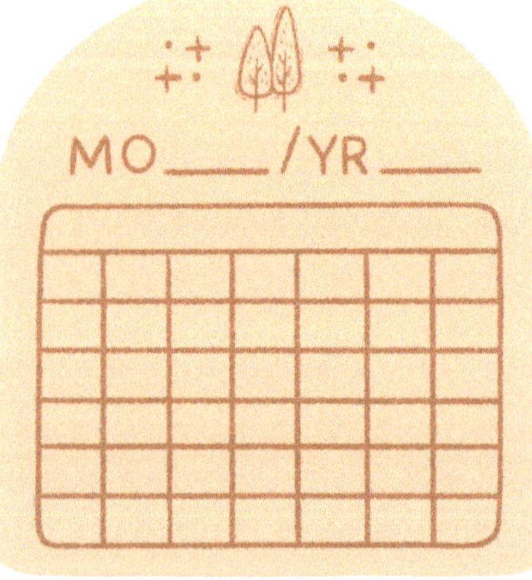

MO____/YR____

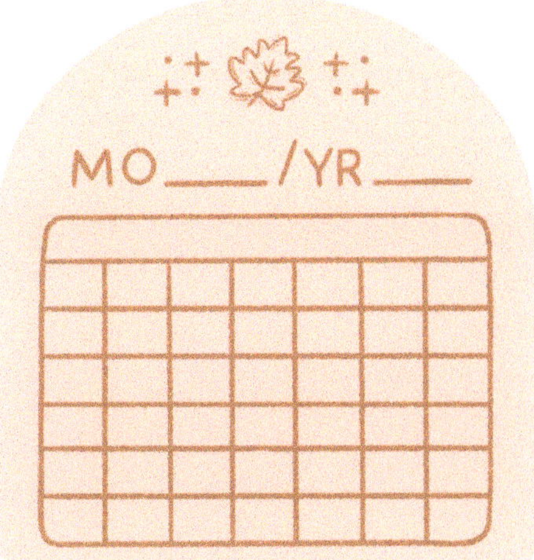
MO____/YR____

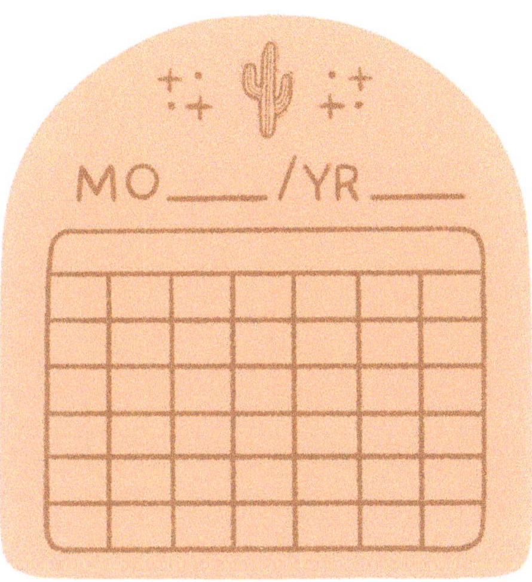
MO____/YR____

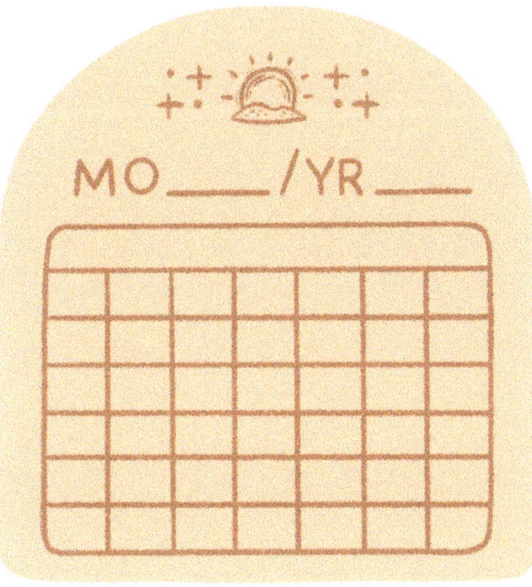
MO____/YR____

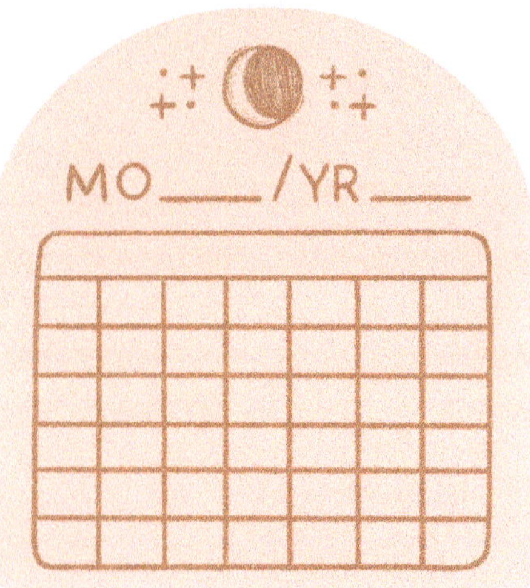
MO____/YR____

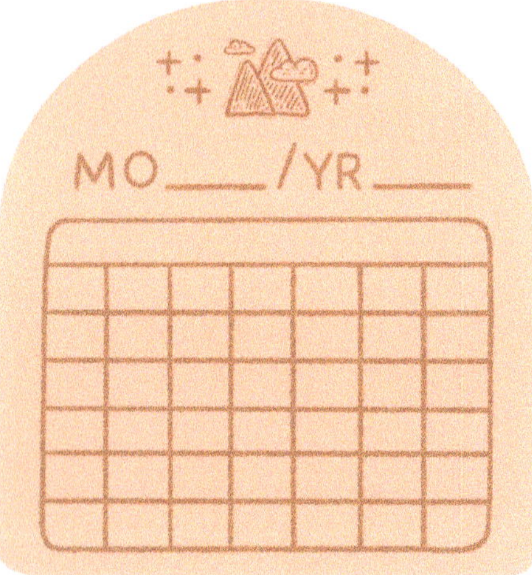
MO____/YR____

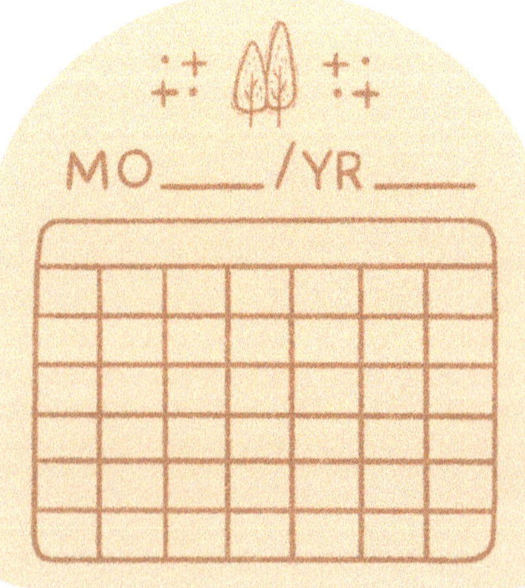
MO____/YR____

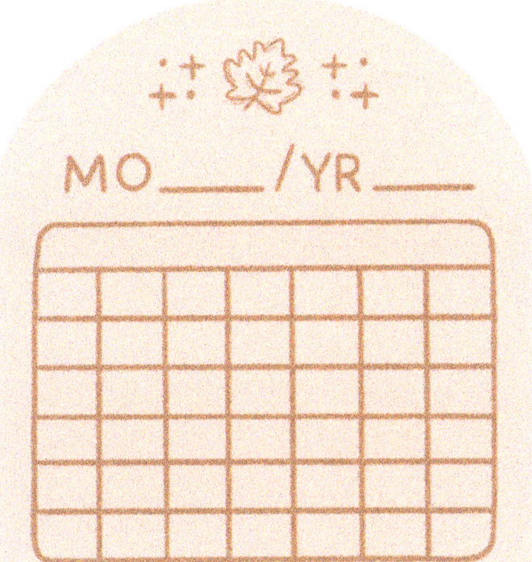

MO____/YR____

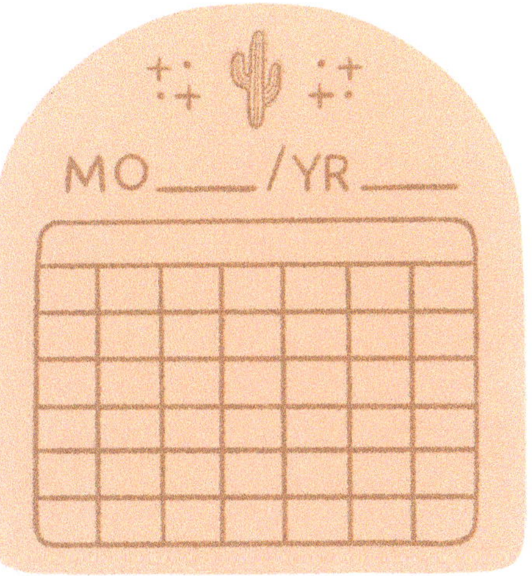

MO____/YR____

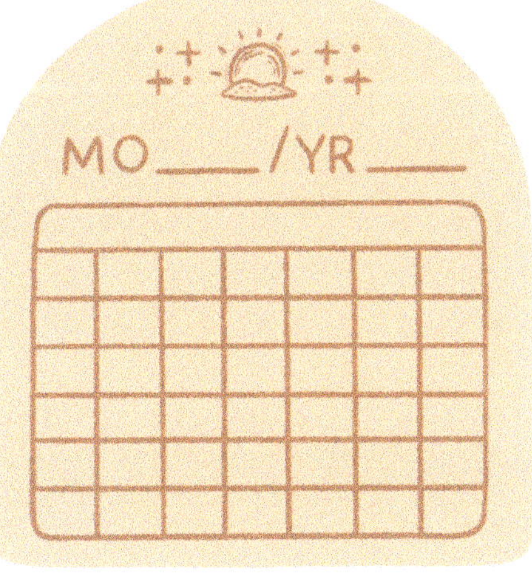

MO____/YR____

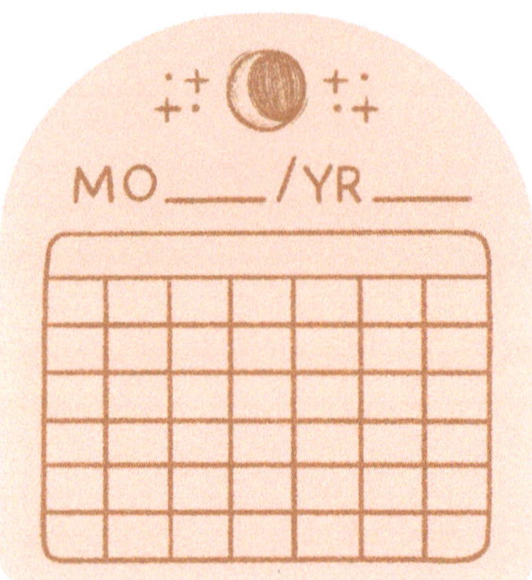

MO____/YR____

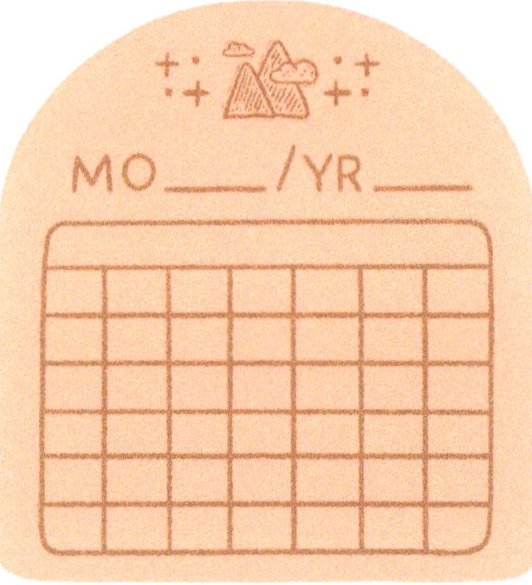

MO____/YR____

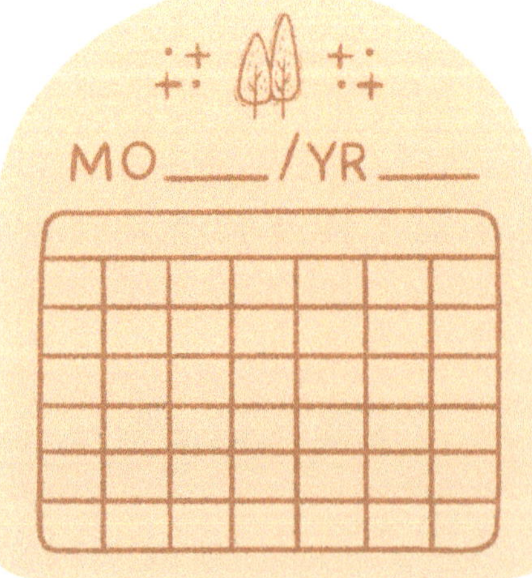

MO____/YR____

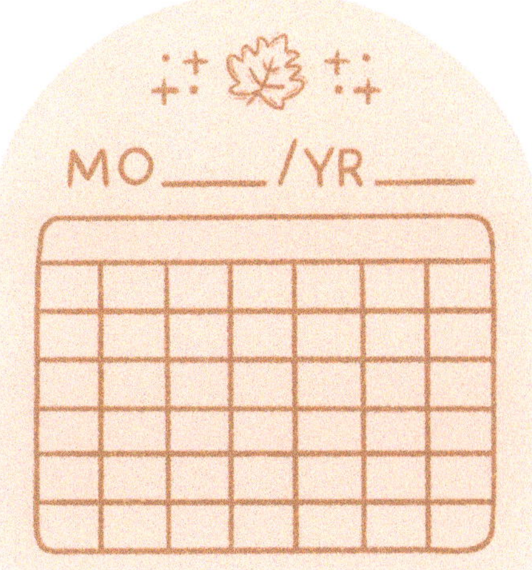

MO____/YR____

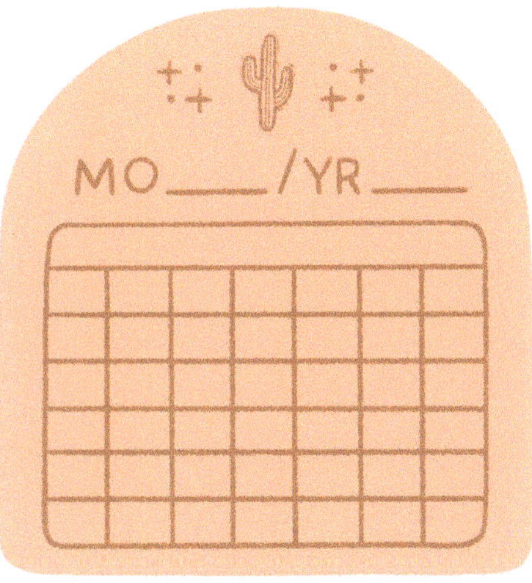

MO____/YR____

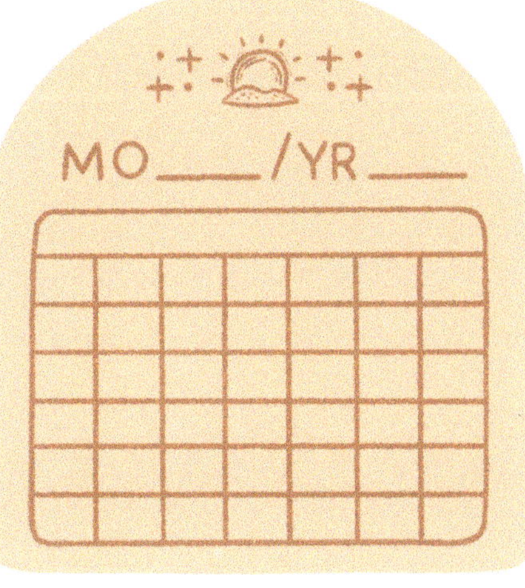

MO____/YR____

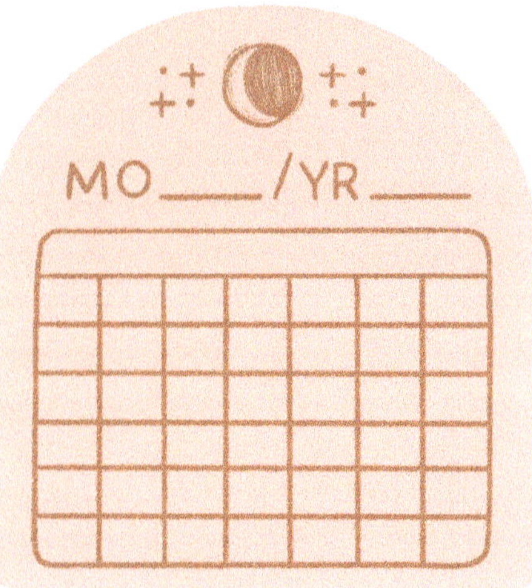

MO____/YR____

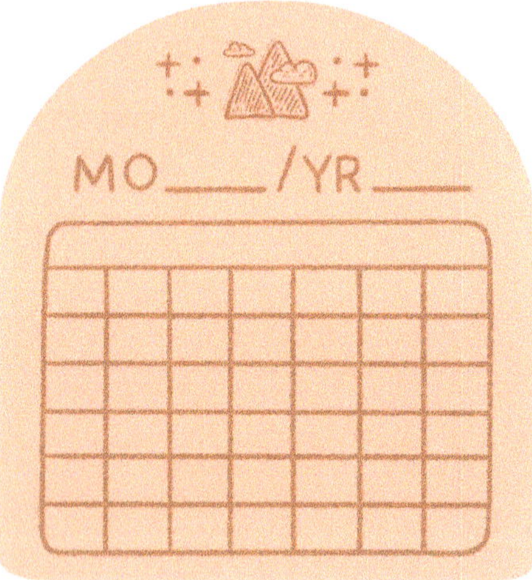

MO____/YR____

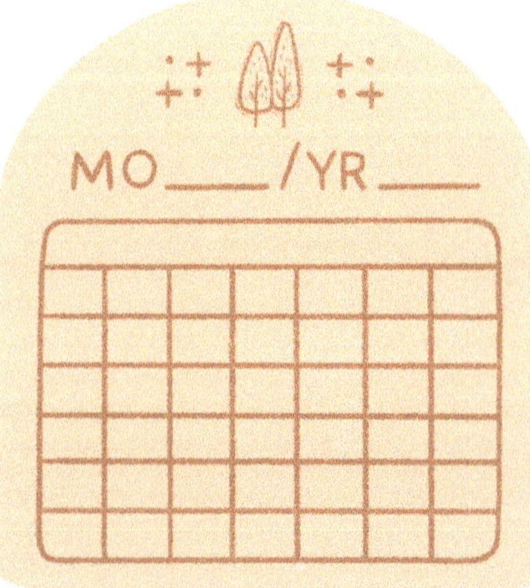

MO____/YR____

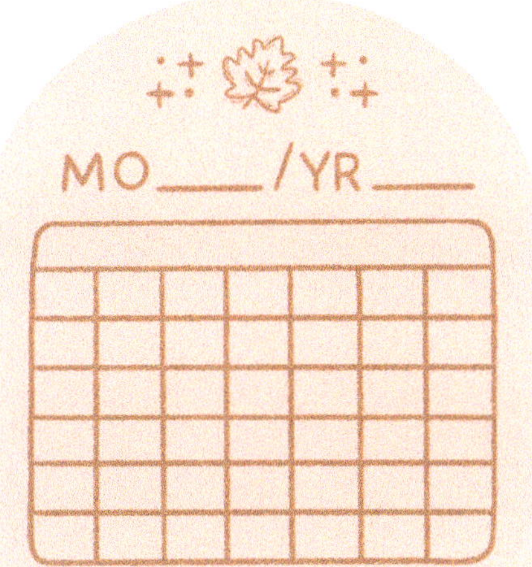

MO_____/YR_____

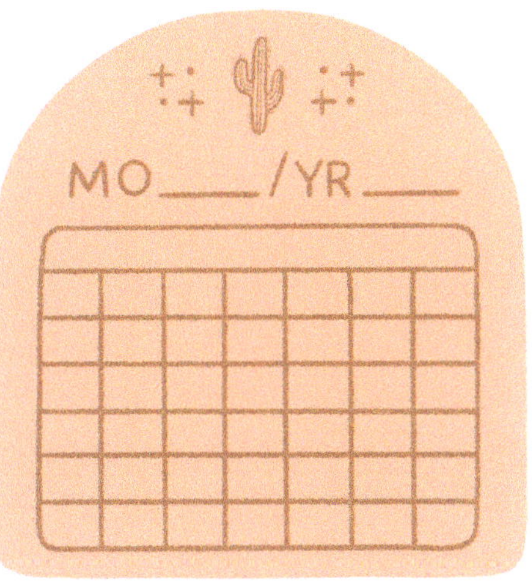

MO_____/YR_____

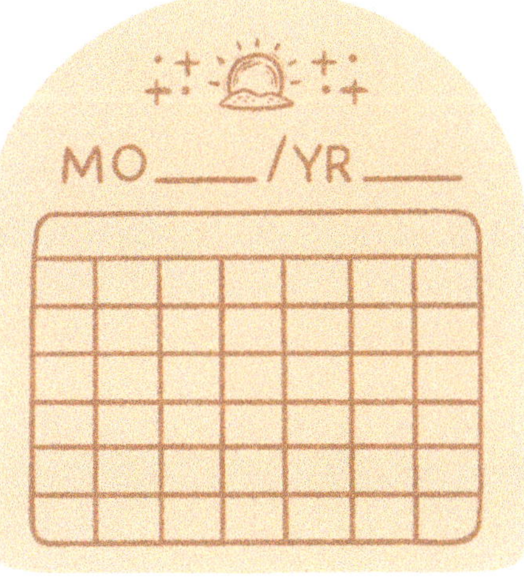

MO_____/YR_____

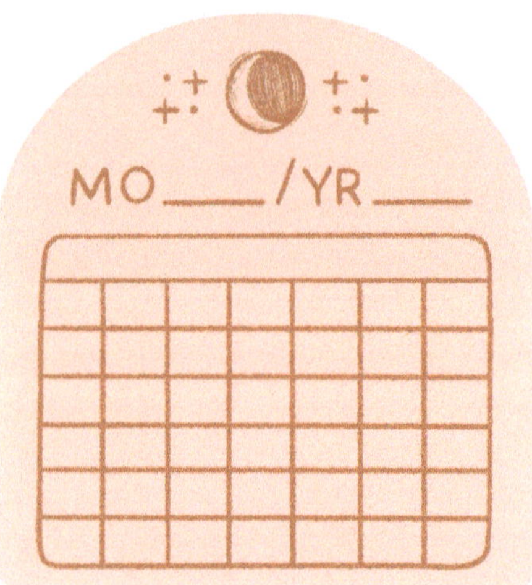

MO____/YR____

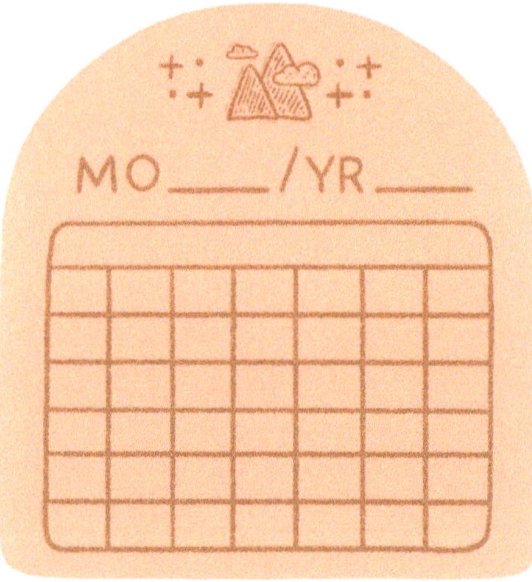

MO____/YR____

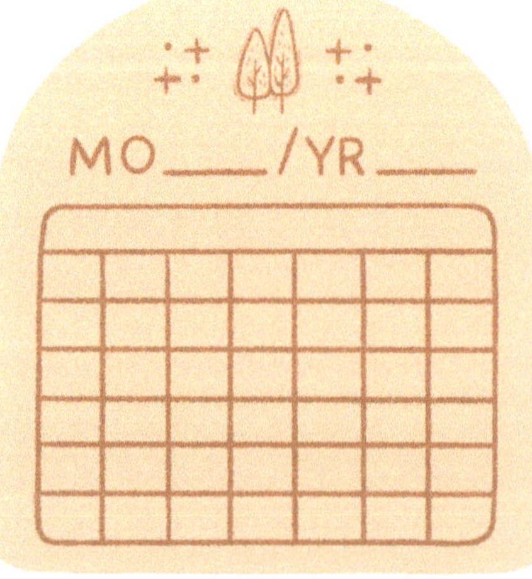

MO____/YR____

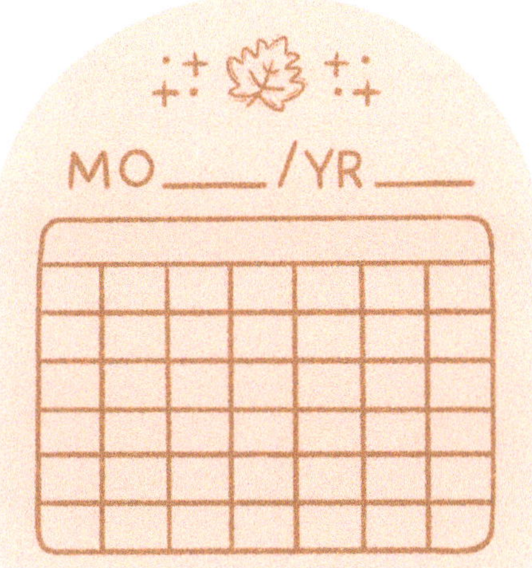

MO___/YR___

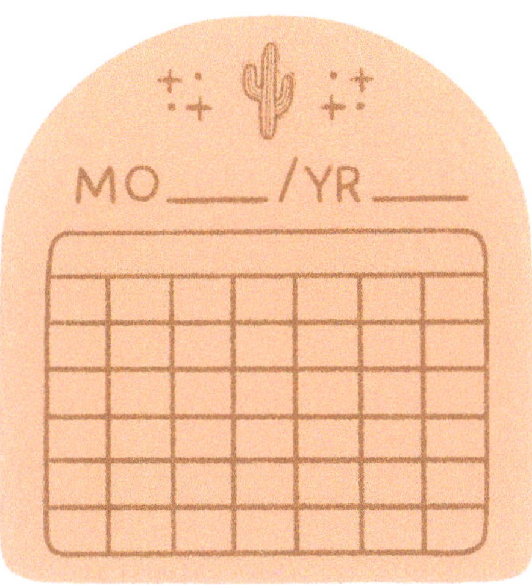

MO___/YR___

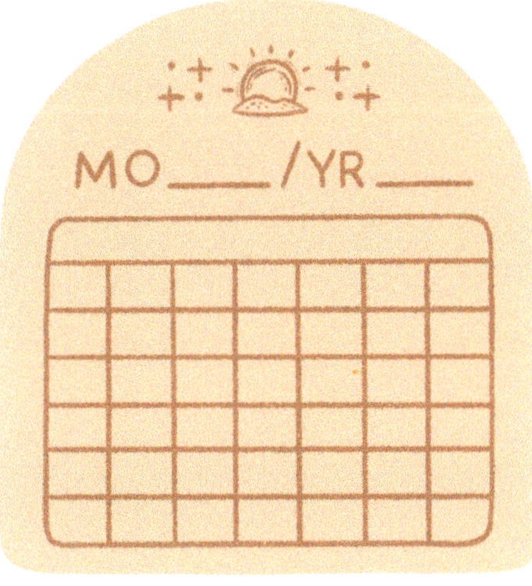

MO___/YR___

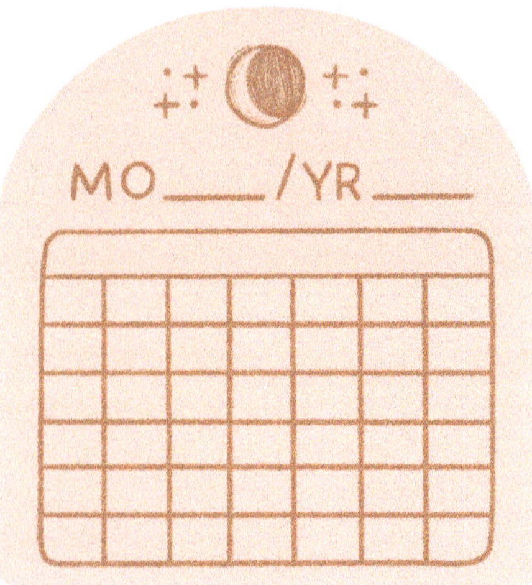
MO____/YR____

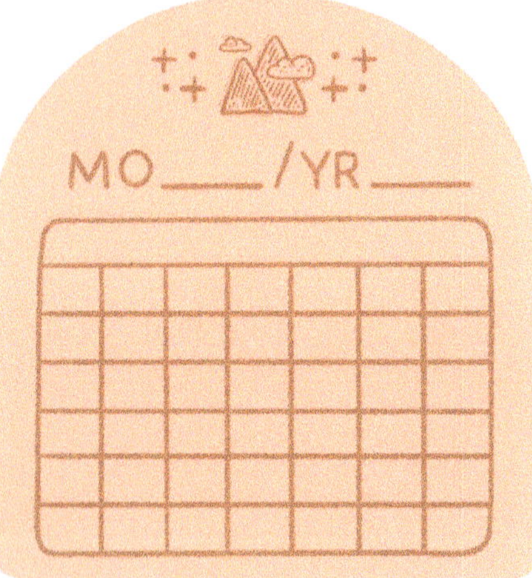
MO____/YR____

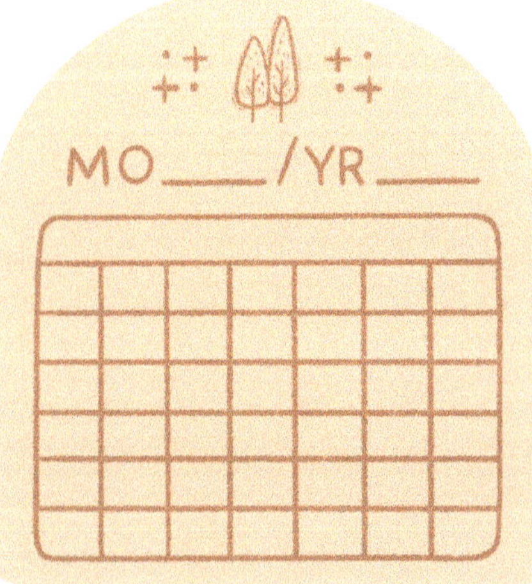
MO____/YR____

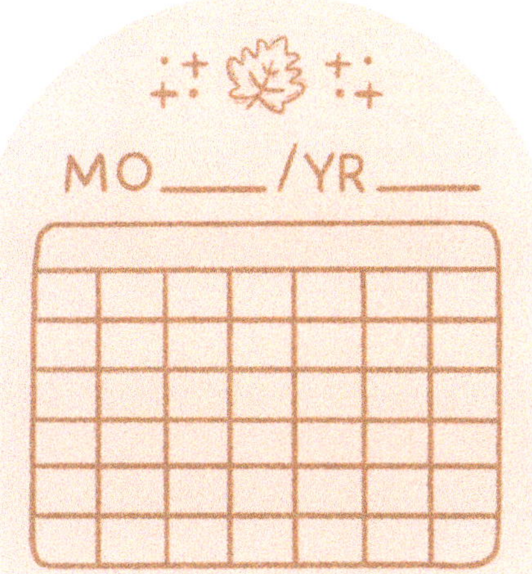

MO____ /YR____

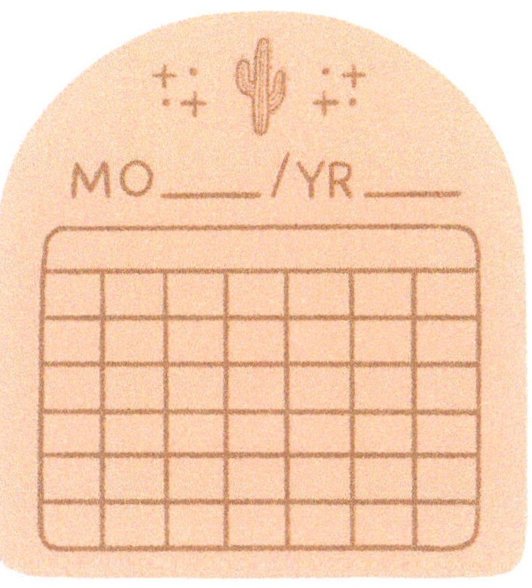

MO____ /YR____

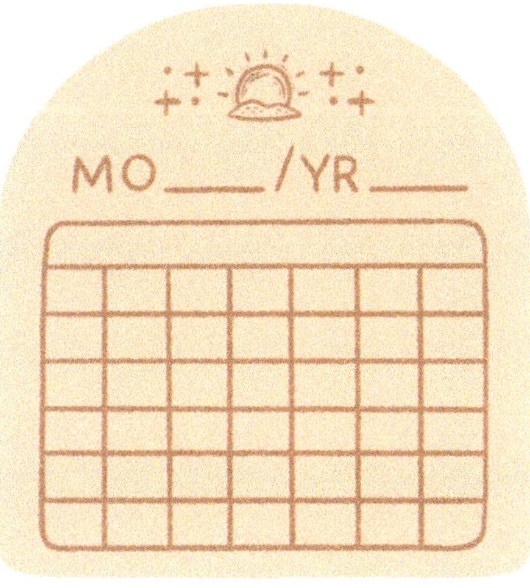

MO____ /YR____

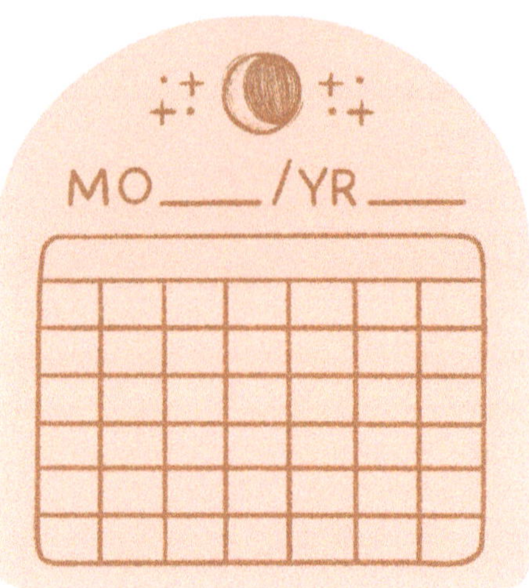

MO_____/YR_____

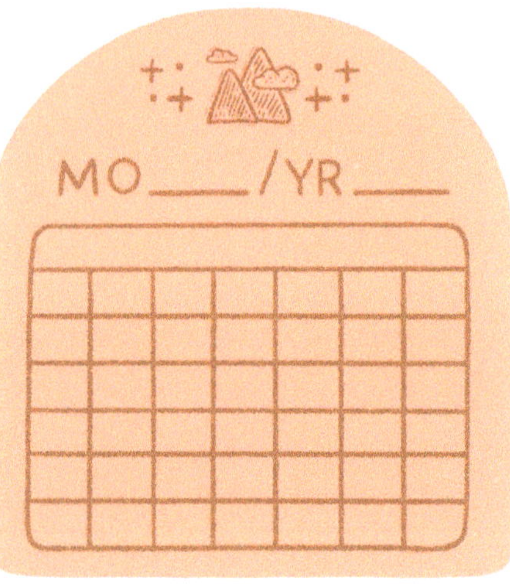

MO_____/YR_____

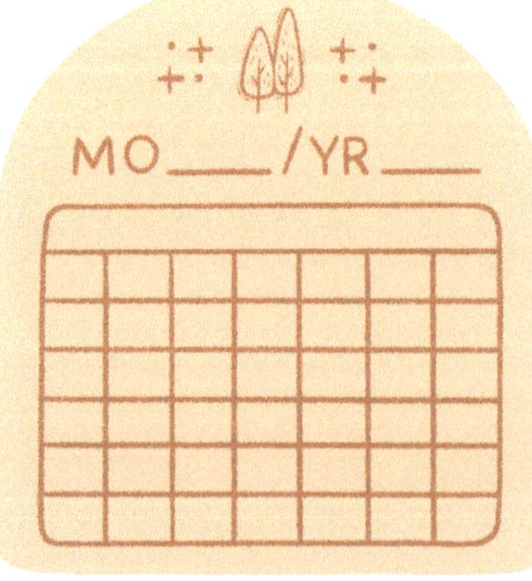

MO_____/YR_____

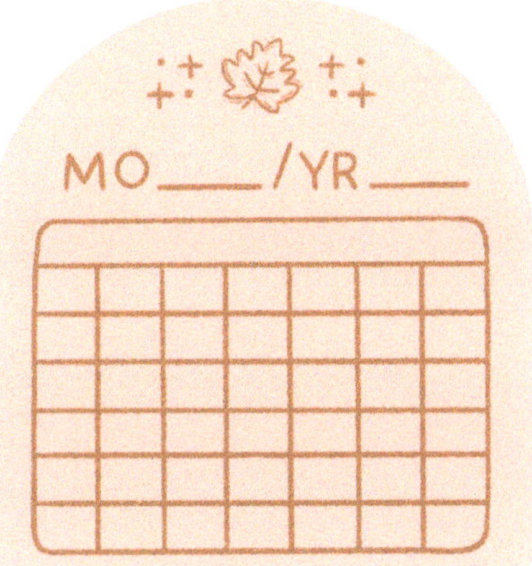
MO____/YR____

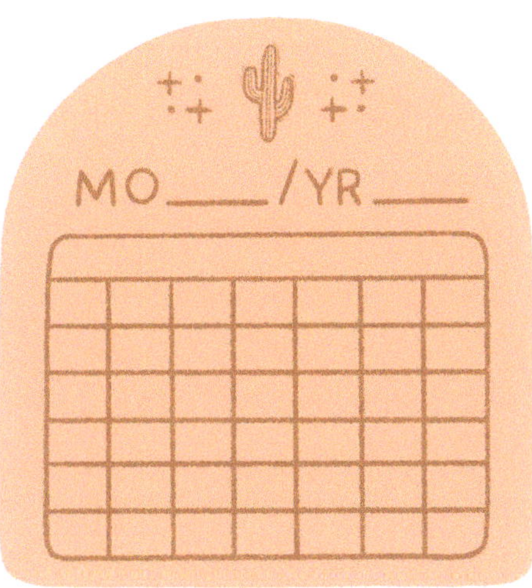
MO____/YR____

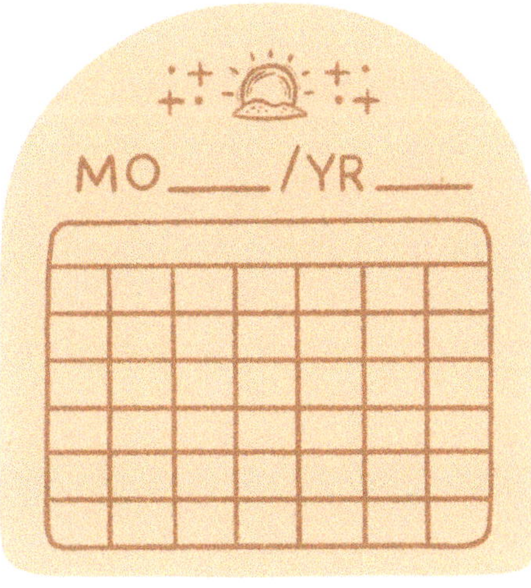
MO____/YR____

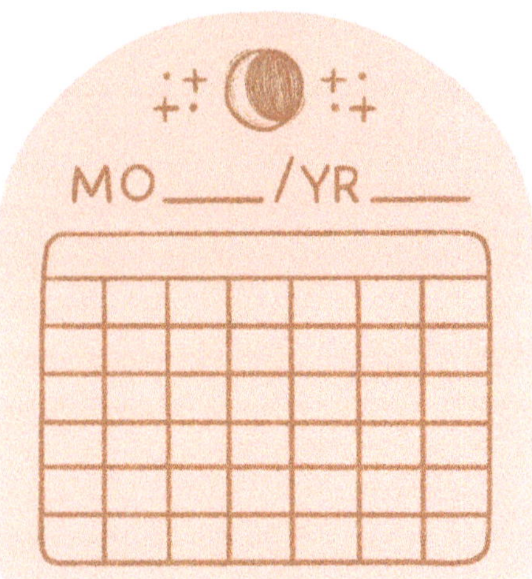

MO_____/YR_____

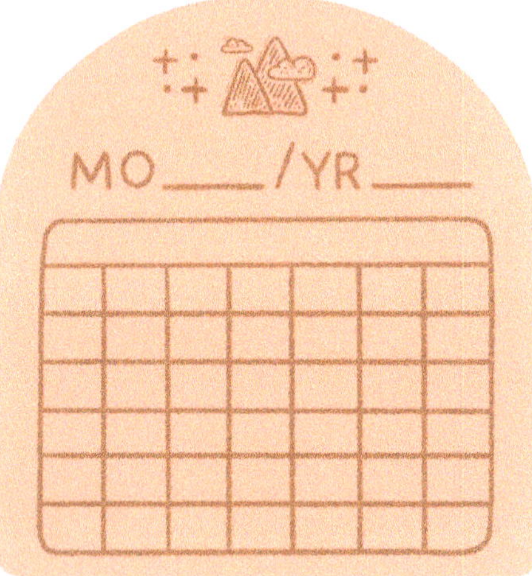

MO_____/YR_____

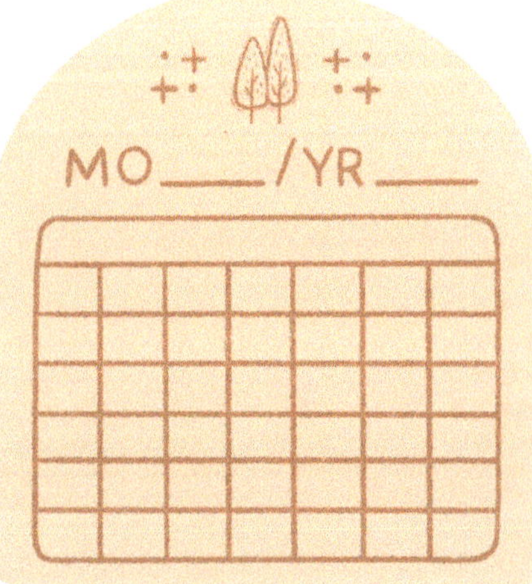

MO_____/YR_____

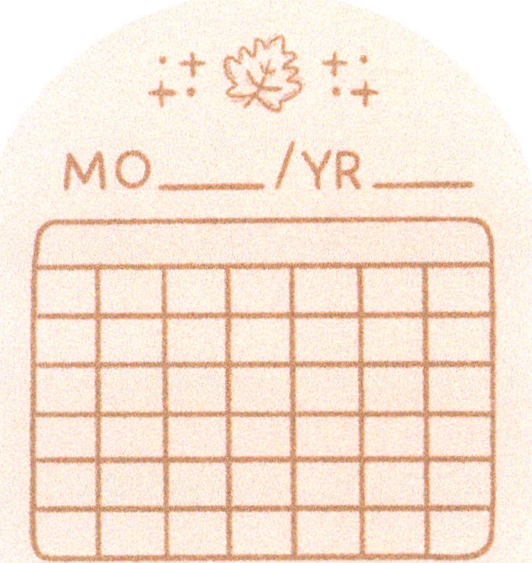
MO_____/YR_____

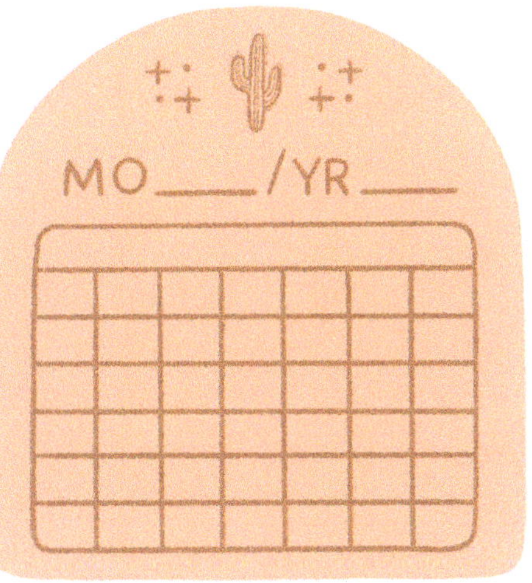
MO_____/YR_____

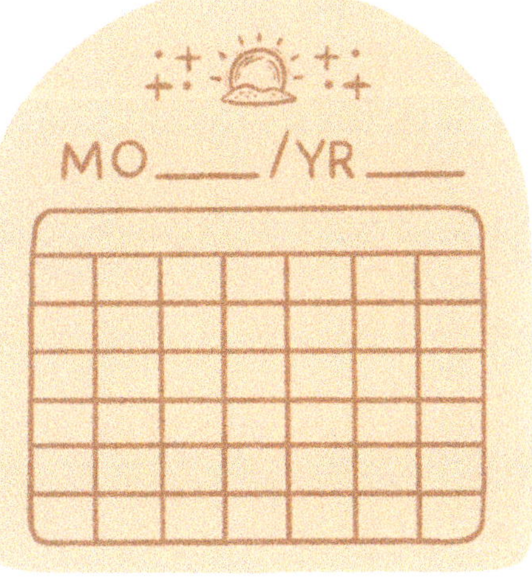
MO_____/YR_____

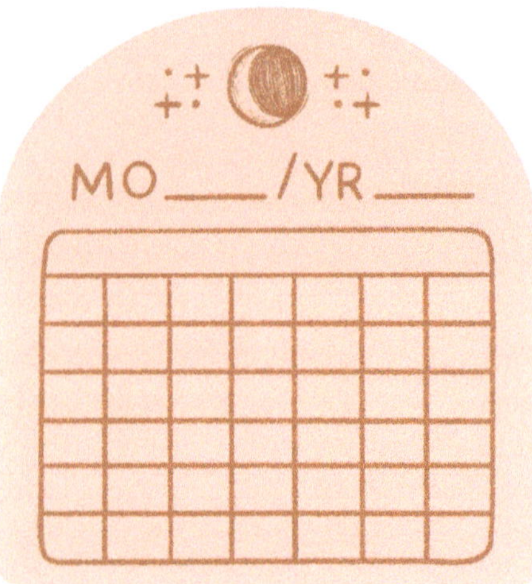
MO_____/YR_____

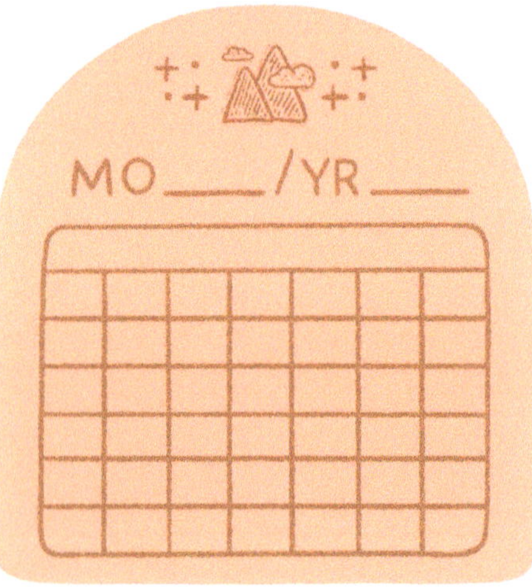
MO_____/YR_____

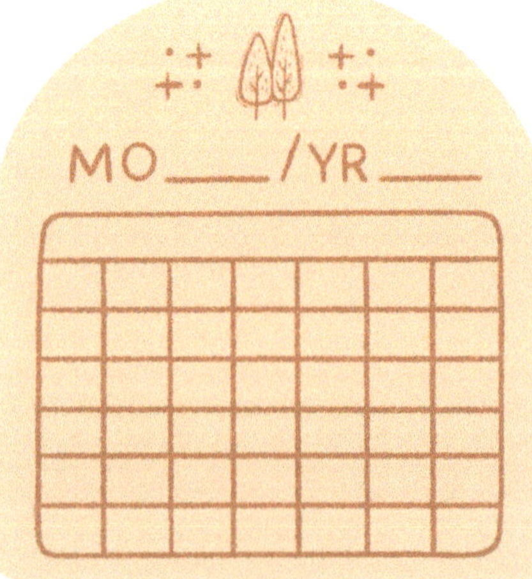
MO_____/YR_____

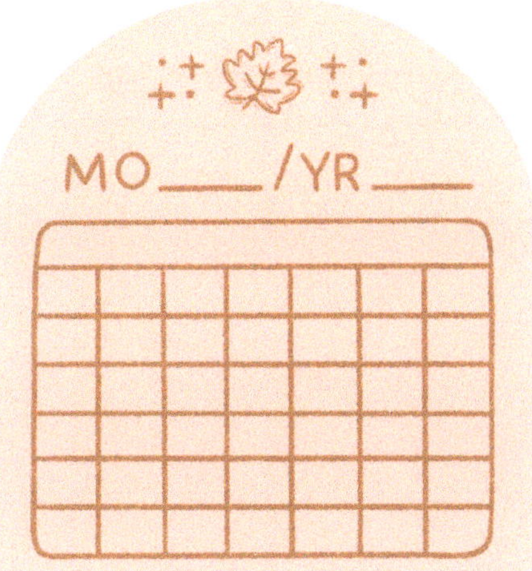

MO____/YR____

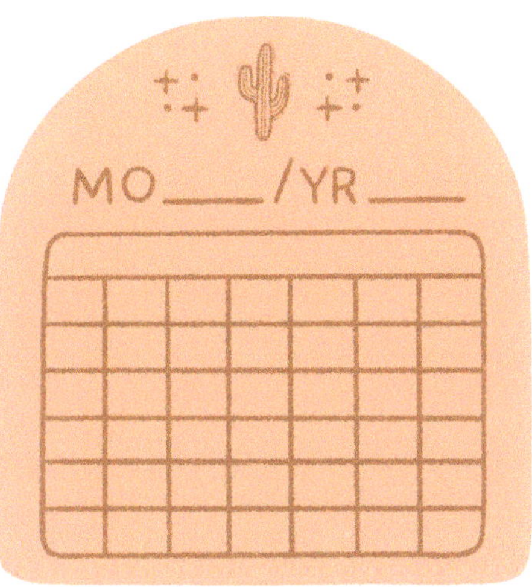

MO____/YR____

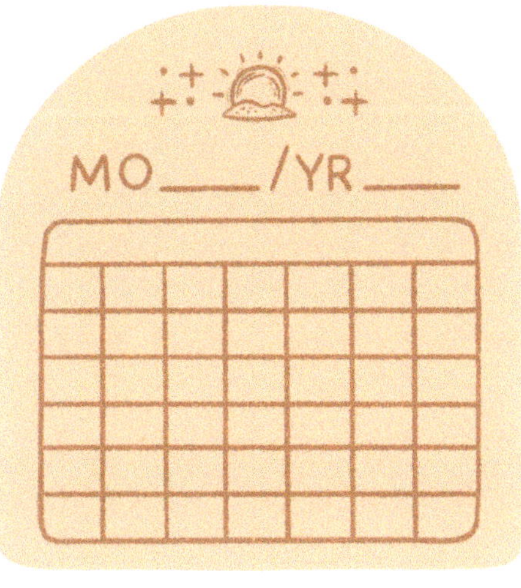

MO____/YR____

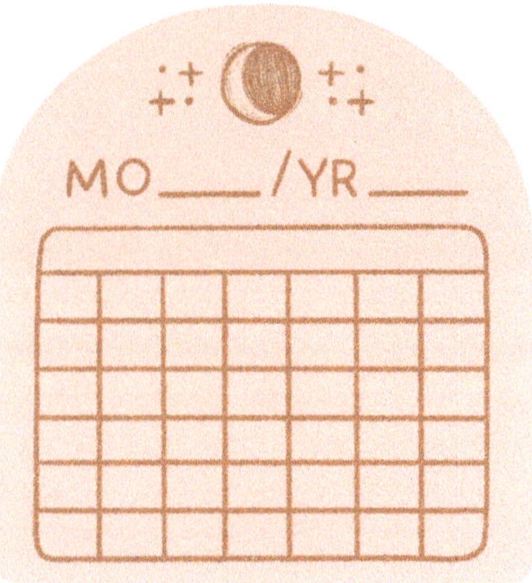

MO_____/YR_____

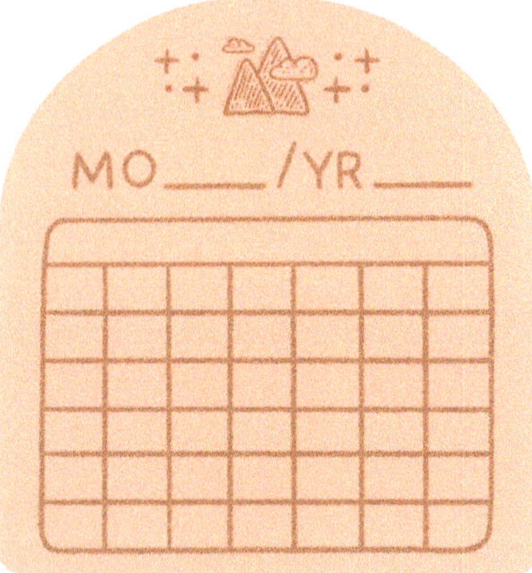

MO_____/YR_____

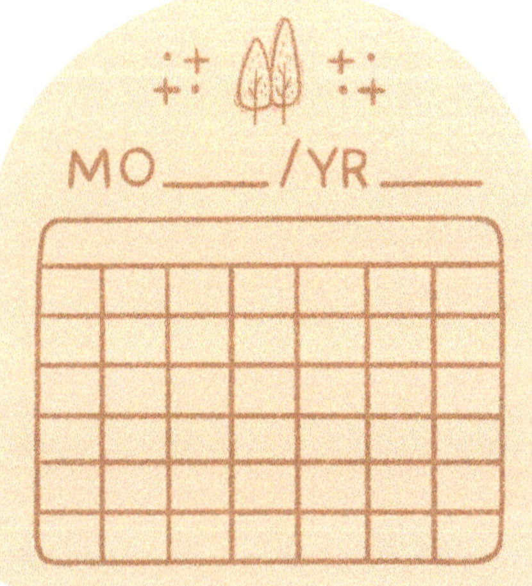

MO_____/YR_____

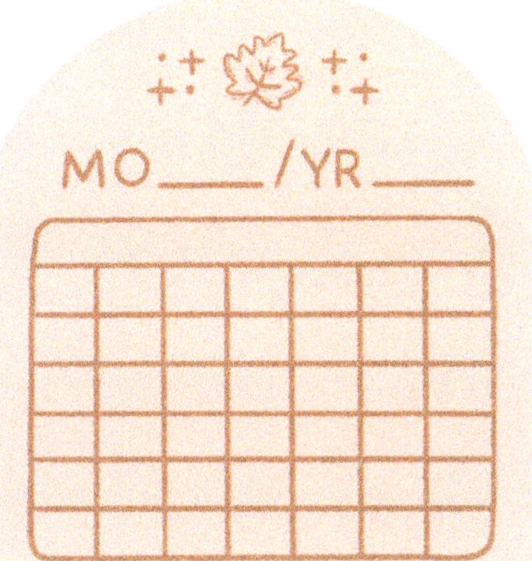

MO____/YR____

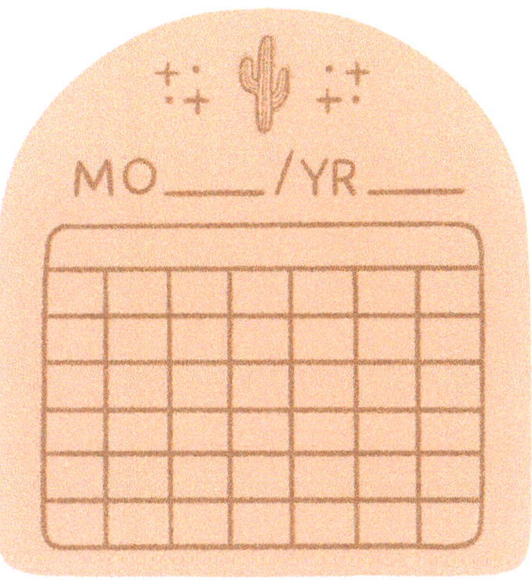

MO____/YR____

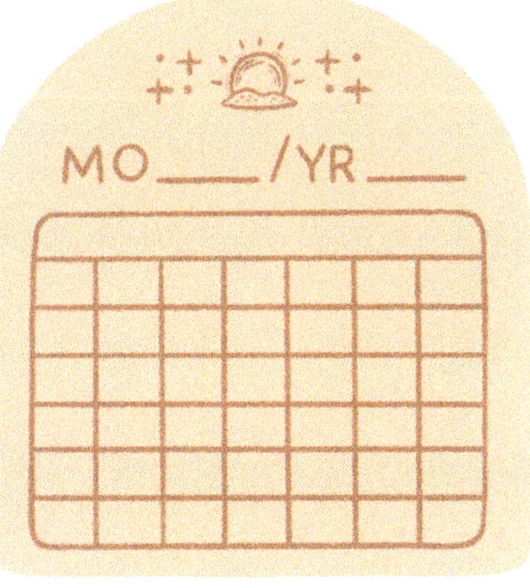

MO____/YR____

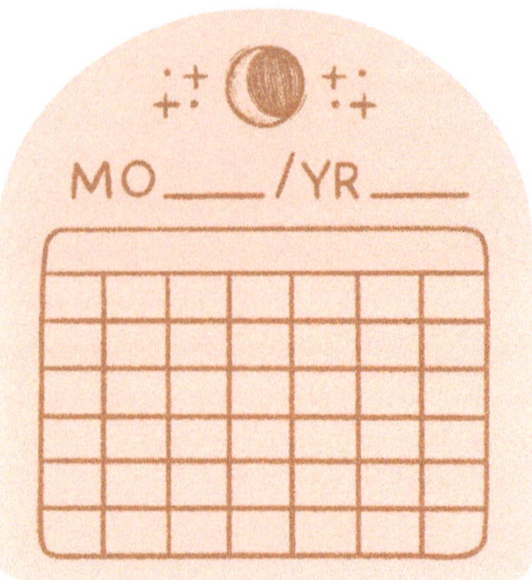

MO____/YR____

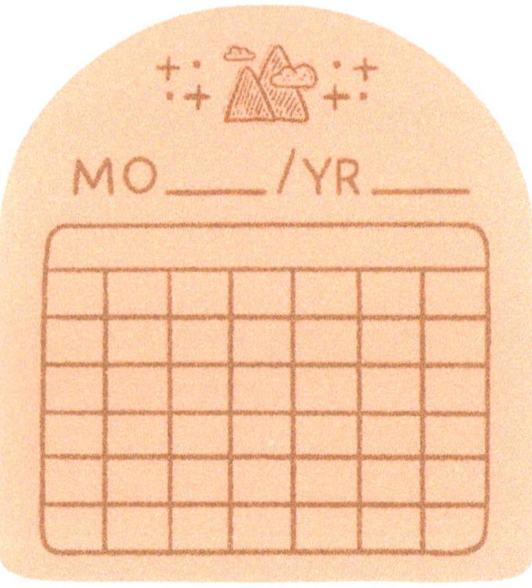

MO____/YR____

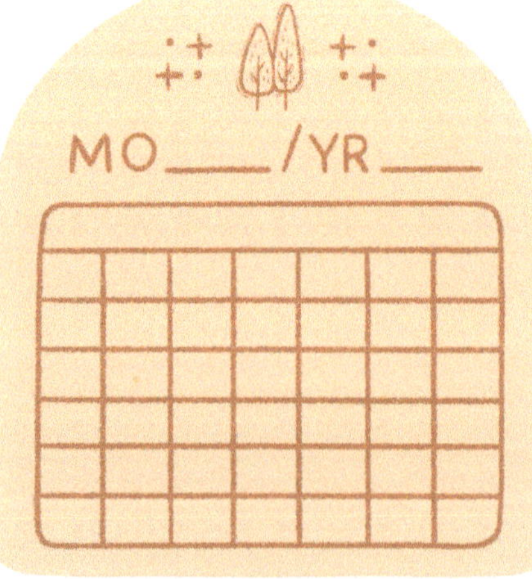

MO____/YR____

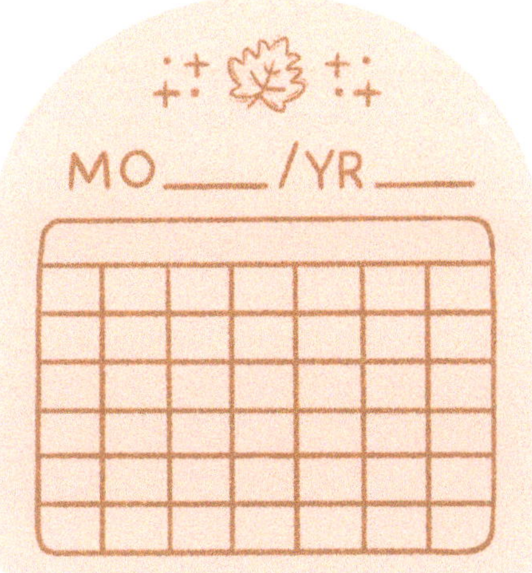

MO____/YR____

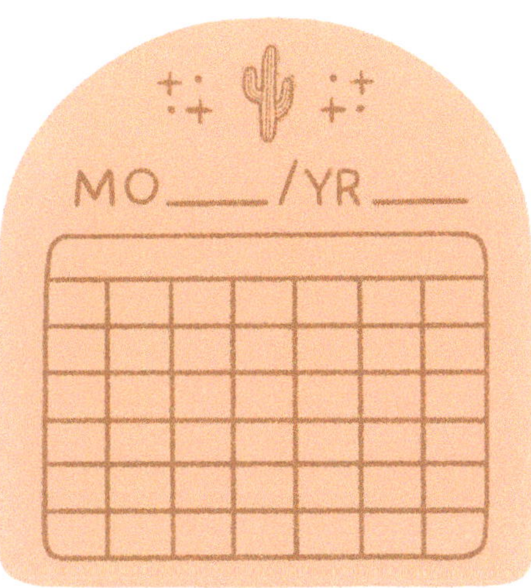

MO____/YR____

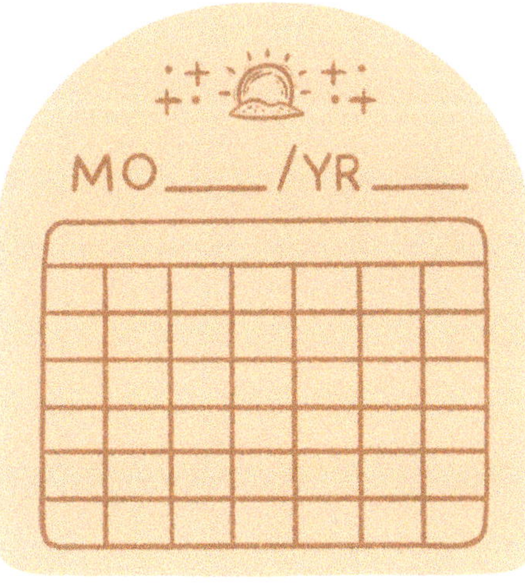

MO____/YR____

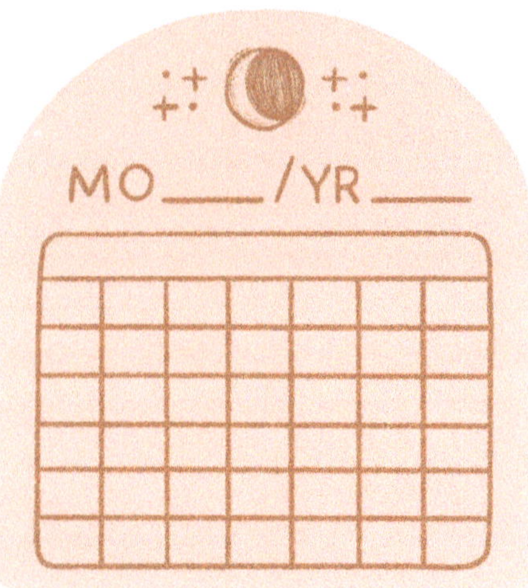

MO____/YR____

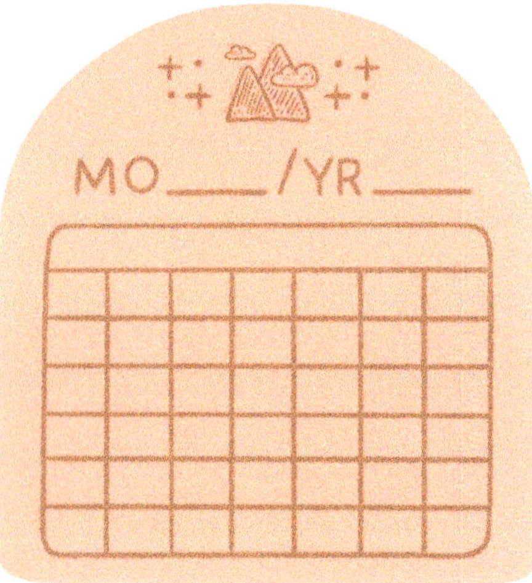

MO____/YR____

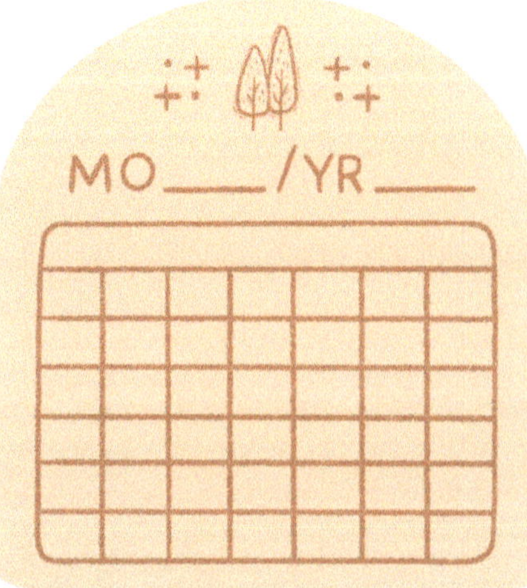

MO____/YR____

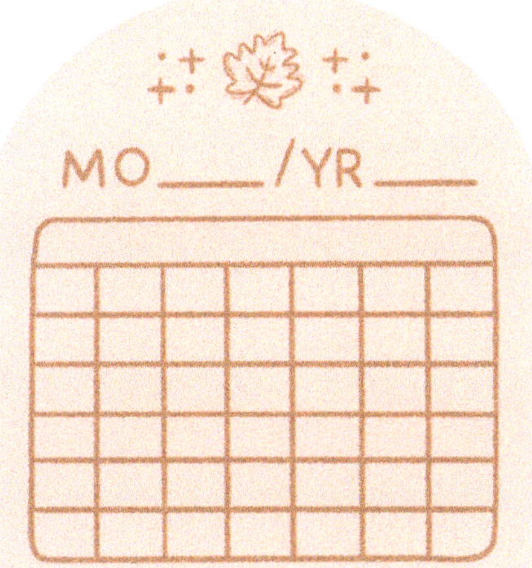

MO____/YR____

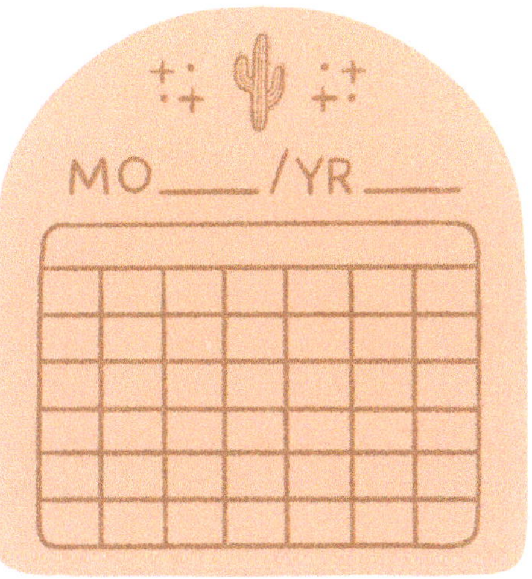

MO____/YR____

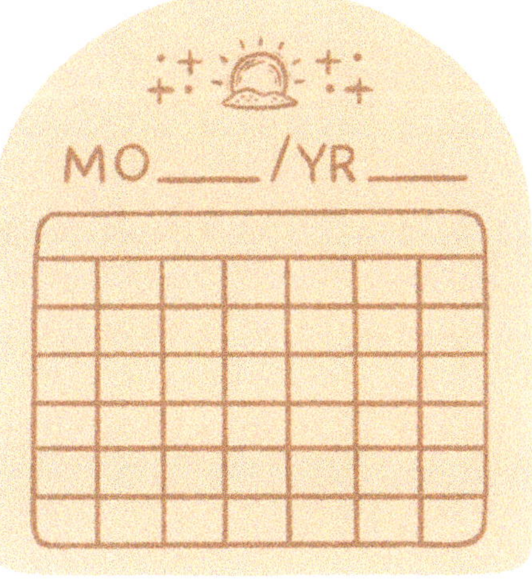

MO____/YR____

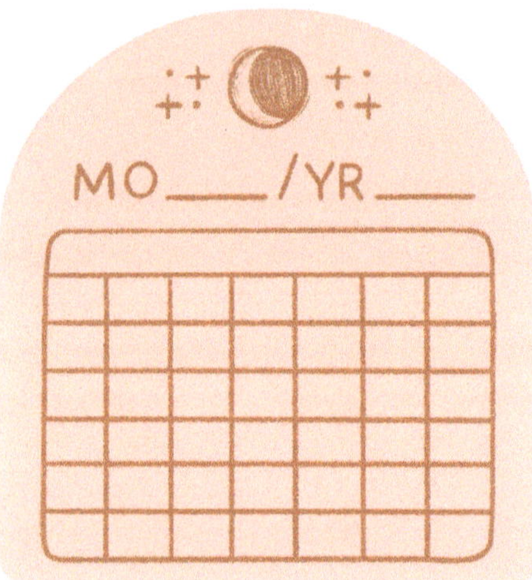

MO____/YR____

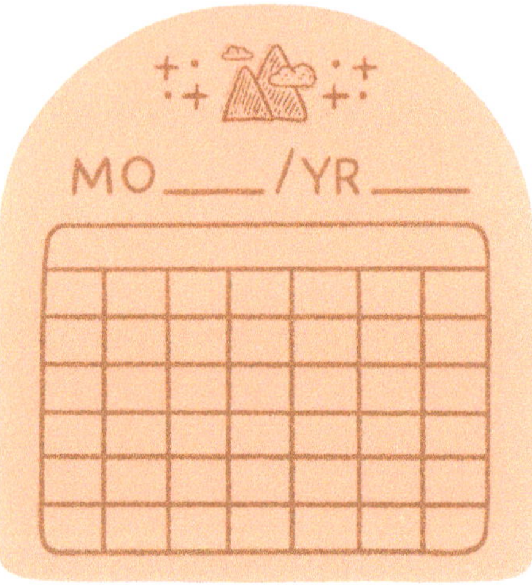

MO____/YR____

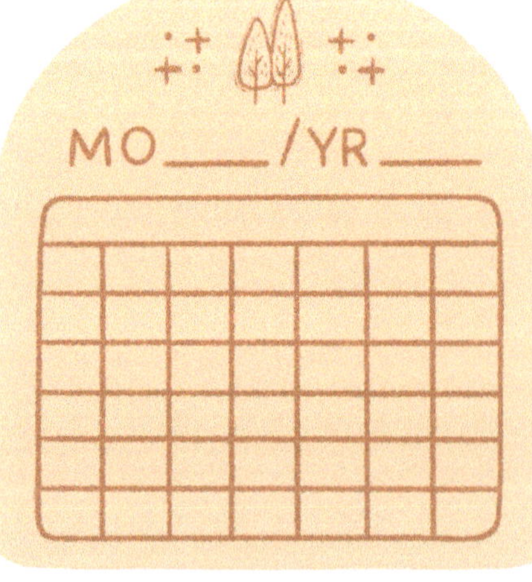

MO____/YR____

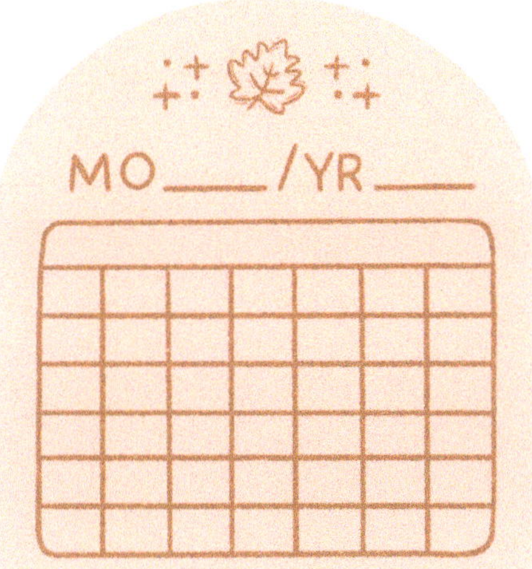
MO____/YR____

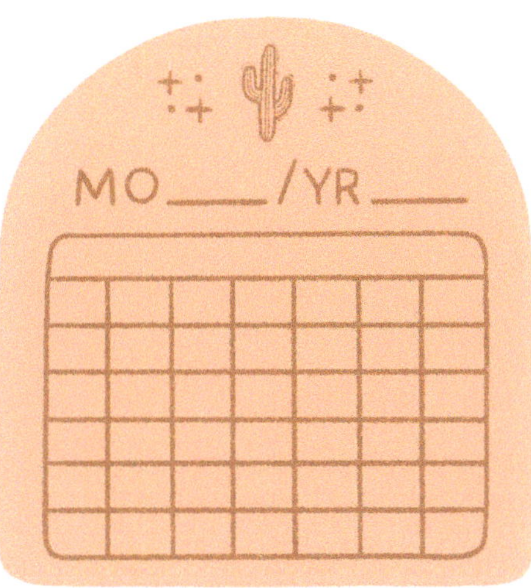
MO____/YR____

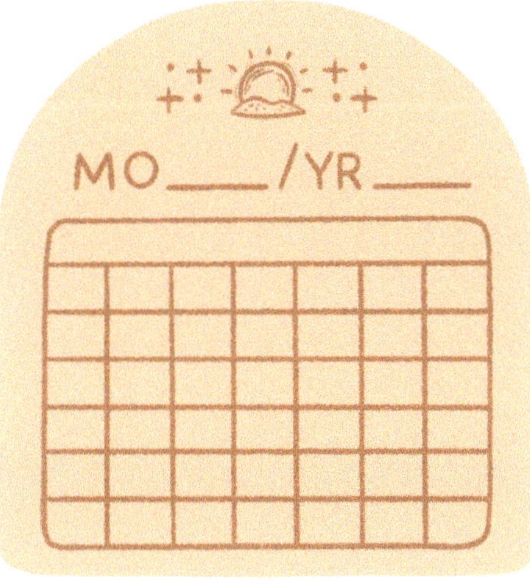
MO____/YR____

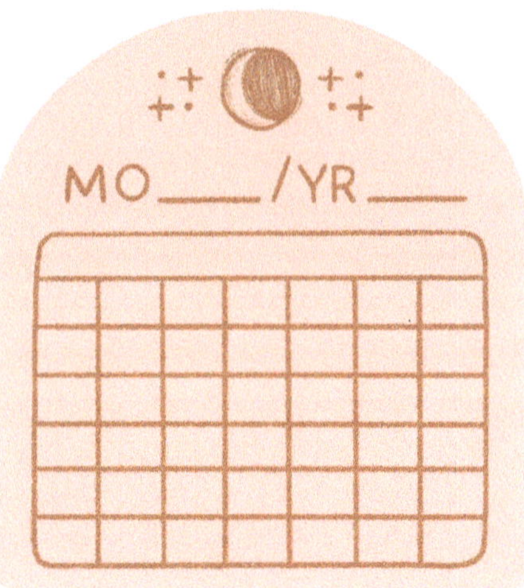

MO____/YR____

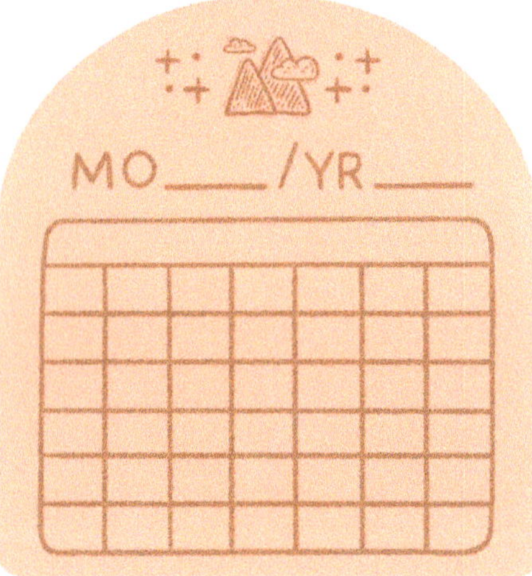

MO____/YR____

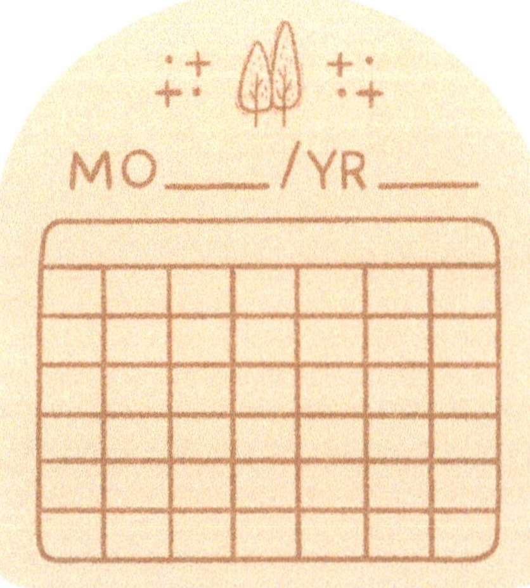

MO____/YR____

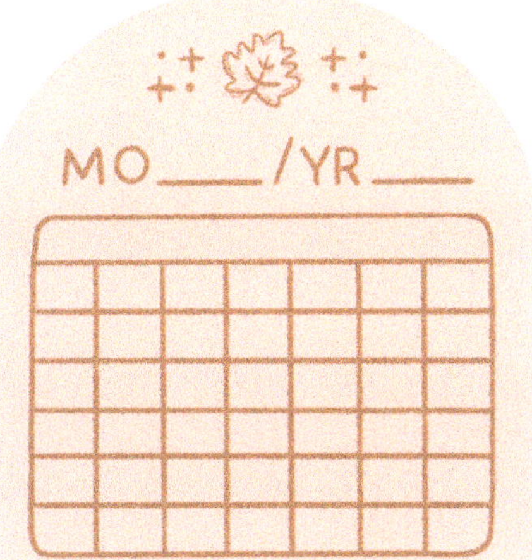
MO____/YR____

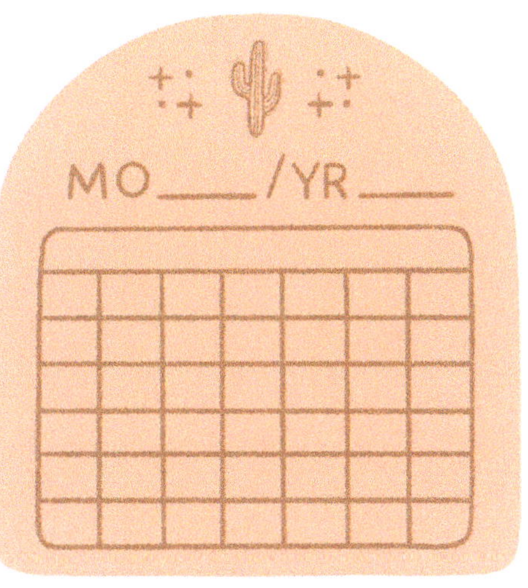
MO____/YR____

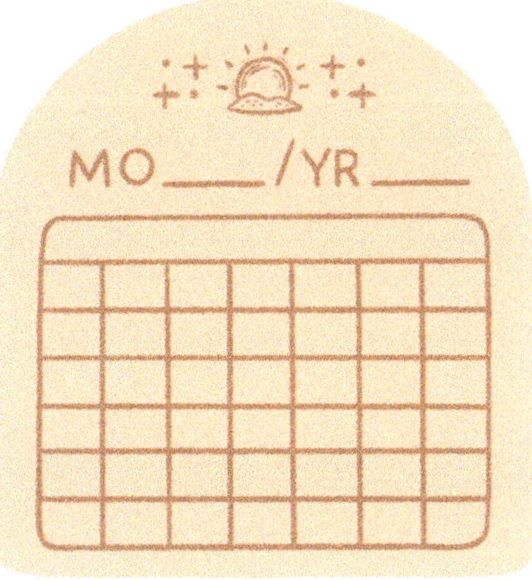
MO____/YR____

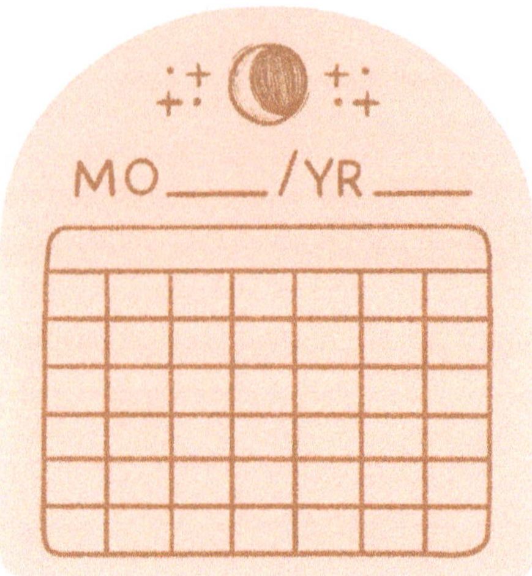

MO ____ / YR ____

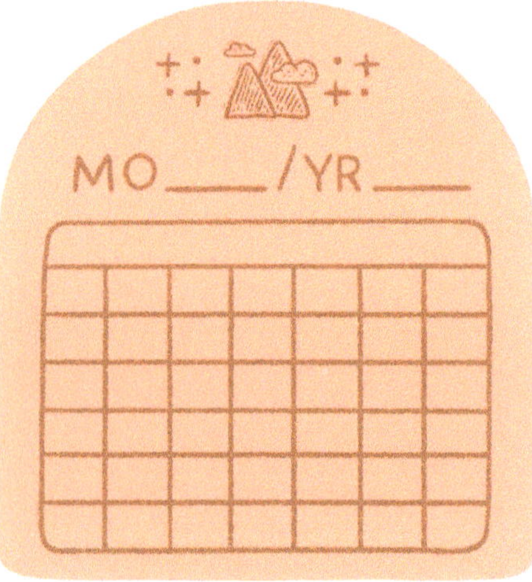

MO ____ / YR ____

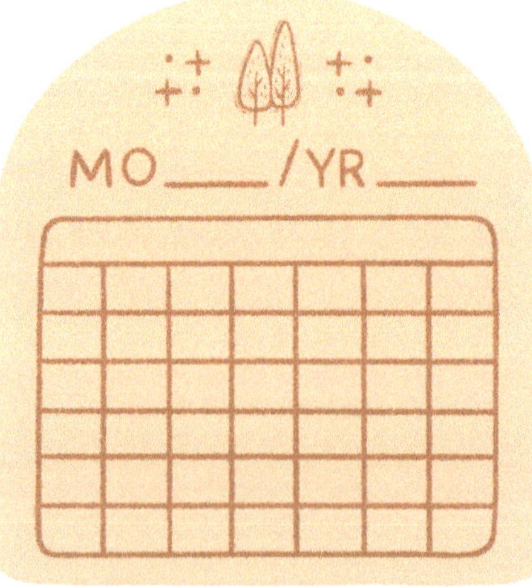

MO ____ / YR ____

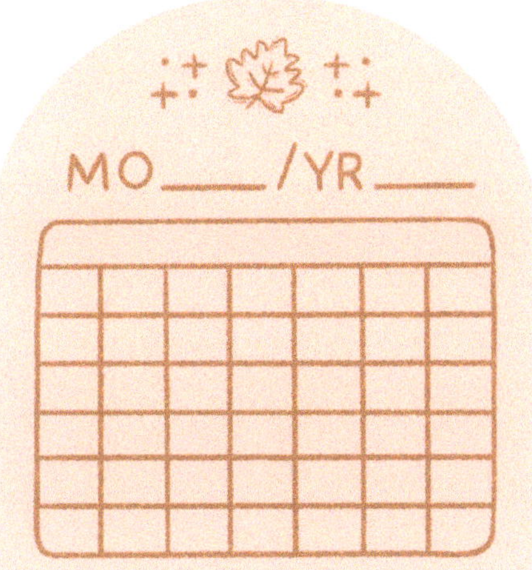
MO____/YR____

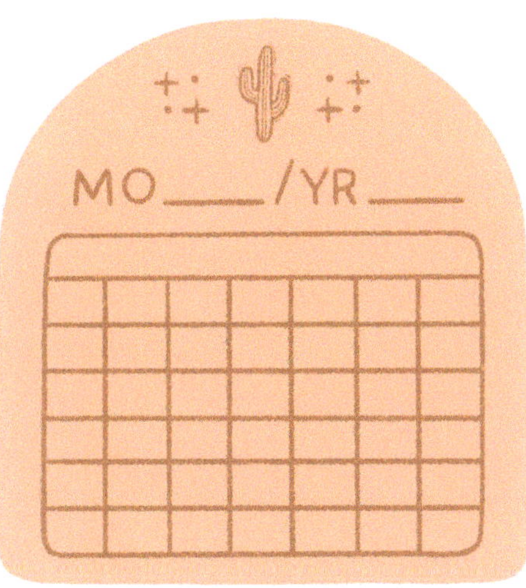
MO____/YR____

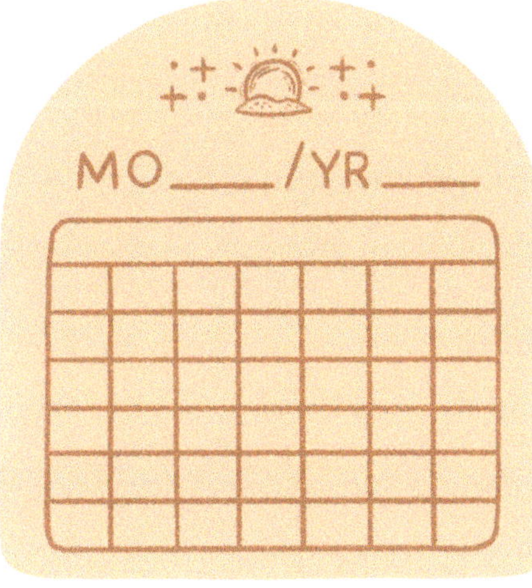
MO____/YR____

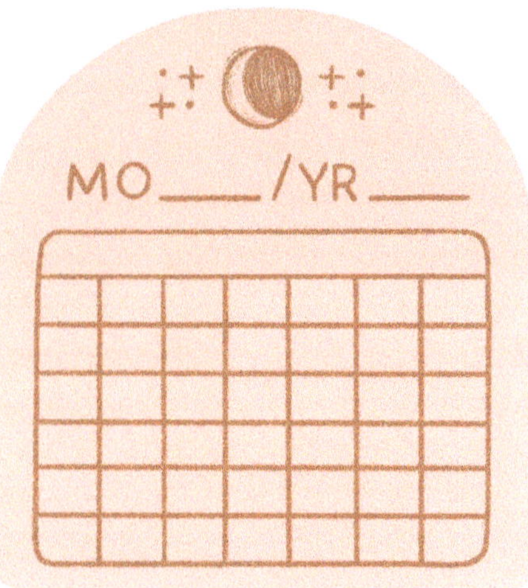
MO_____/YR_____

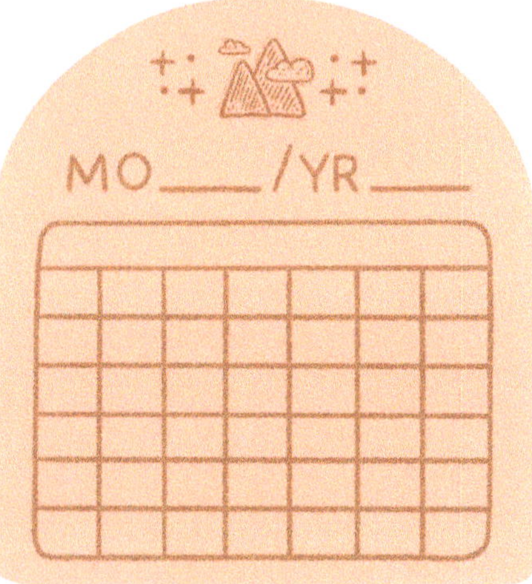
MO_____/YR_____

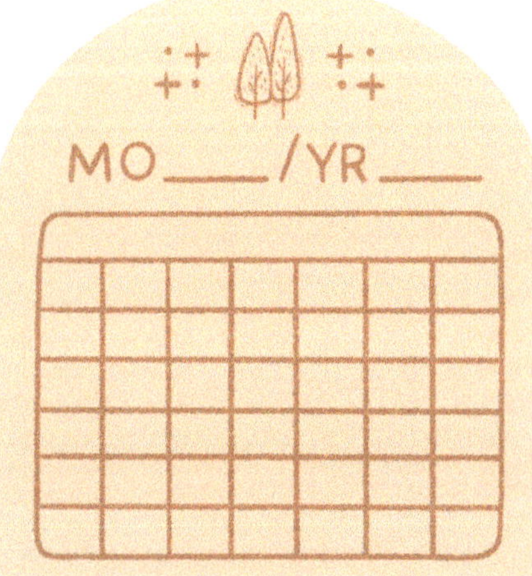
MO_____/YR_____

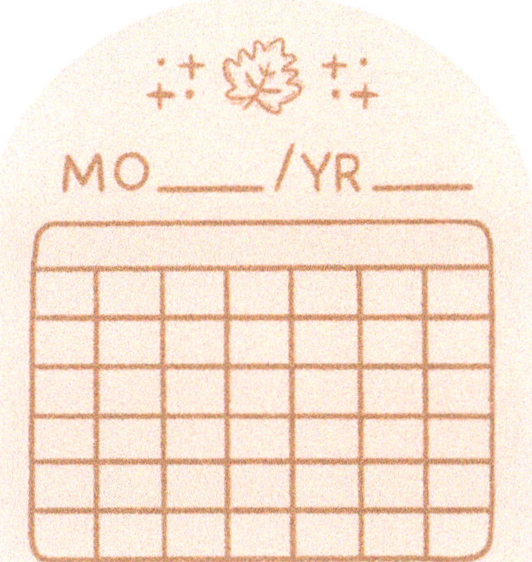

MO____/YR____

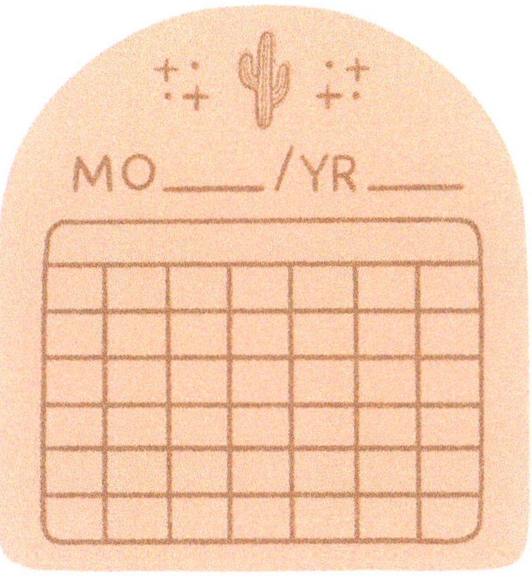

MO____/YR____

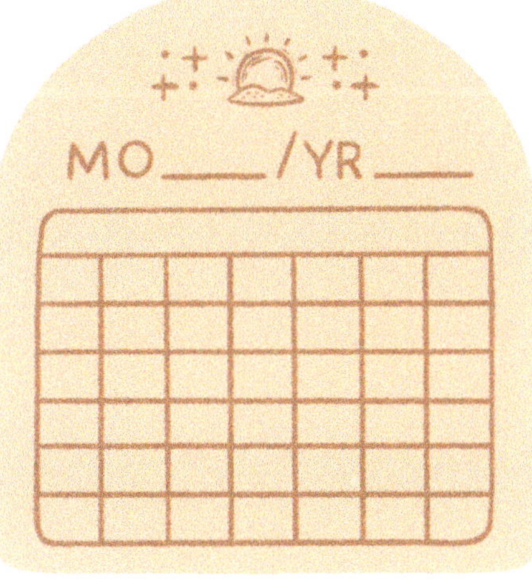

MO____/YR____

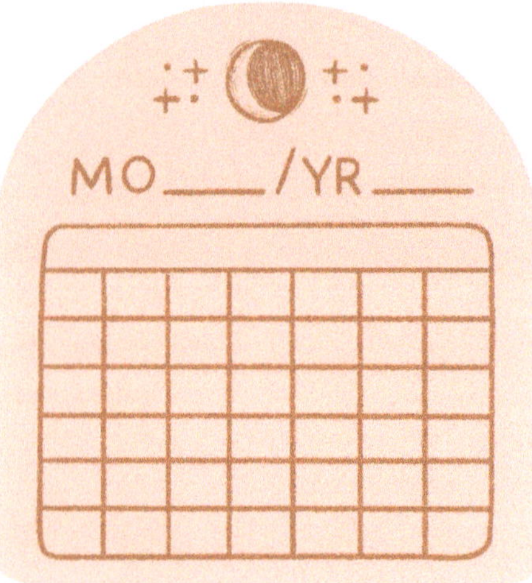

MO____/YR____

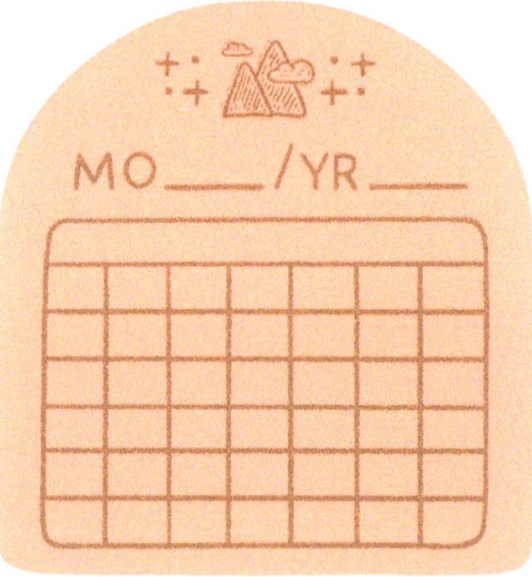

MO____/YR____

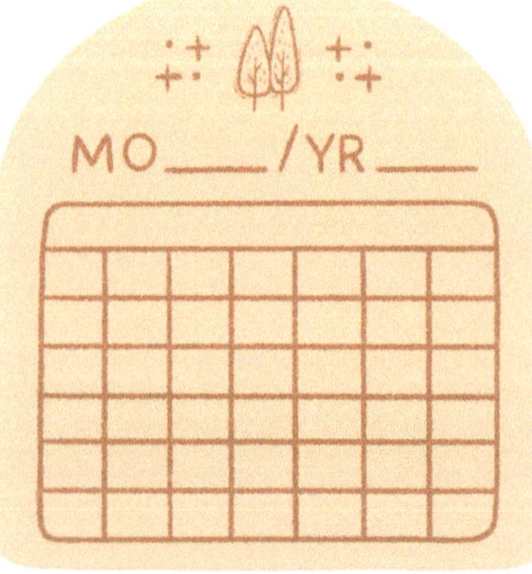

MO____/YR____

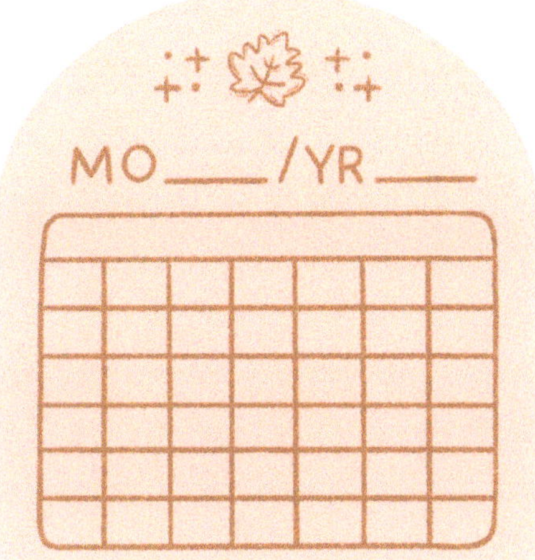
MO____/YR____

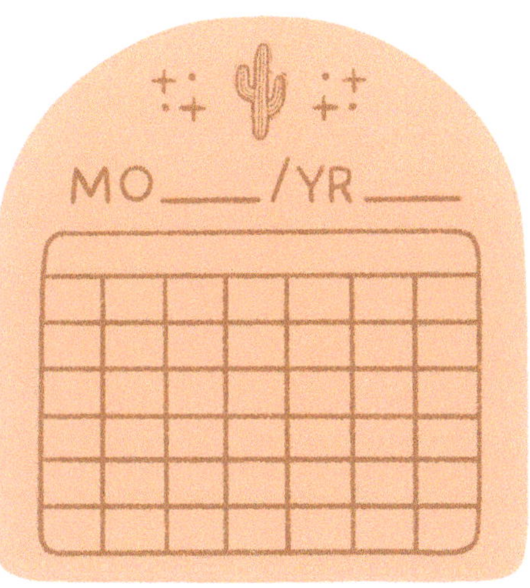
MO____/YR____

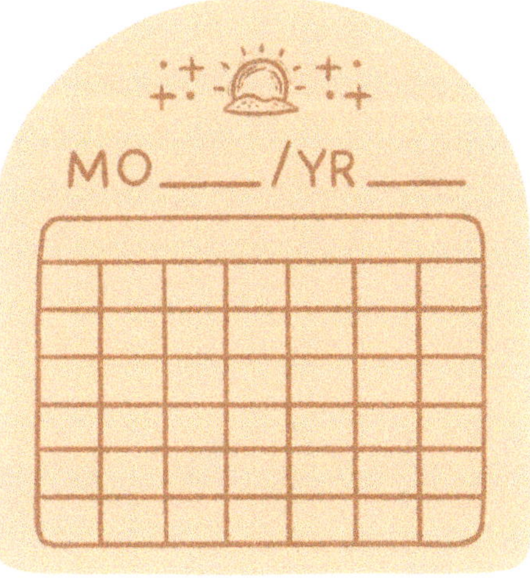
MO____/YR____

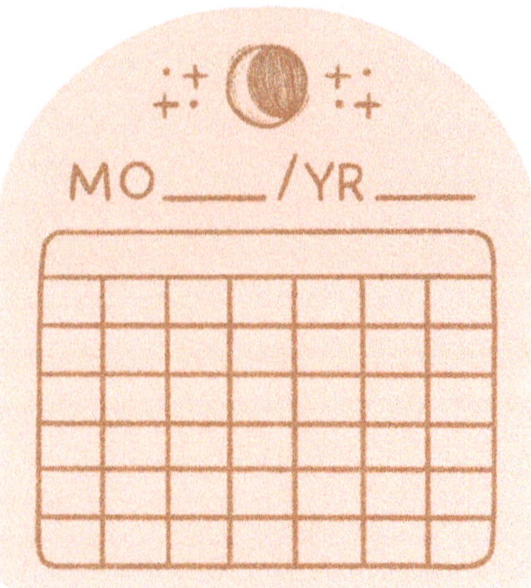

MO____/YR____

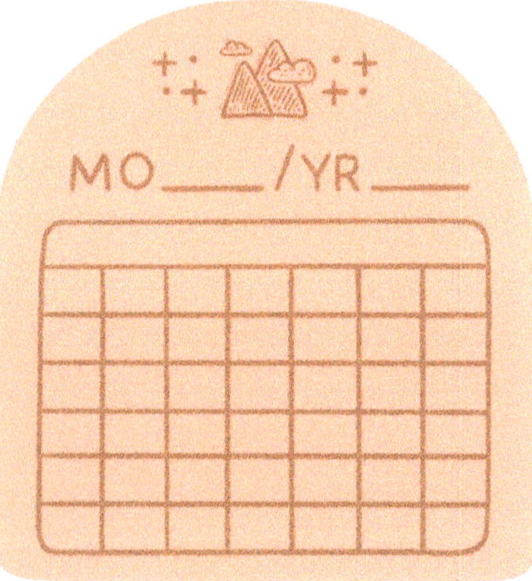

MO____/YR____

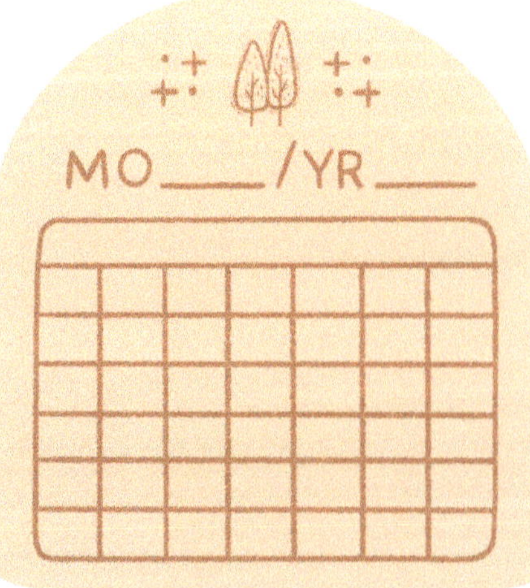

MO____/YR____

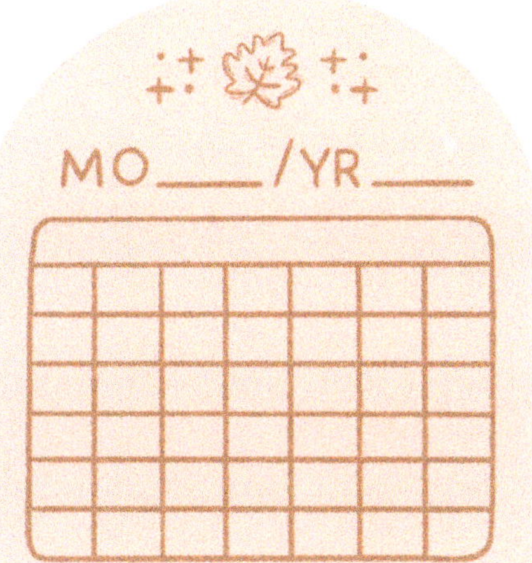
MO____/YR____

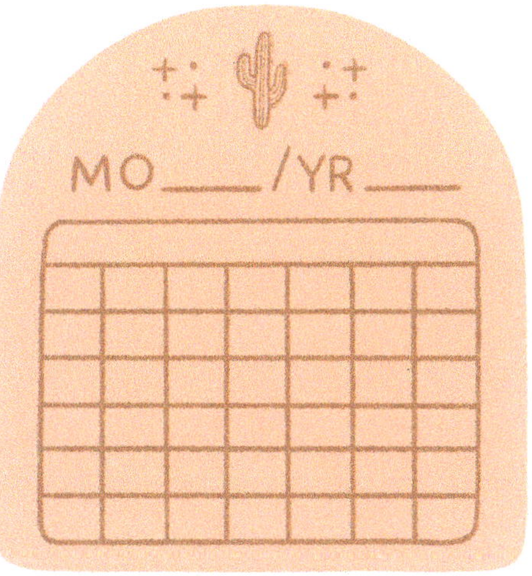
MO____/YR____

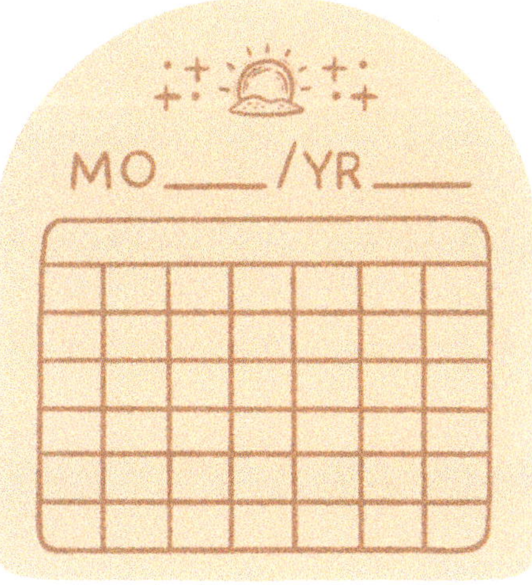
MO____/YR____

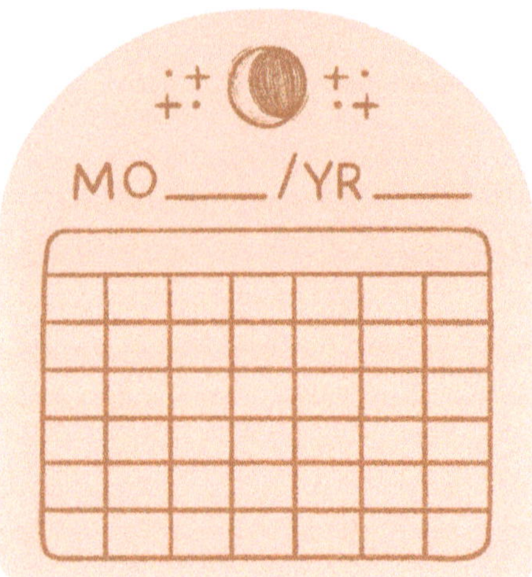
MO ____ /YR ____

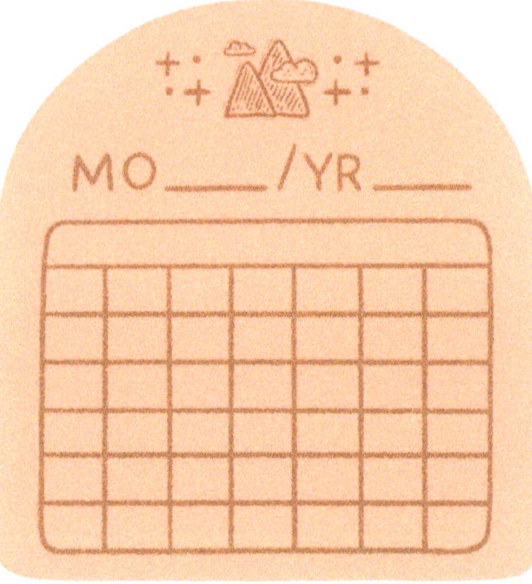
MO ____ /YR ____

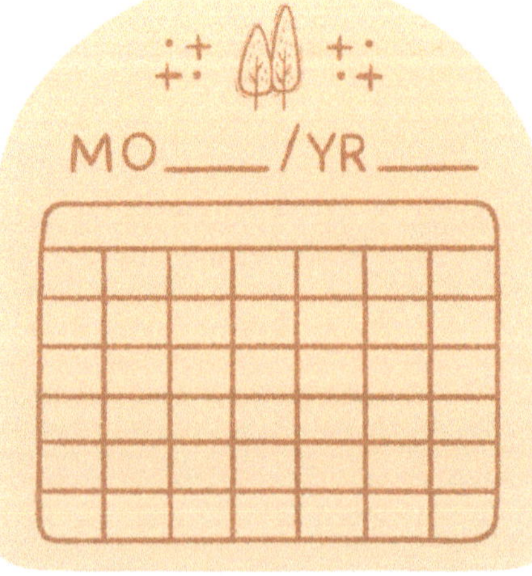
MO ____ /YR ____

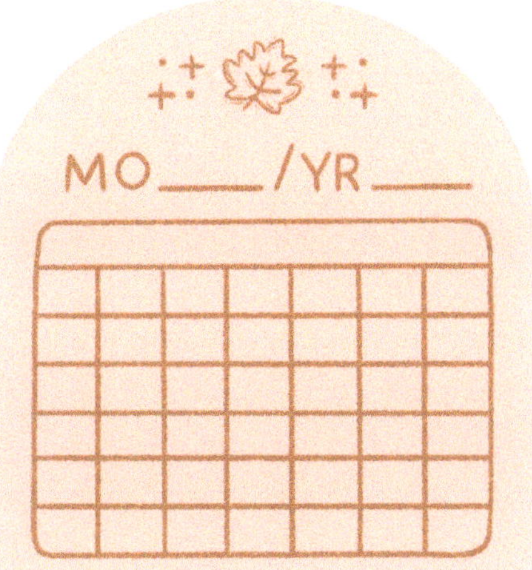
MO____/YR____

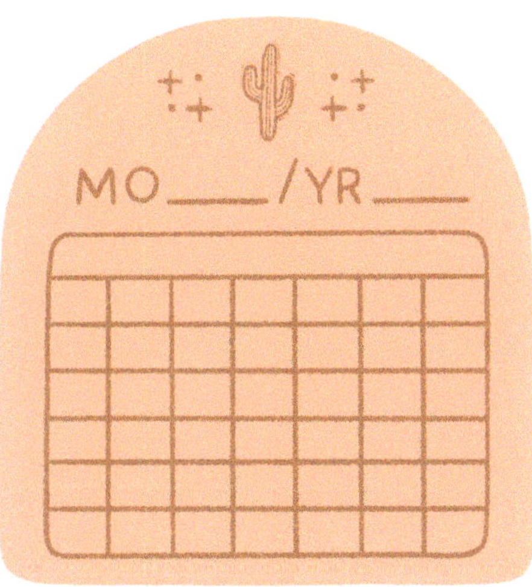
MO____/YR____

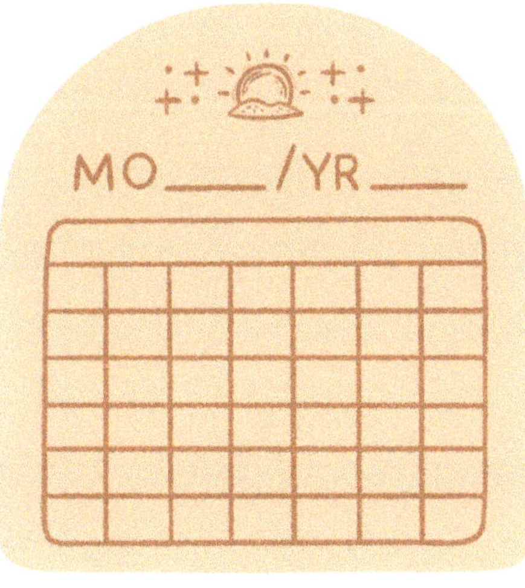
MO____/YR____

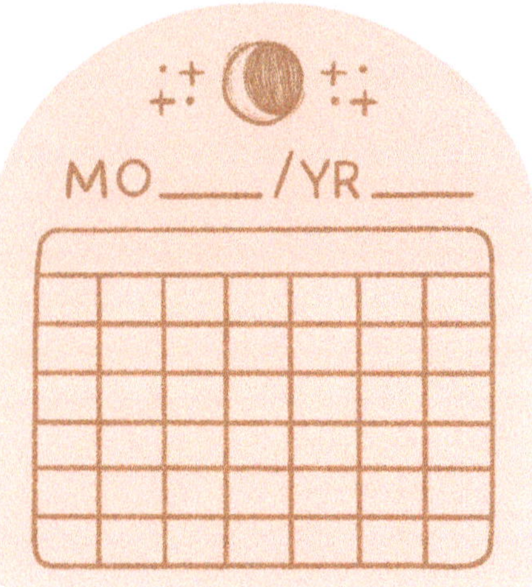

MO____/YR____

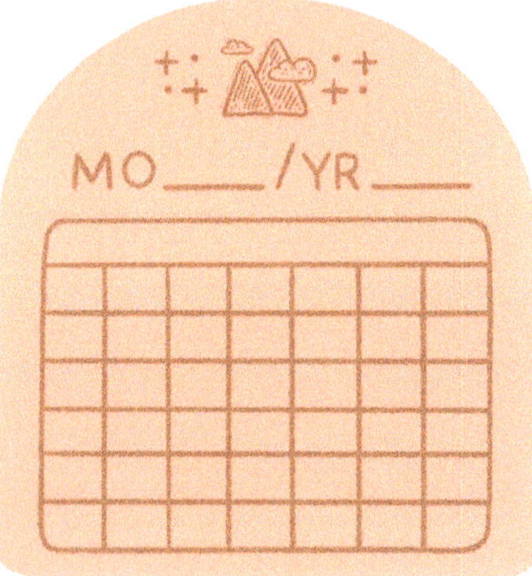

MO____/YR____

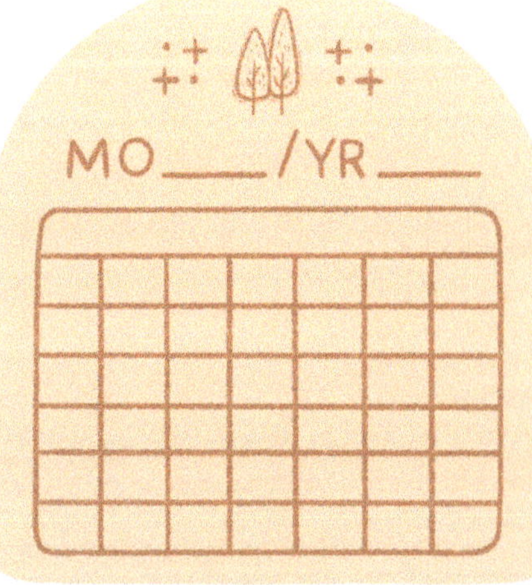

MO____/YR____

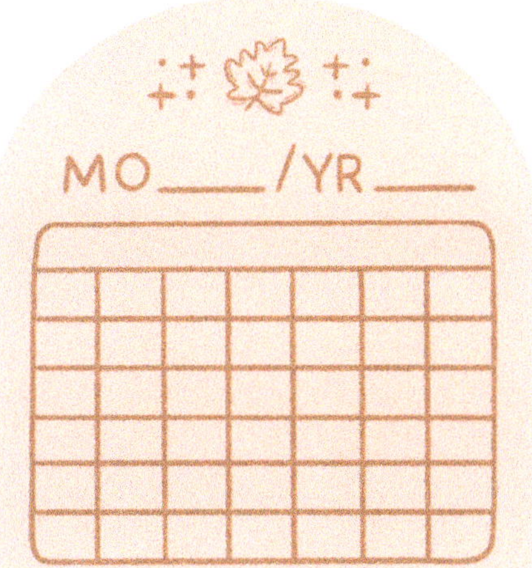

MO_____/YR_____

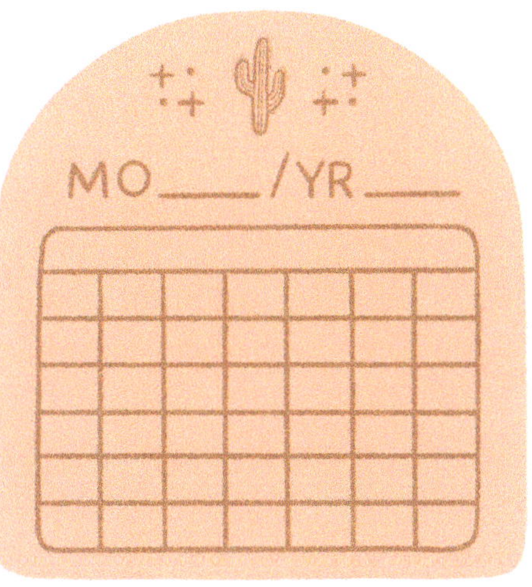

MO_____/YR_____

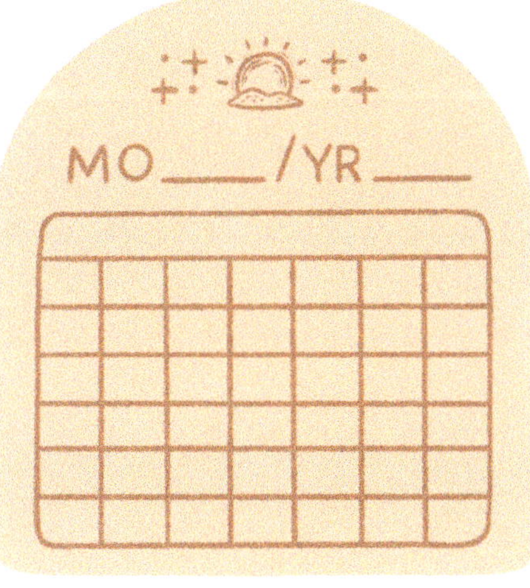

MO_____/YR_____

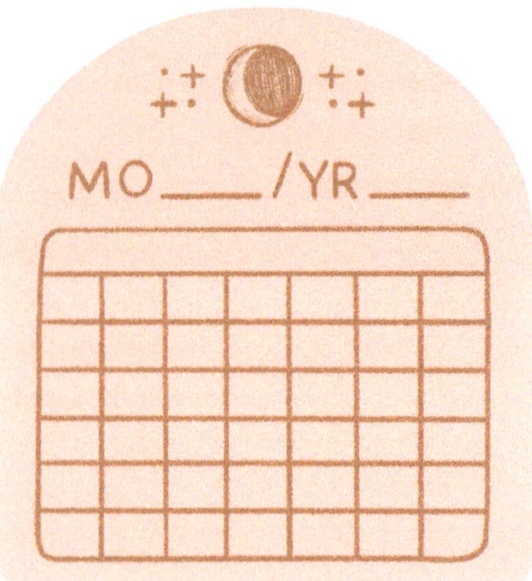

MO____/YR____

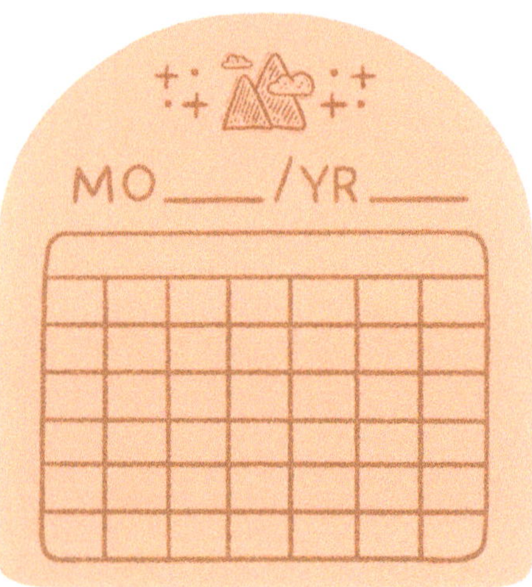

MO____/YR____

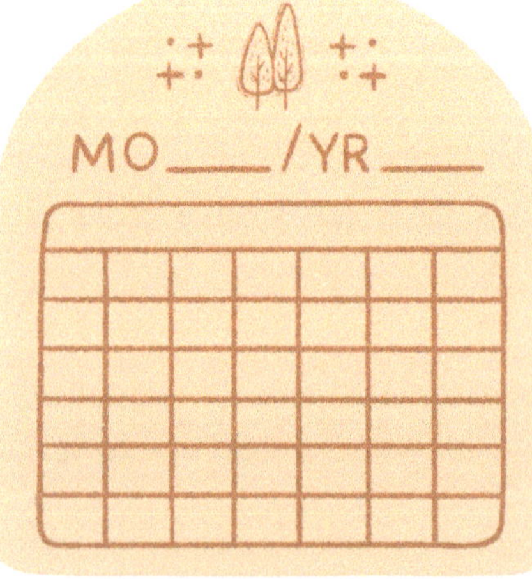

MO____/YR____

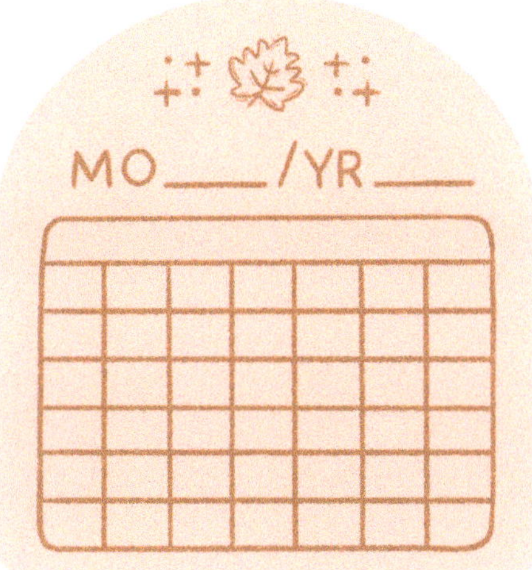

MO____/YR____

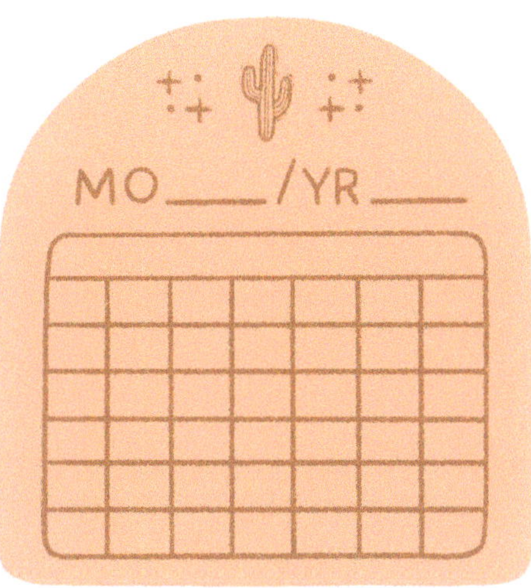

MO____/YR____

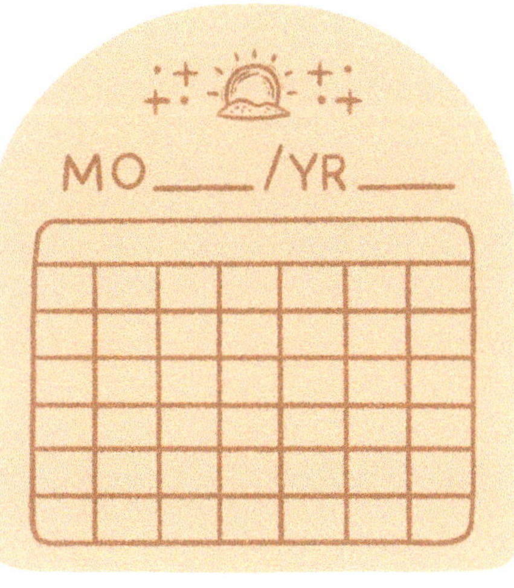

MO____/YR____

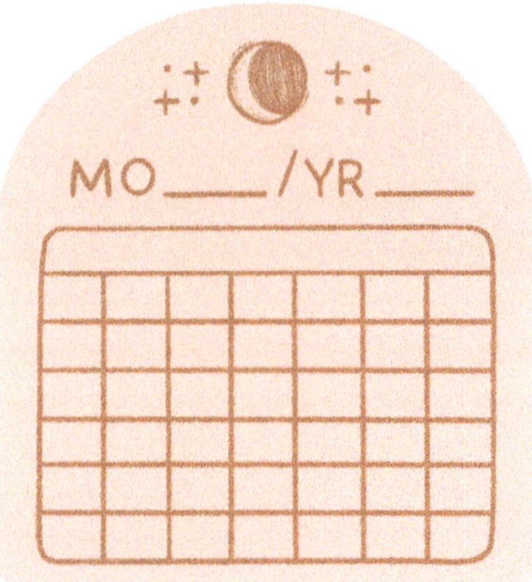
MO____/YR____

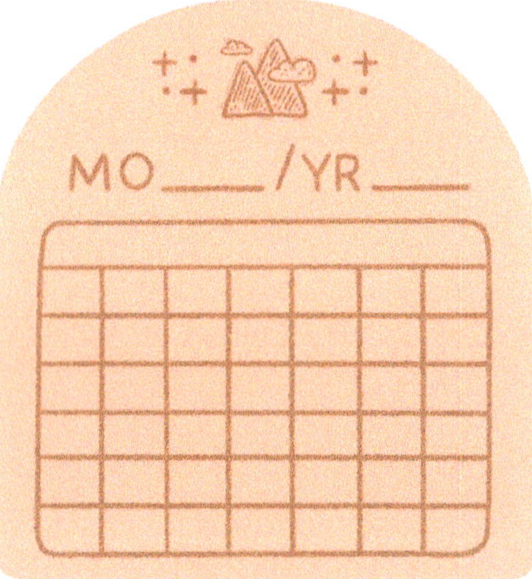
MO____/YR____

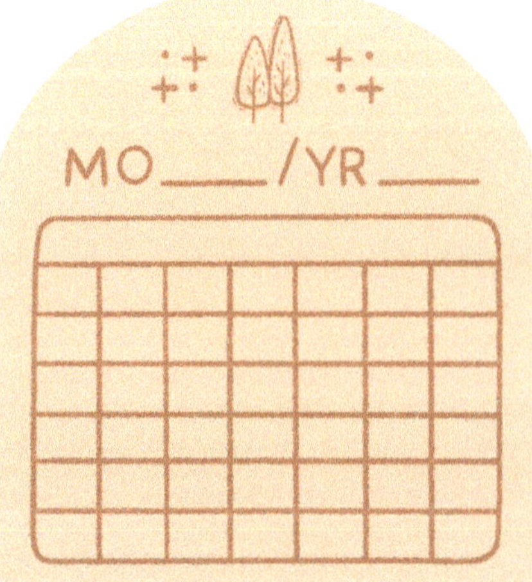
MO____/YR____

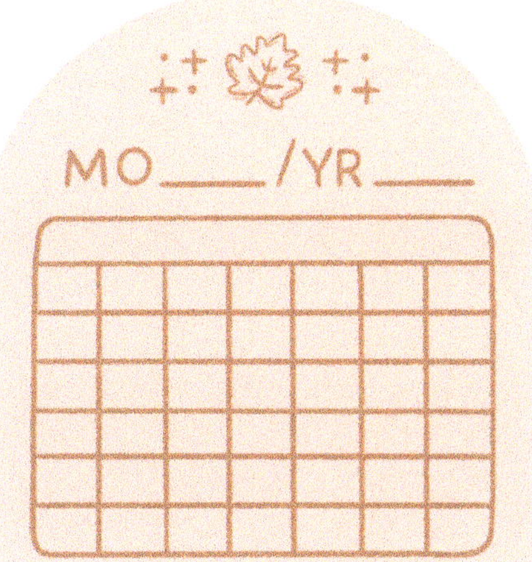

MO____/YR____

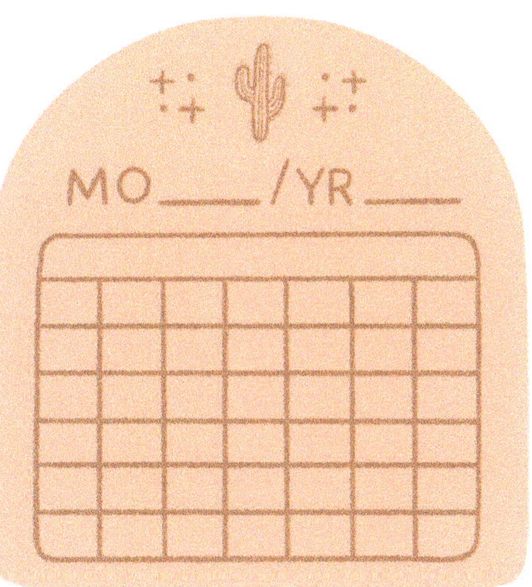

MO____/YR____

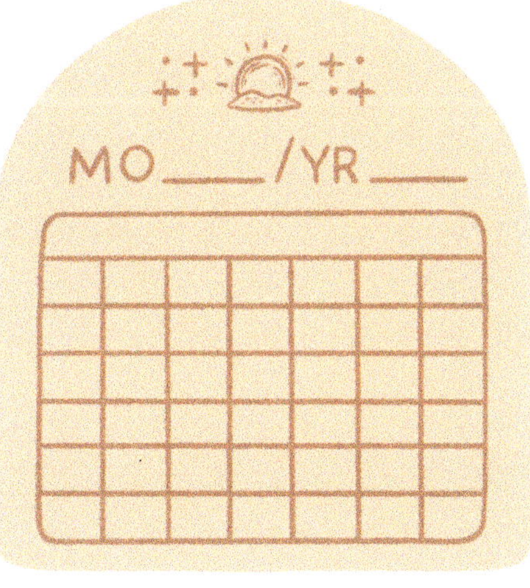

MO____/YR____

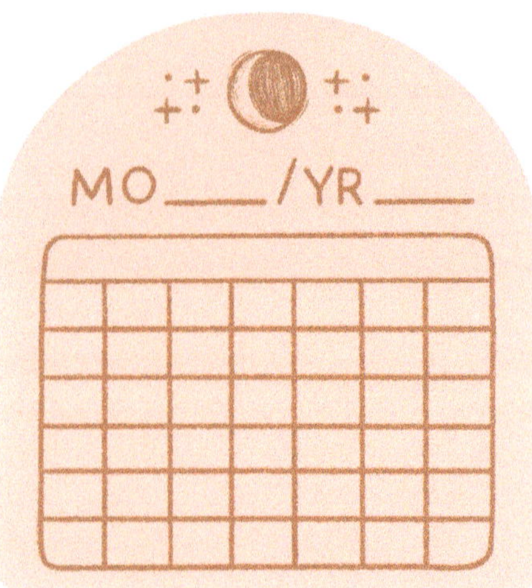

MO____/YR____

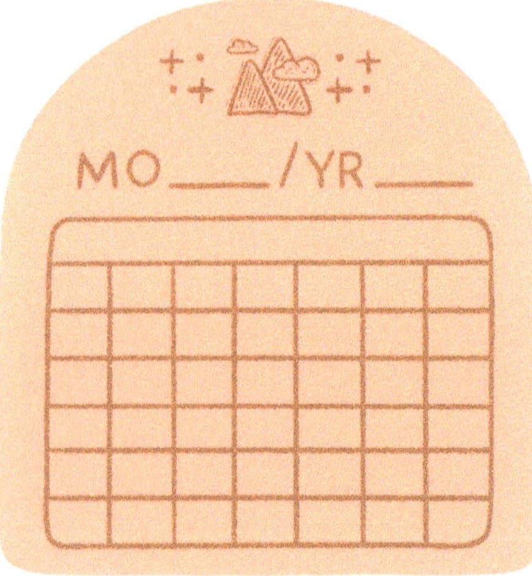

MO____/YR____

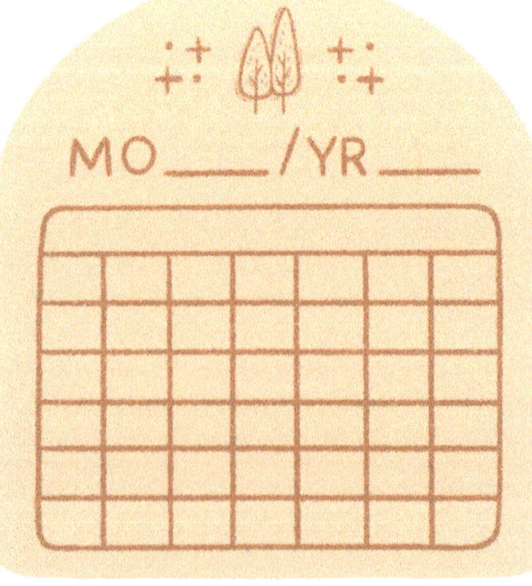

MO____/YR____

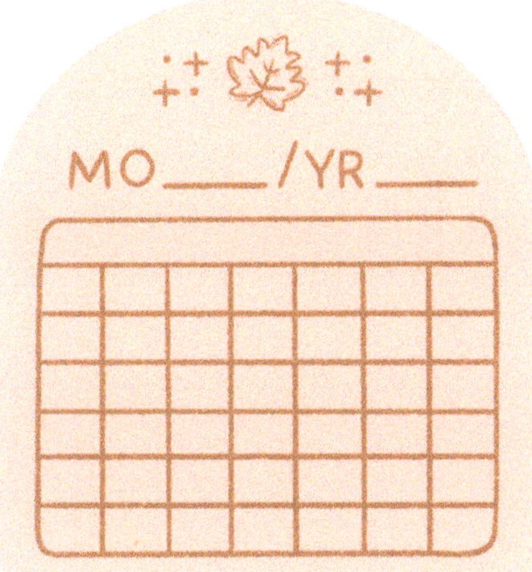

MO____/YR____

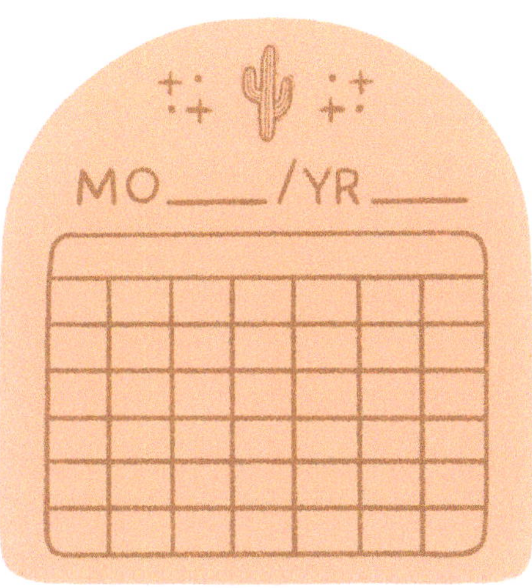

MO____/YR____

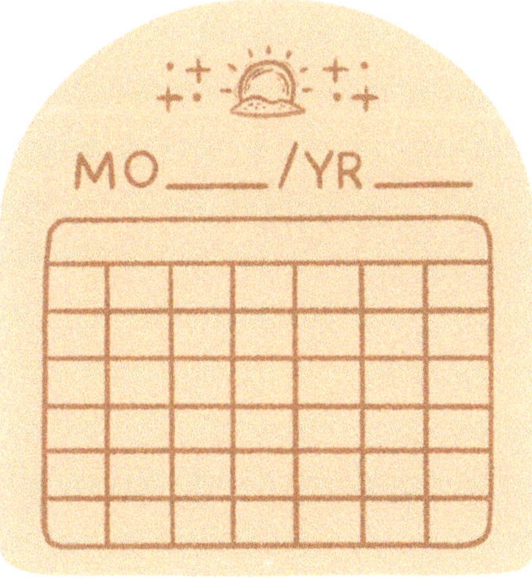

MO____/YR____

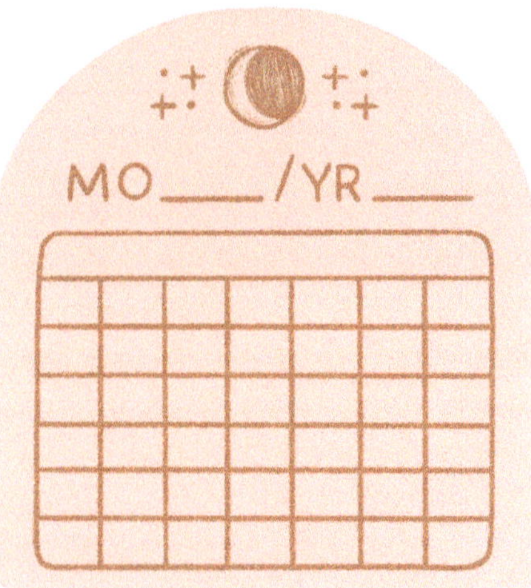
MO_____/YR_____

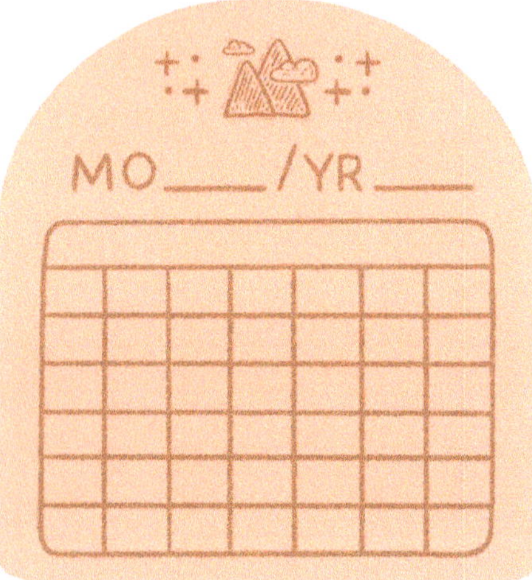
MO_____/YR_____

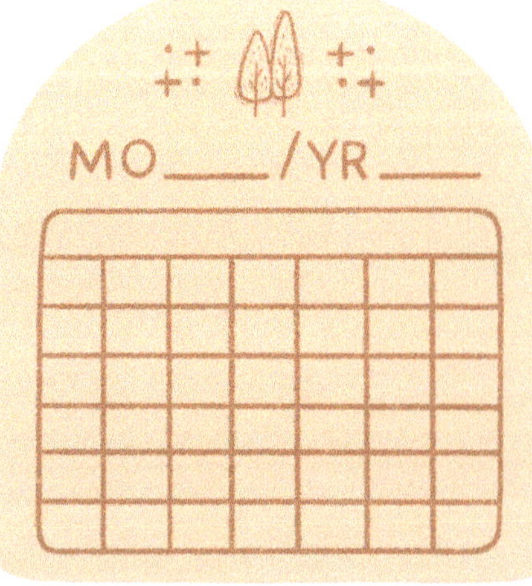
MO_____/YR_____

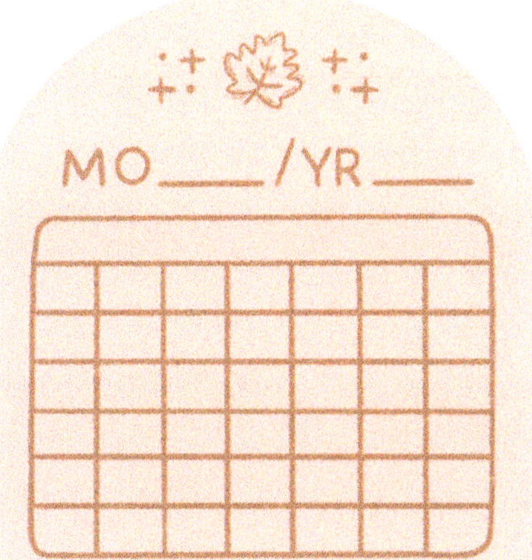

MO____/YR____

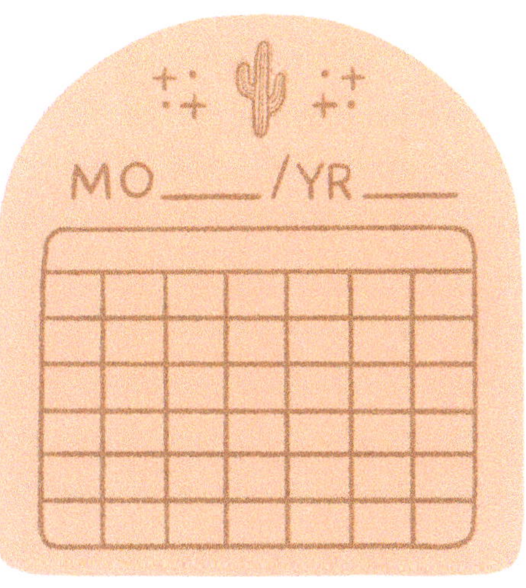

MO____/YR____

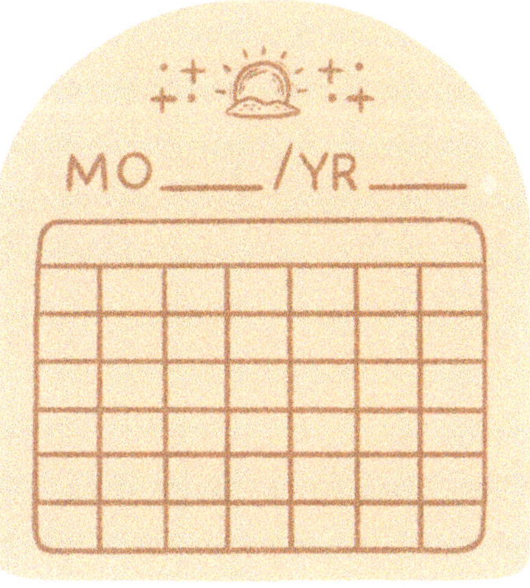

MO____/YR____

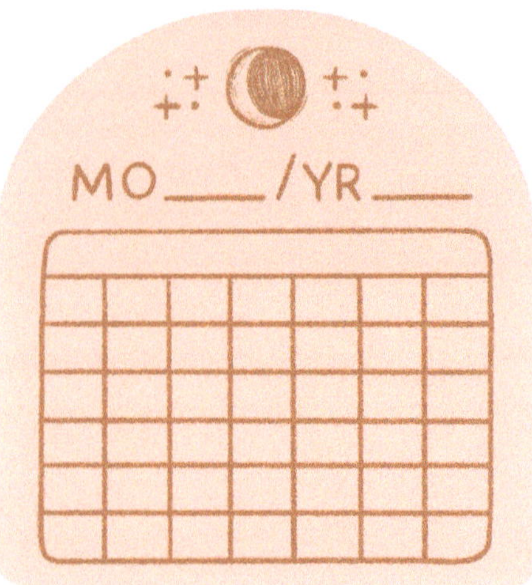

MO____/YR____

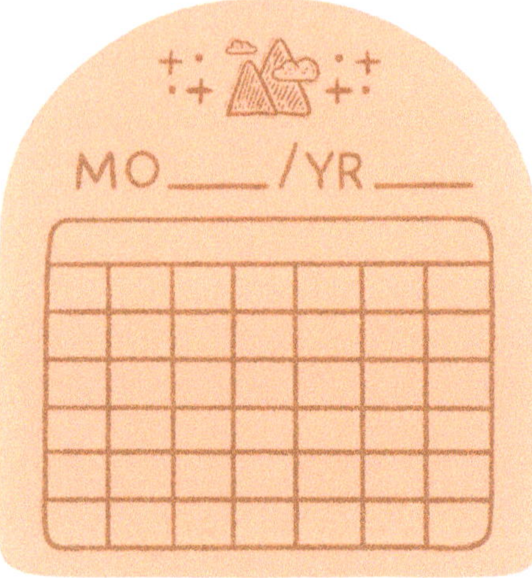

MO____/YR____

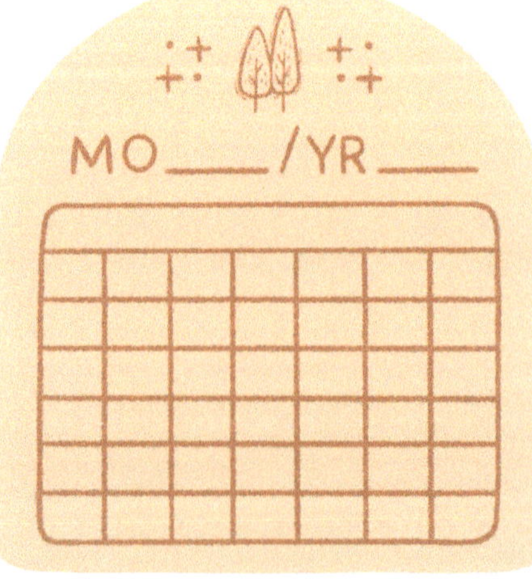

MO____/YR____

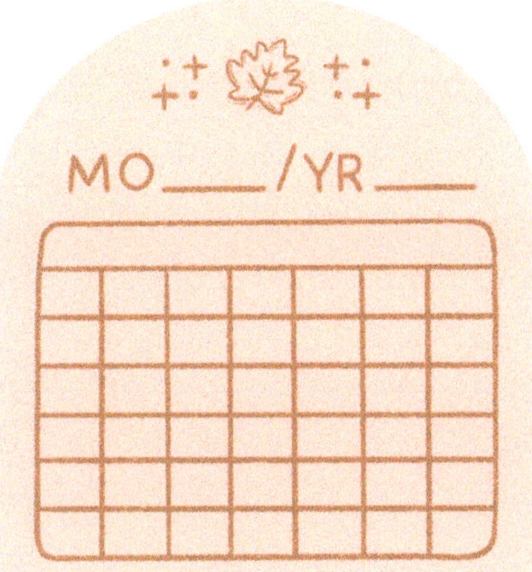

MO____/YR____

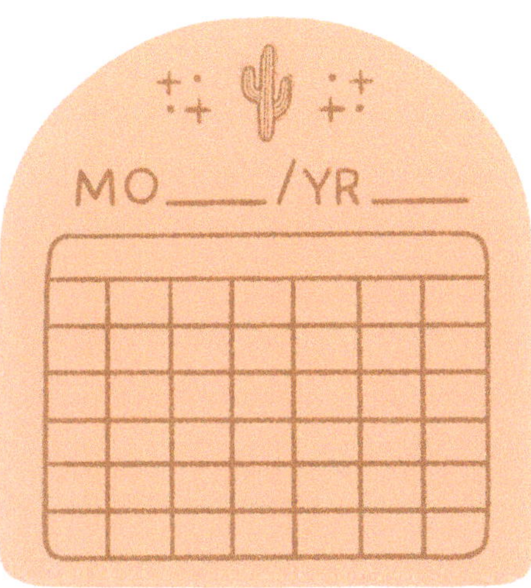

MO____/YR____

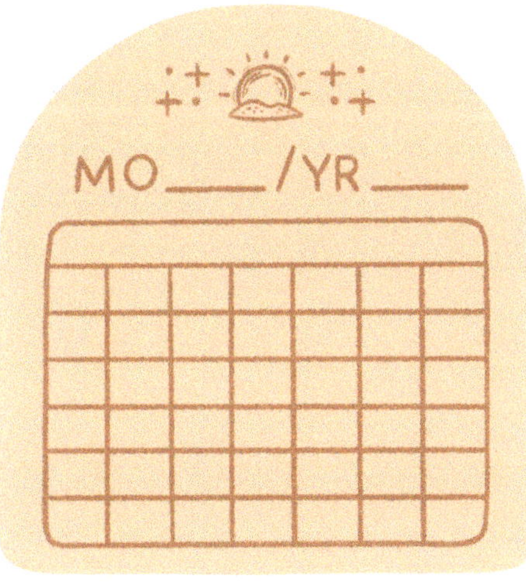

MO____/YR____

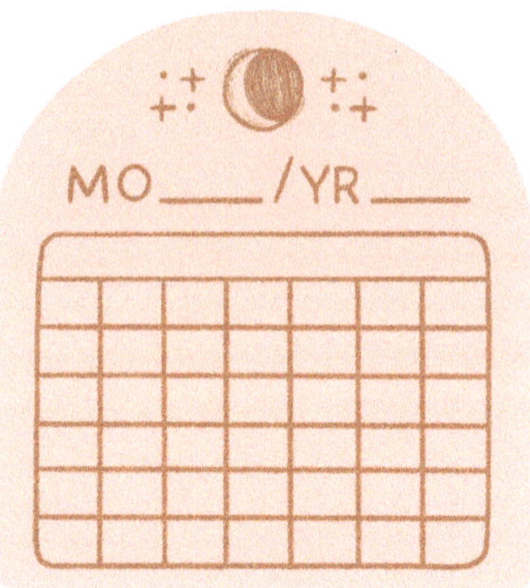

MO_____/YR_____

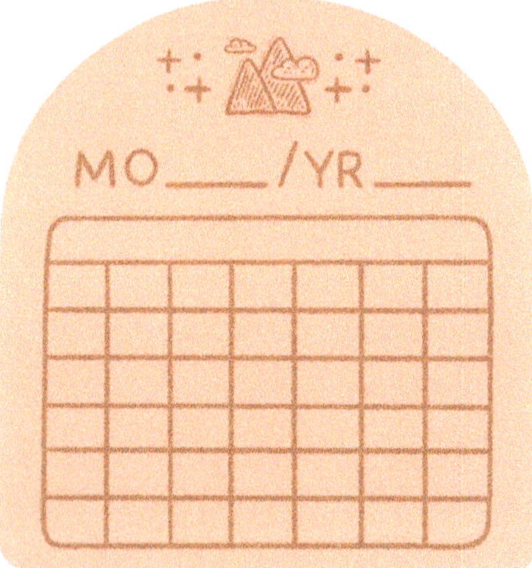

MO_____/YR_____

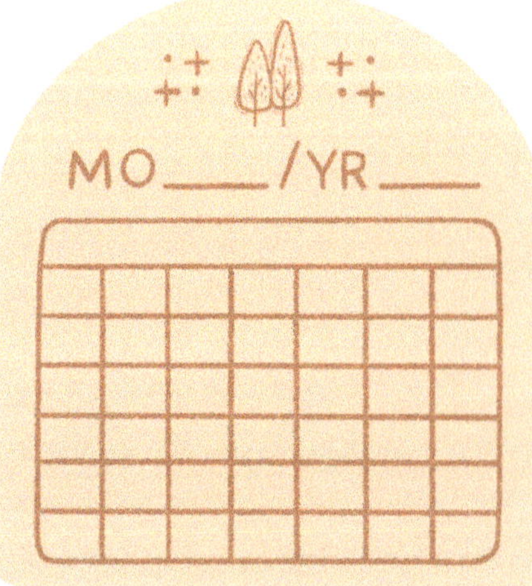

MO_____/YR_____

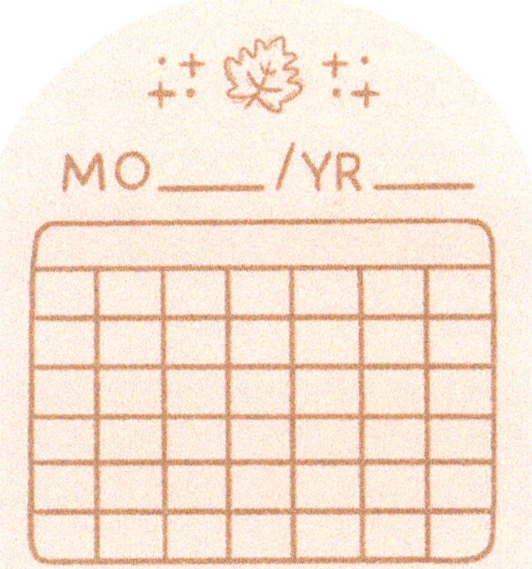

MO_____/YR_____

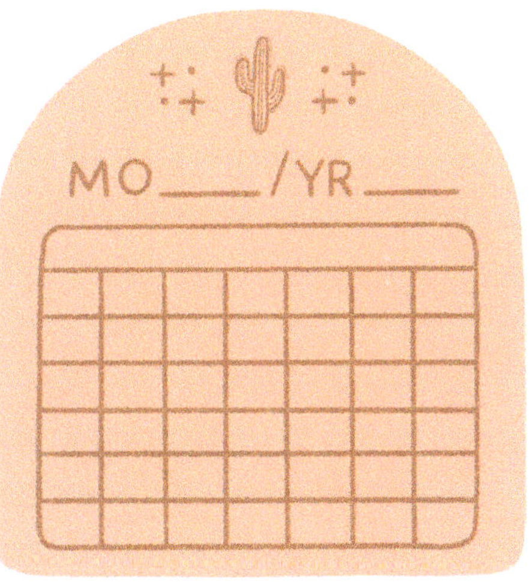

MO_____/YR_____

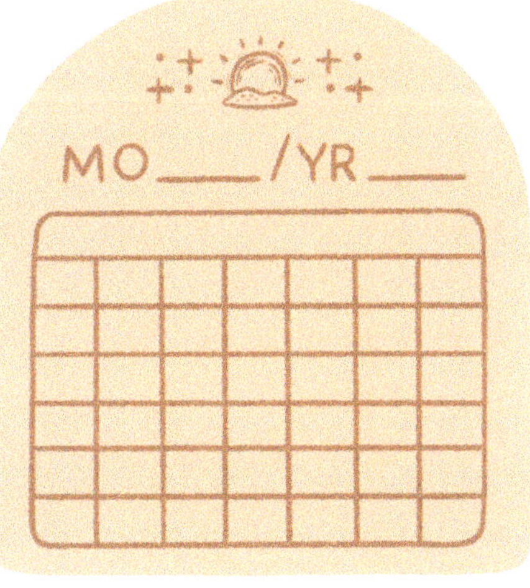

MO_____/YR_____

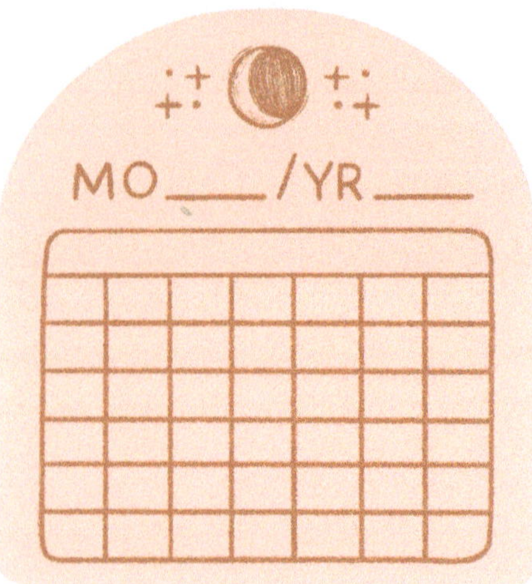
MO ____ /YR ____

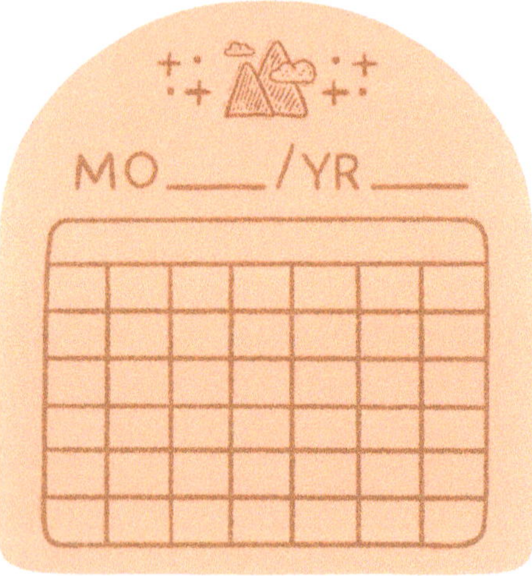
MO ____ /YR ____

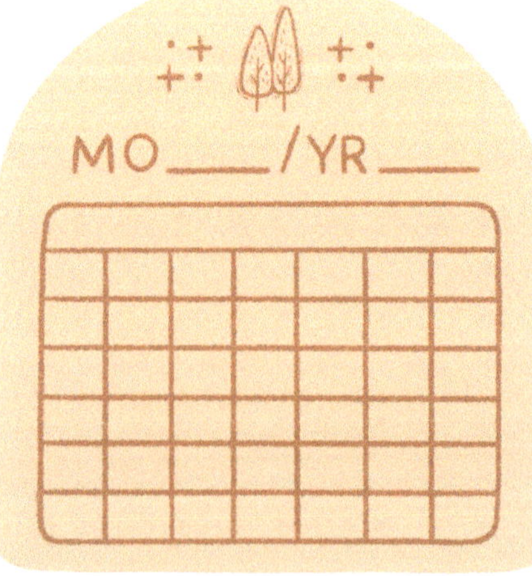
MO ____ /YR ____

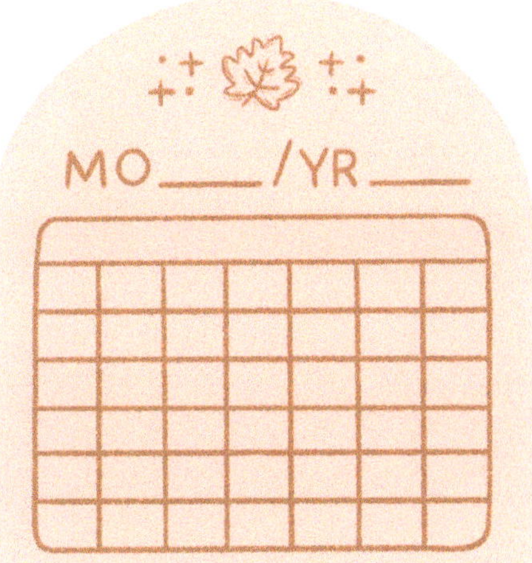

MO____/YR____

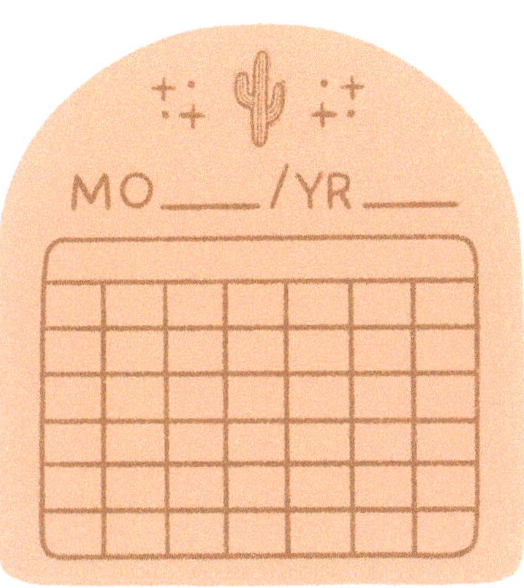

MO____/YR____

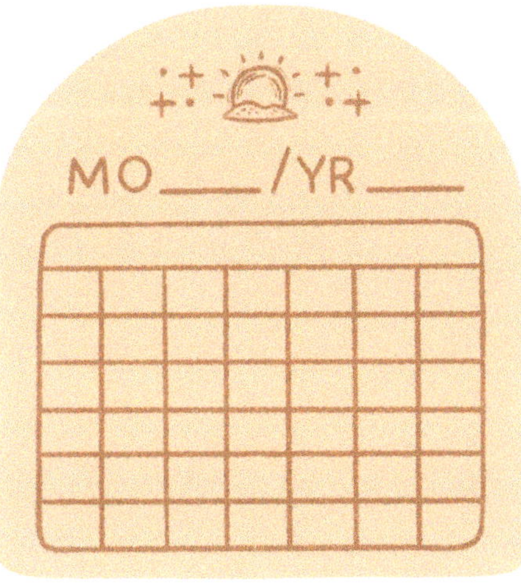

MO____/YR____

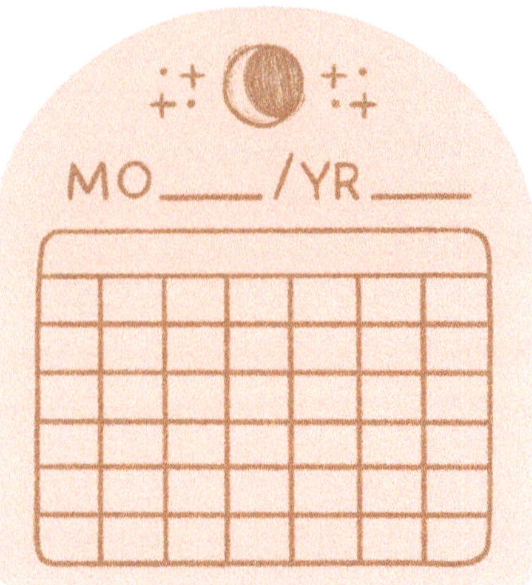
MO_____/YR_____

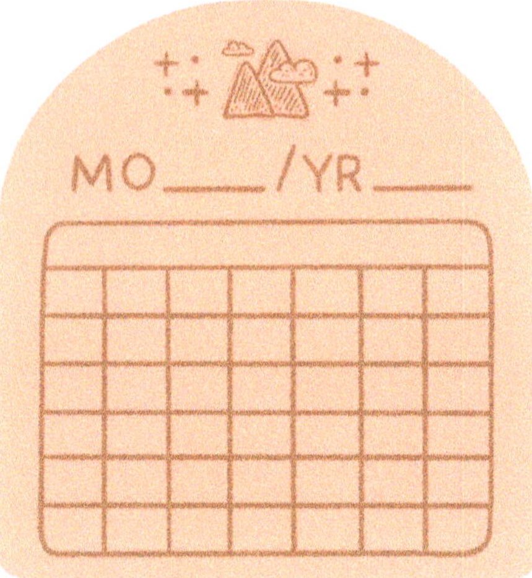
MO_____/YR_____

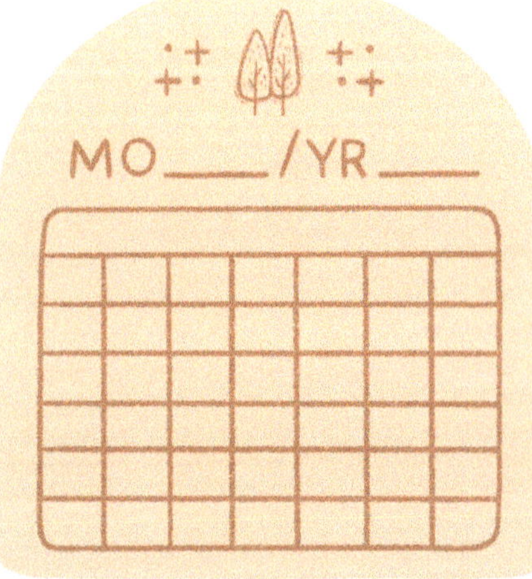
MO_____/YR_____

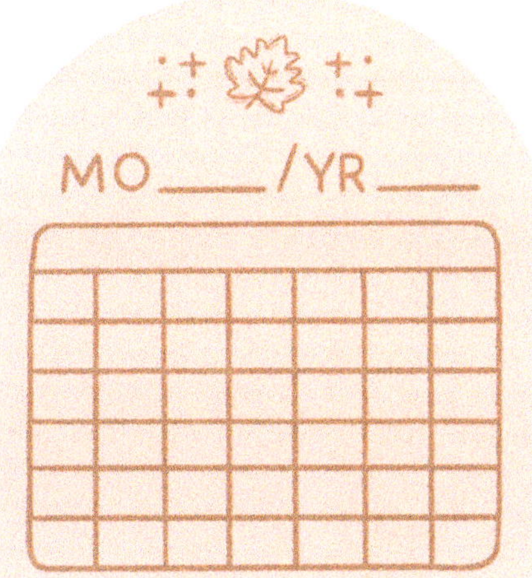

MO____/YR____

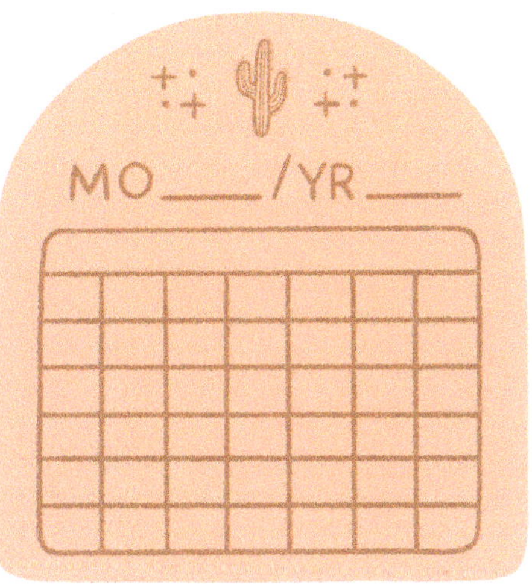

MO____/YR____

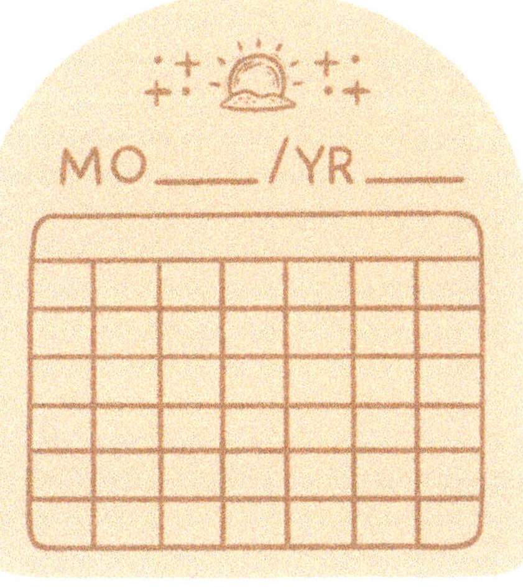

MO____/YR____

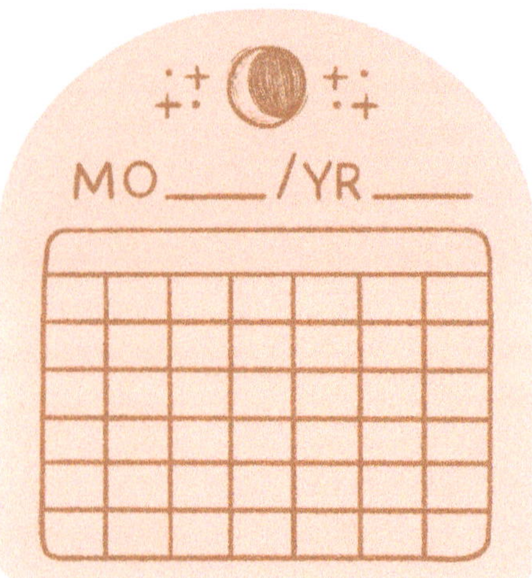

MO____/YR____

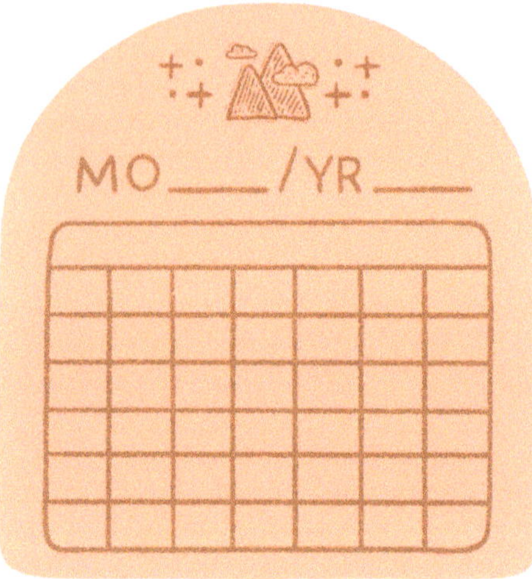

MO____/YR____

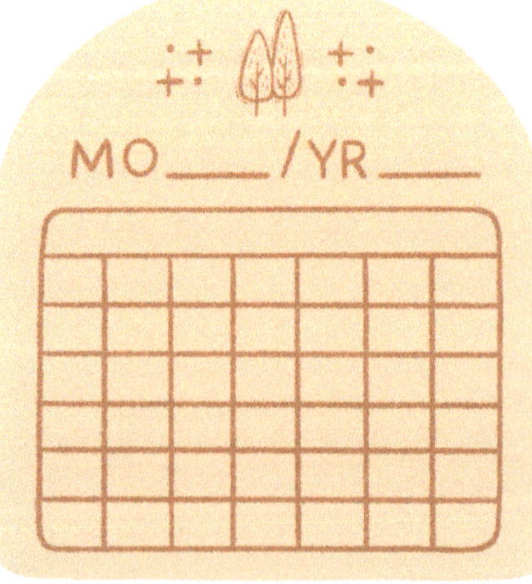

MO____/YR____

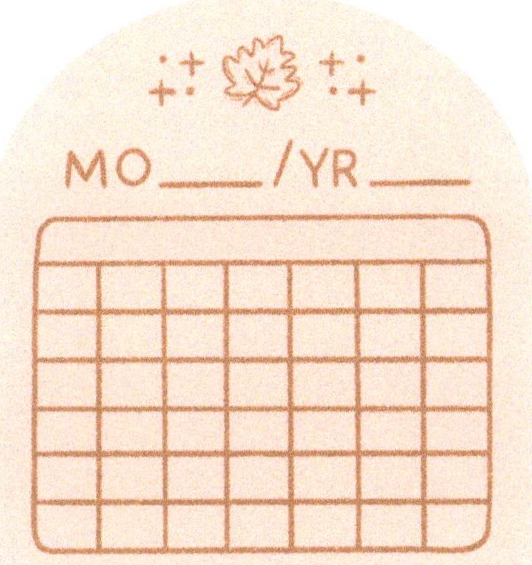
MO____/YR____
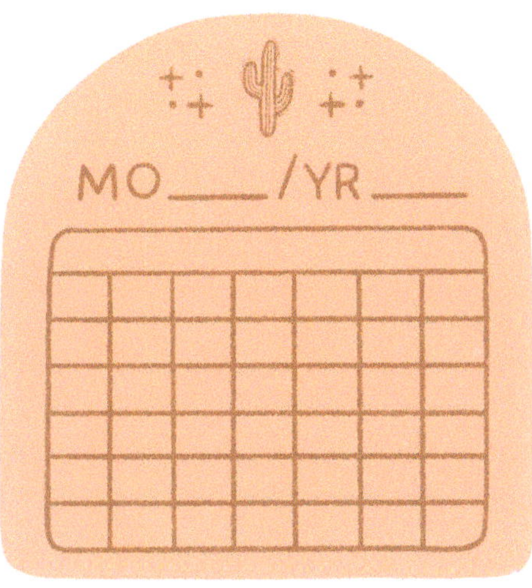
MO____/YR____
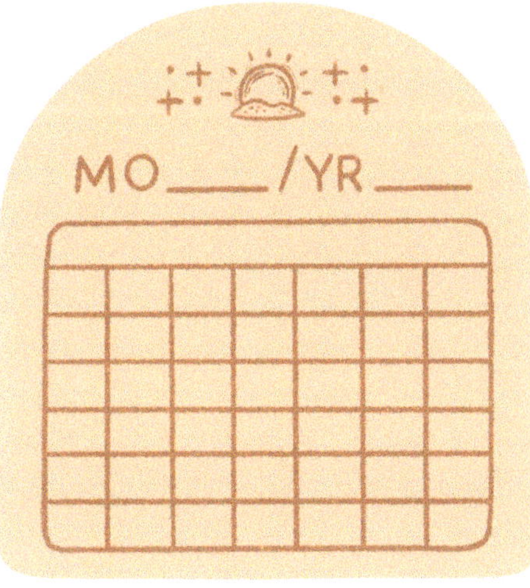
MO____/YR____

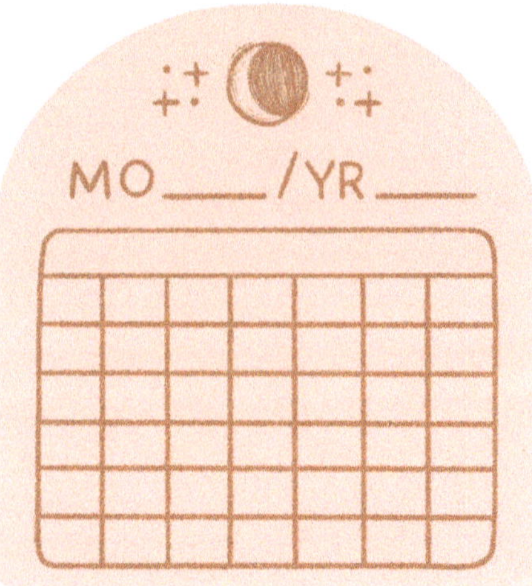
MO____ /YR____

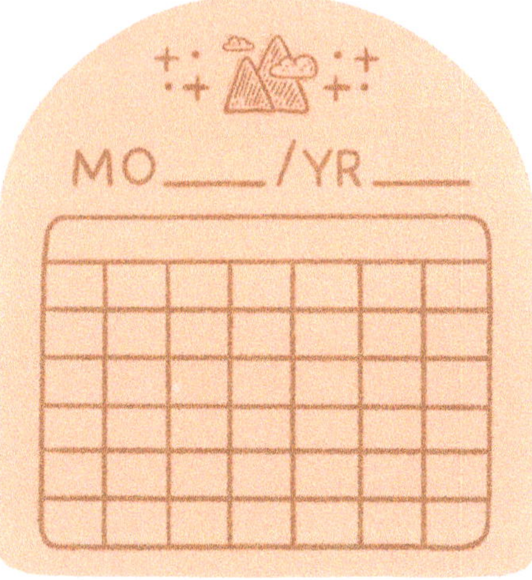
MO____ /YR____

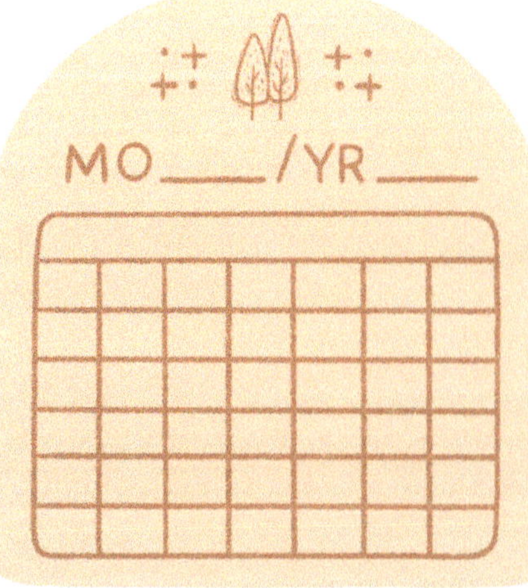
MO____ /YR____

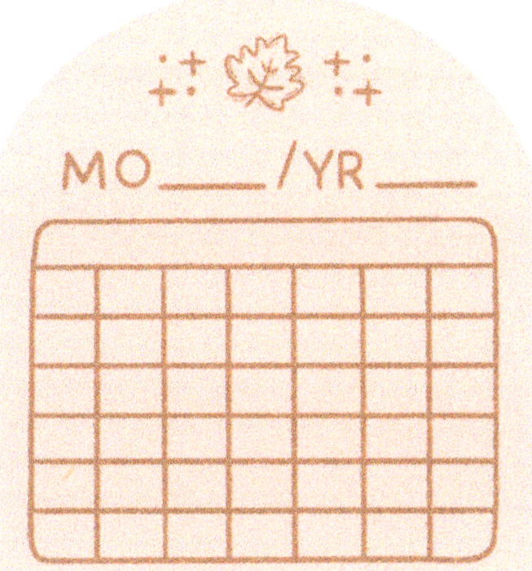
MO_____/YR_____

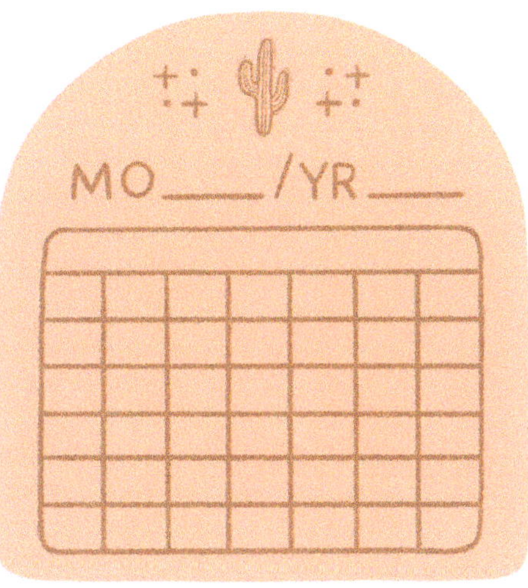
MO_____/YR_____

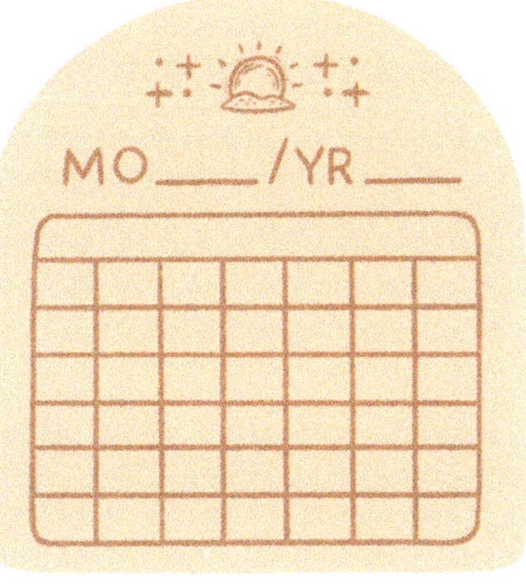
MO_____/YR_____

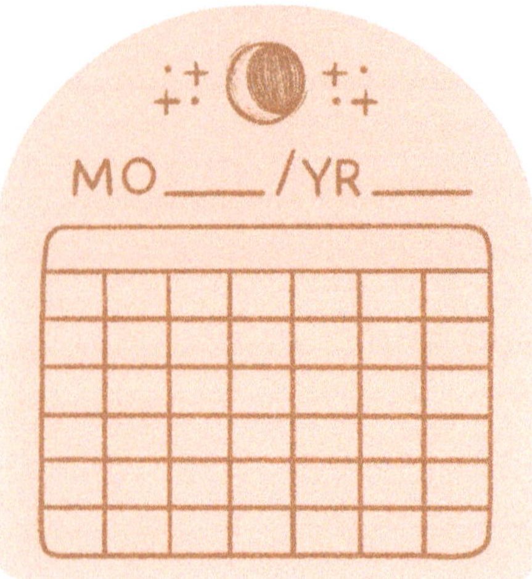

MO____/YR____

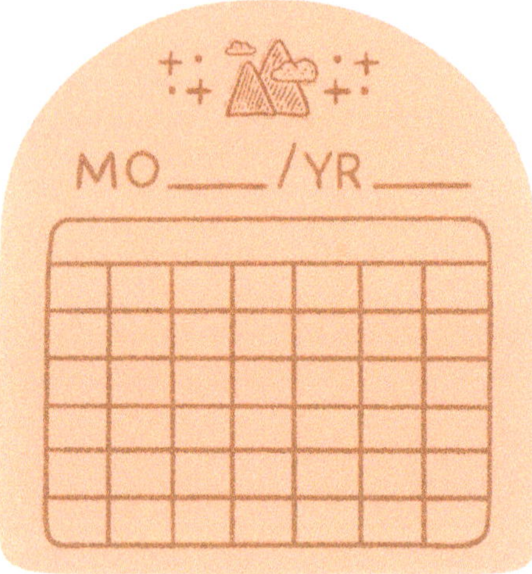

MO____/YR____

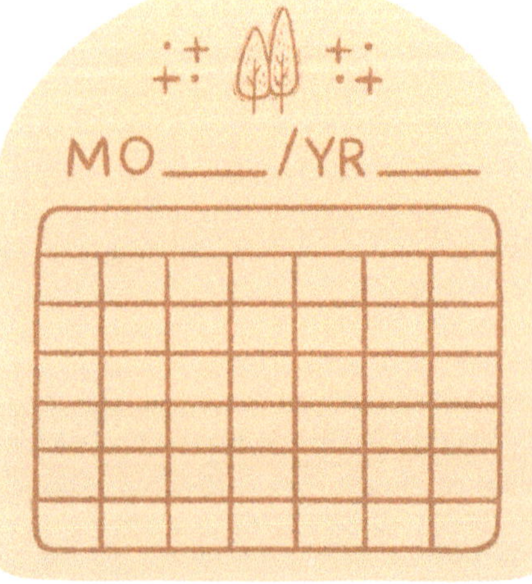

MO____/YR____

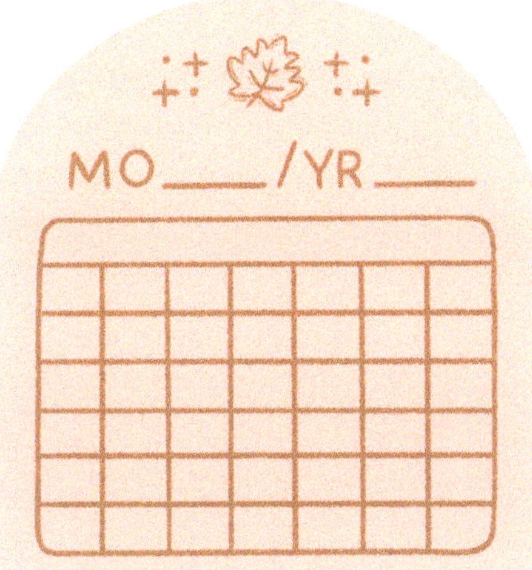

MO_____/YR_____

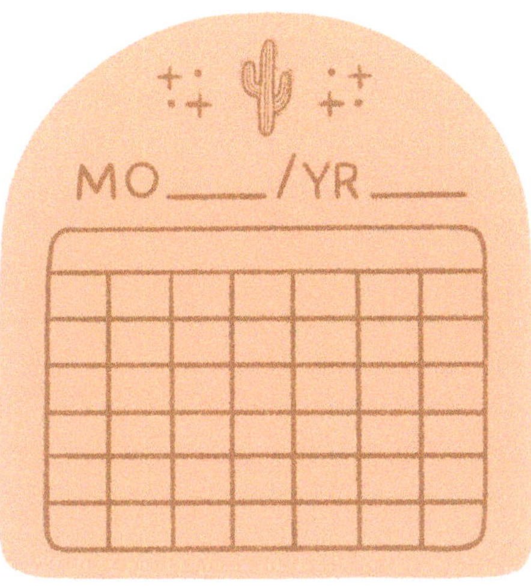

MO_____/YR_____

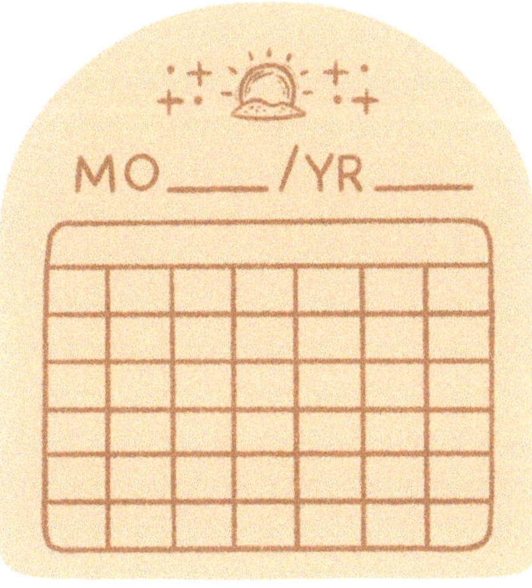

MO_____/YR_____

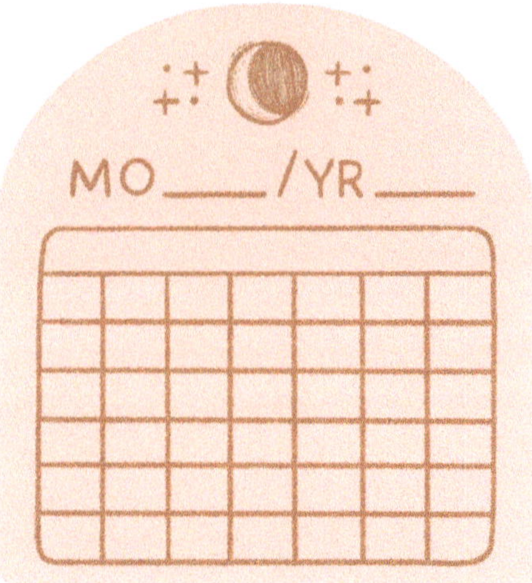

MO_____/YR_____

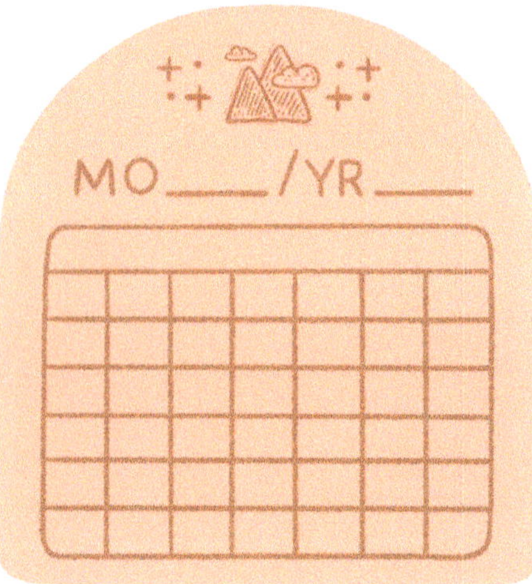

MO_____/YR_____

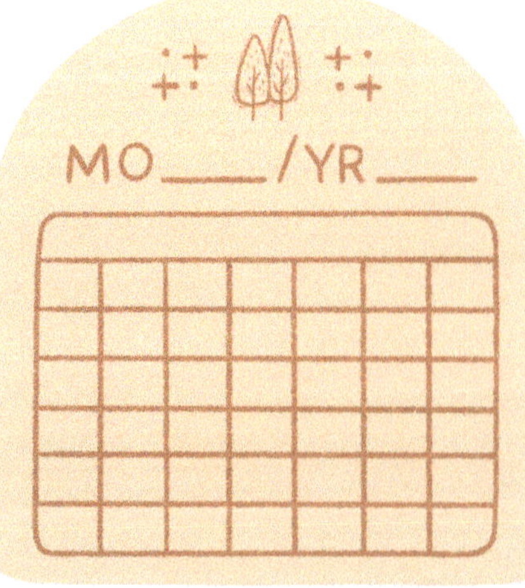

MO_____/YR_____

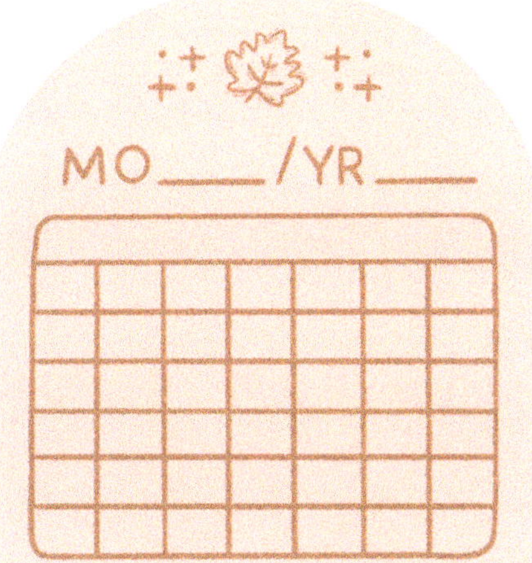
MO____/YR____

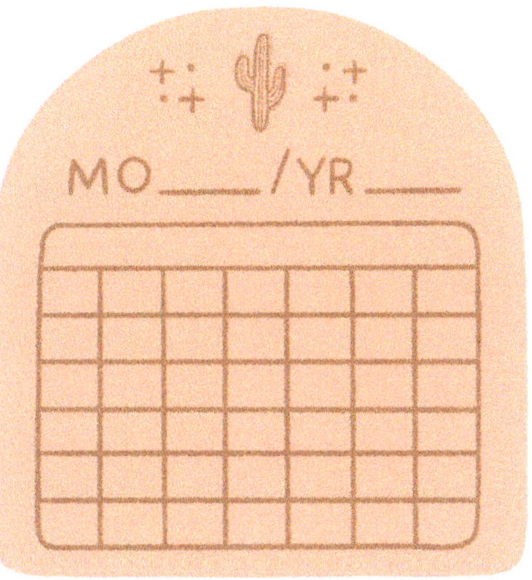
MO____/YR____

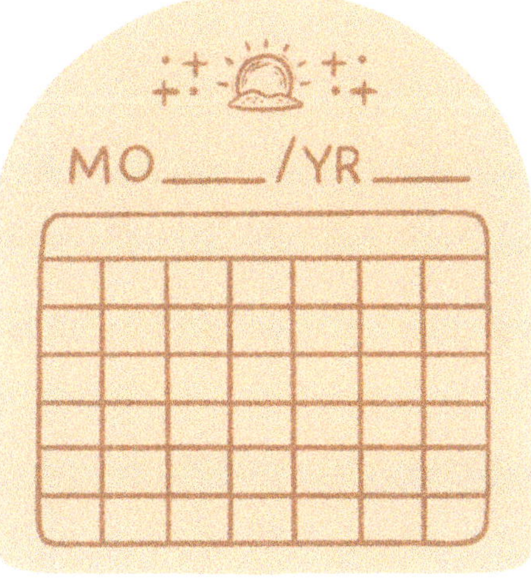
MO____/YR____

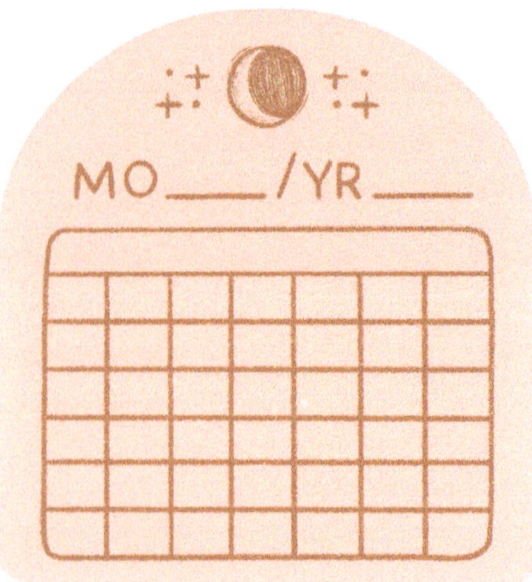
MO____/YR____

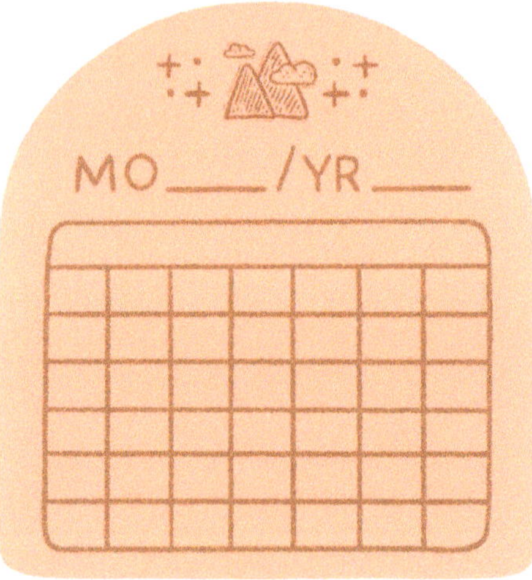
MO____/YR____

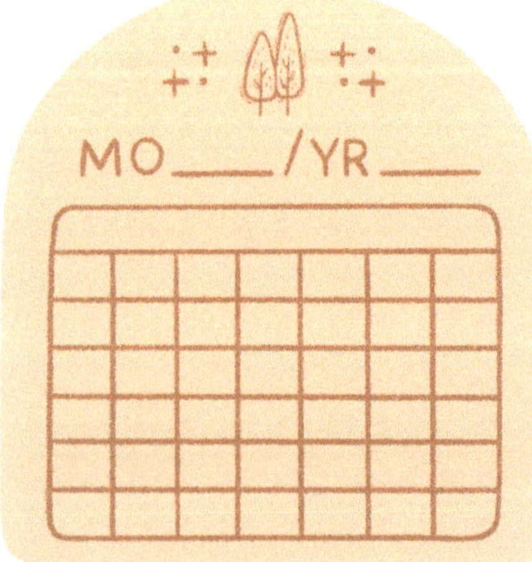
MO____/YR____

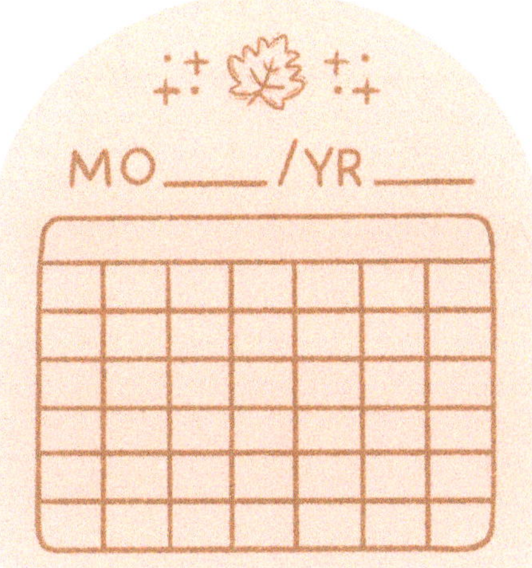

MO_____/YR_____

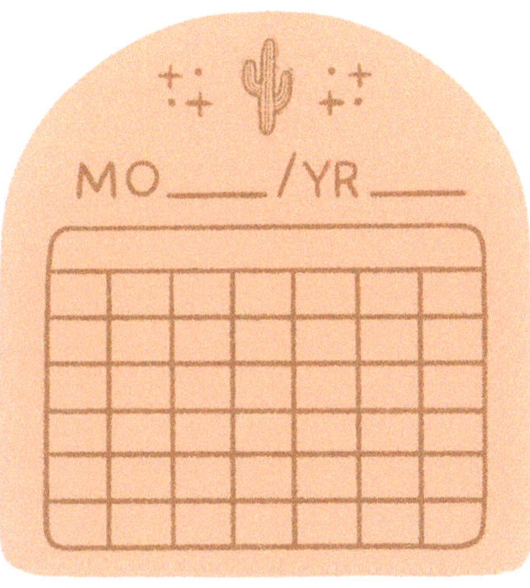

MO_____/YR_____

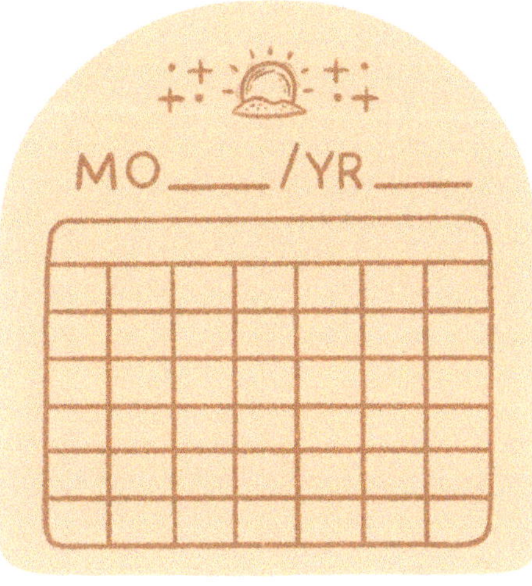

MO_____/YR_____

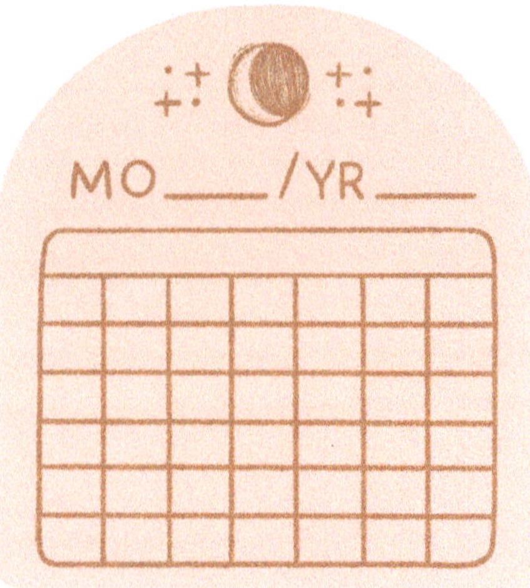

MO_____/YR_____

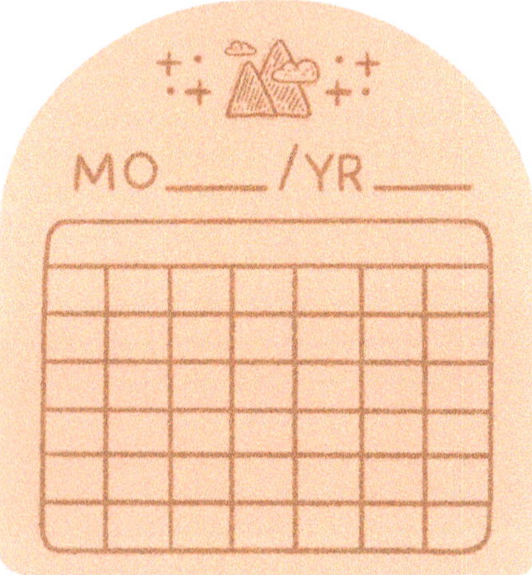

MO_____/YR_____

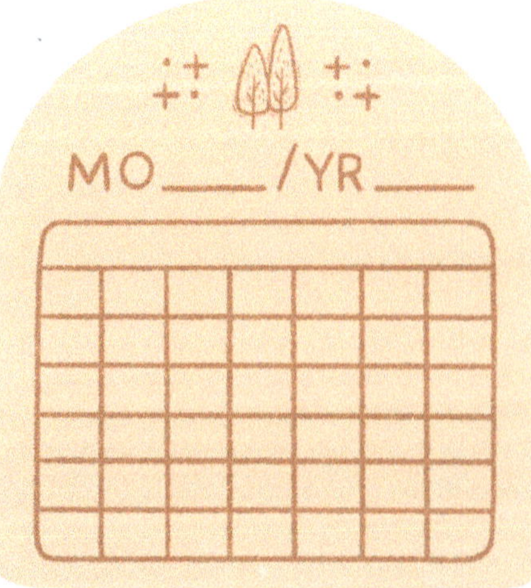

MO_____/YR_____

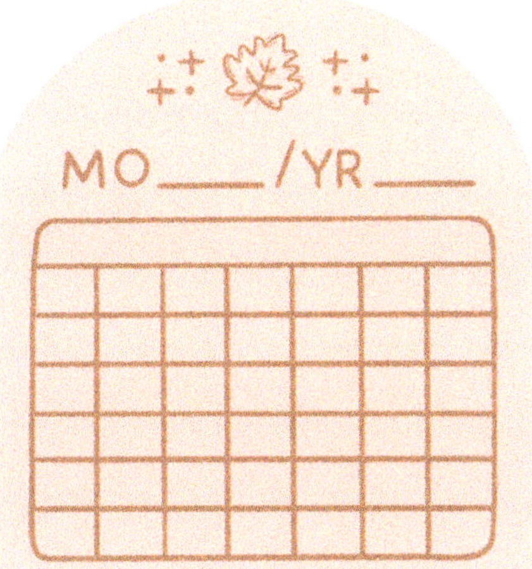

MO____ /YR____

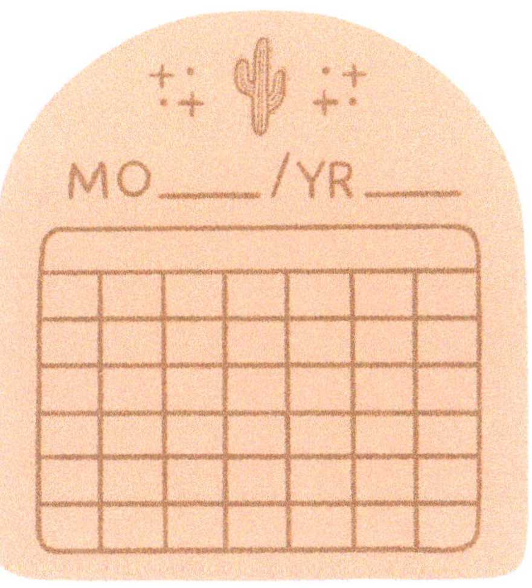

MO____ /YR____

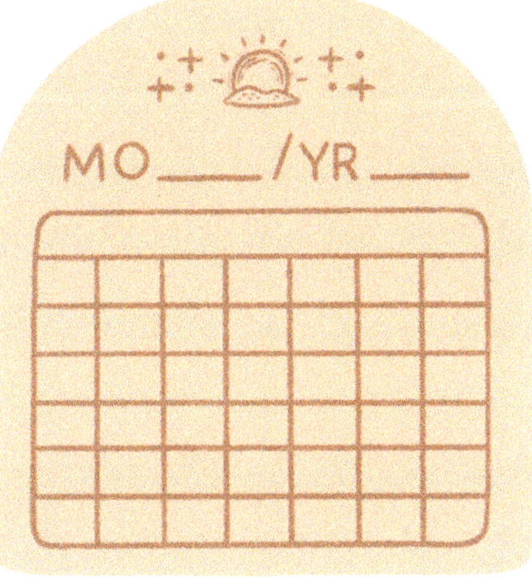

MO____ /YR____

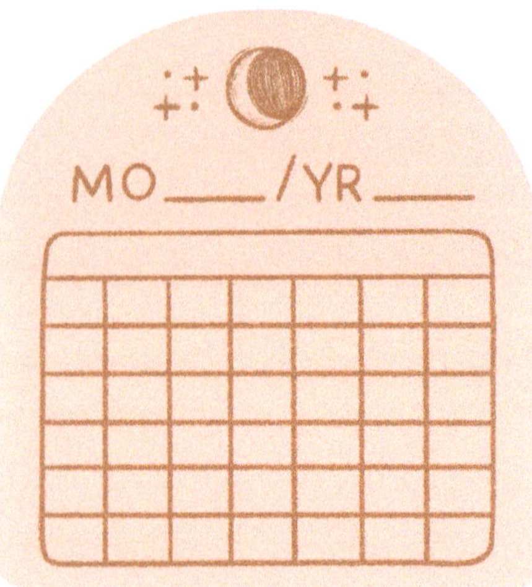

MO_____/YR_____

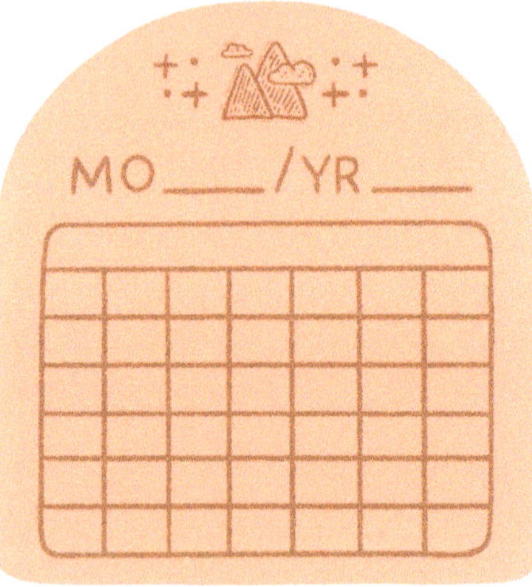

MO_____/YR_____

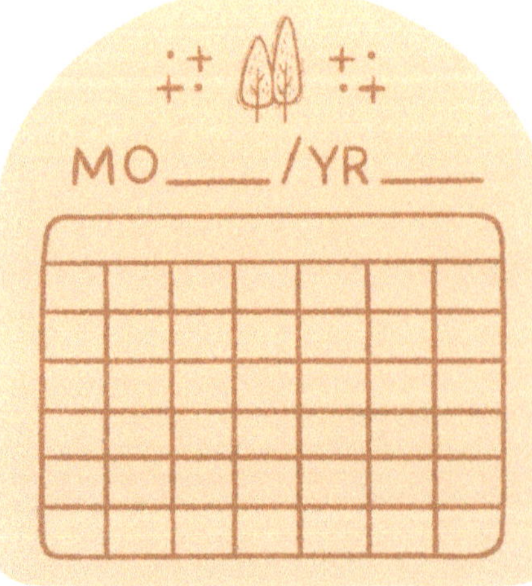

MO_____/YR_____

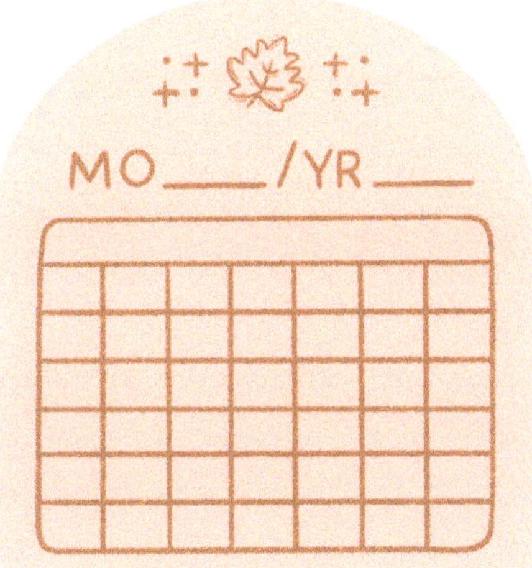
MO____/YR____

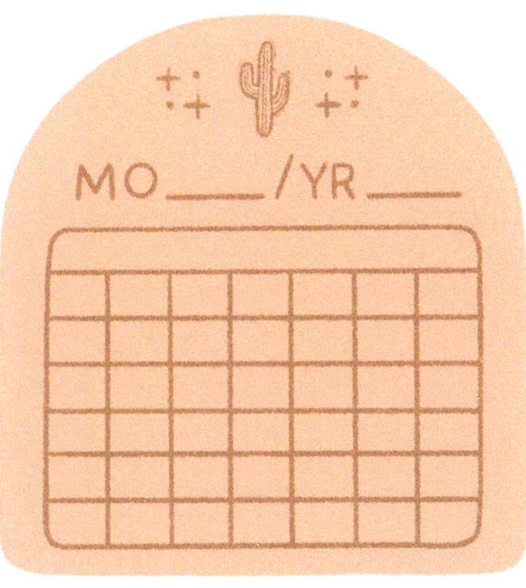
MO____/YR____

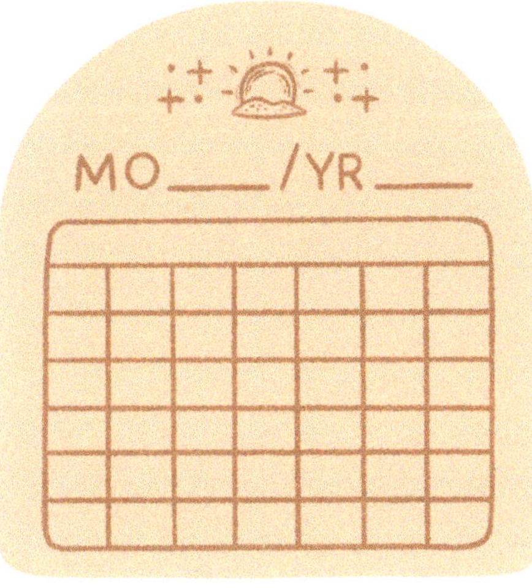
MO____/YR____

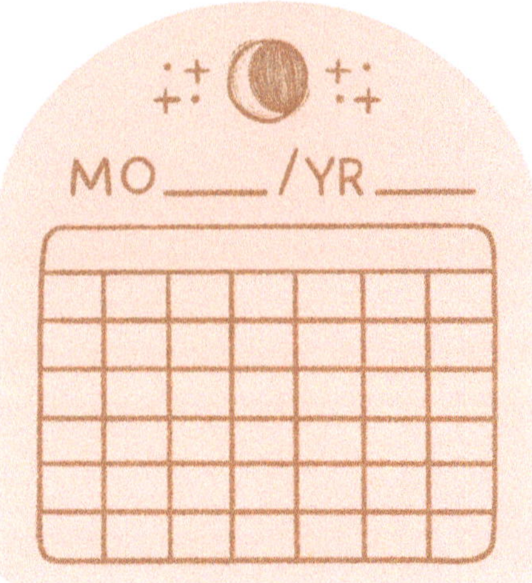
MO____/YR____

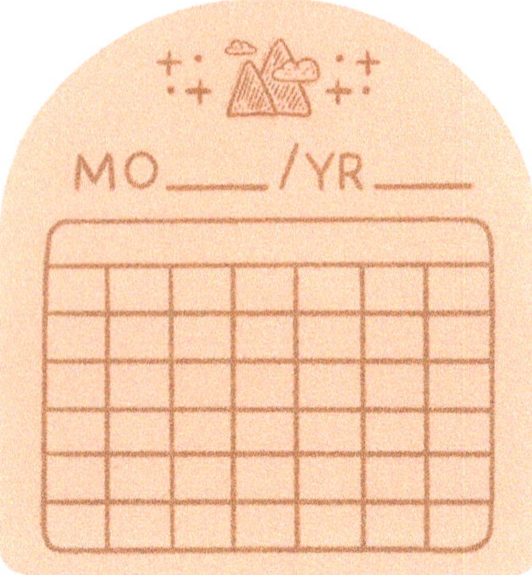
MO____/YR____

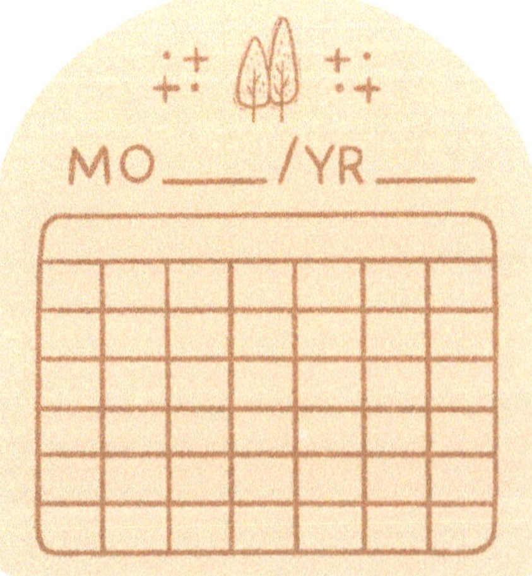
MO____/YR____

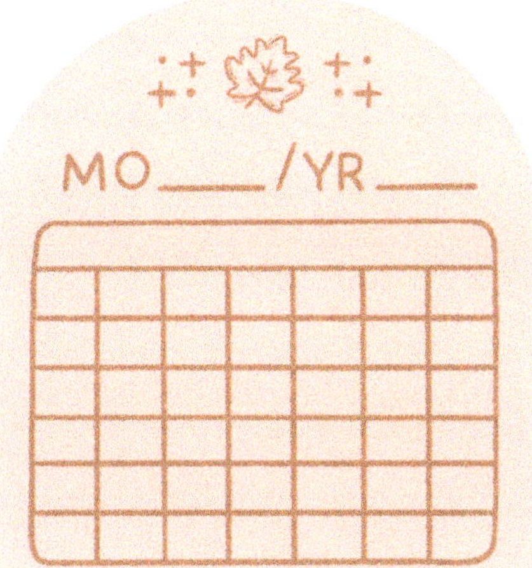

MO ____ /YR ____

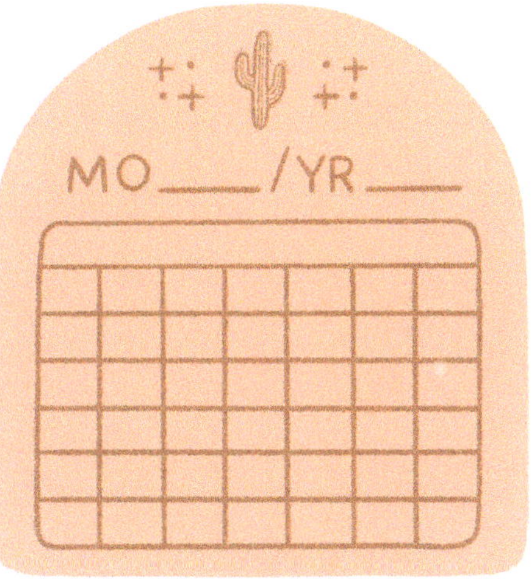

MO ____ /YR ____

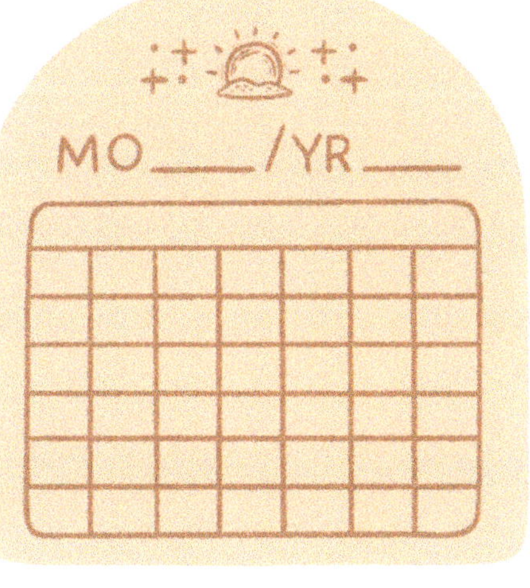

MO ____ /YR ____

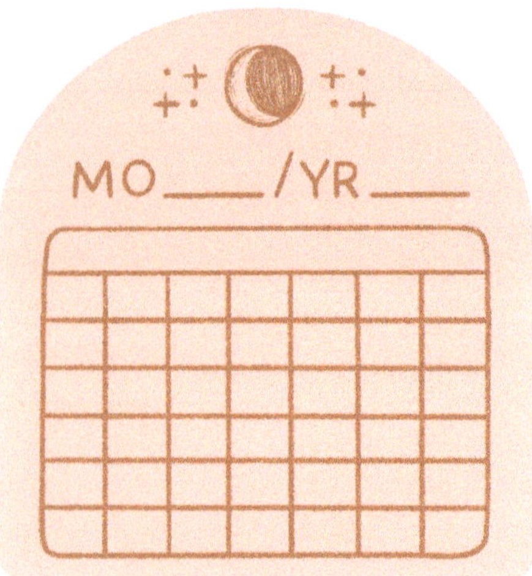

MO_____/YR_____

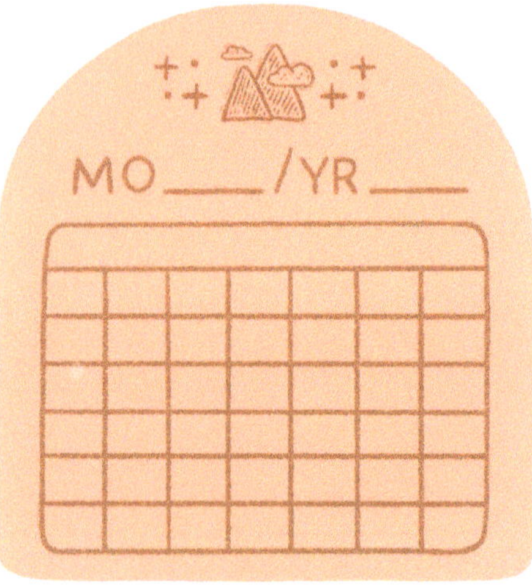

MO_____/YR_____

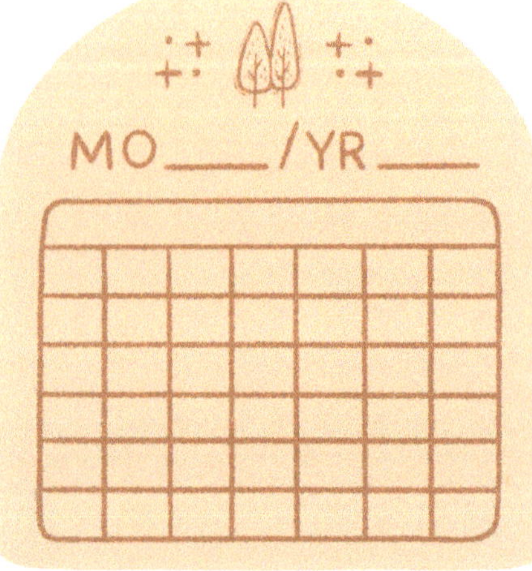

MO_____/YR_____

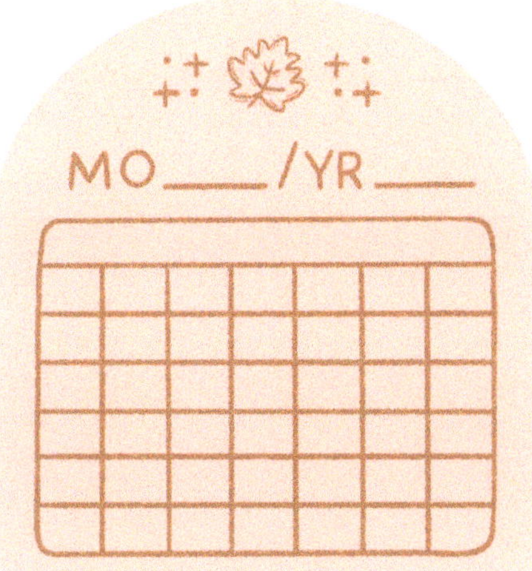

MO____/YR____

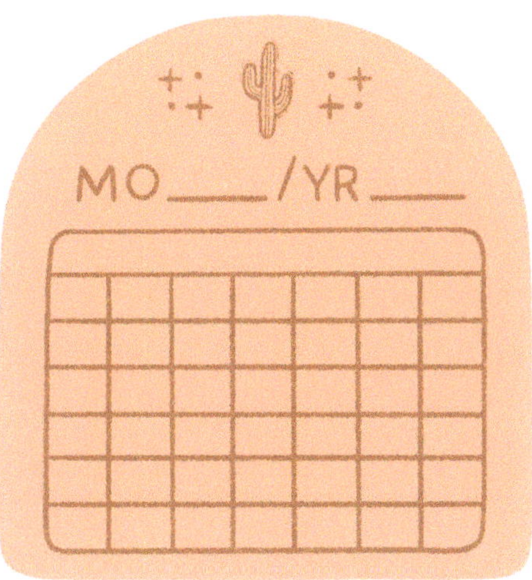

MO____/YR____

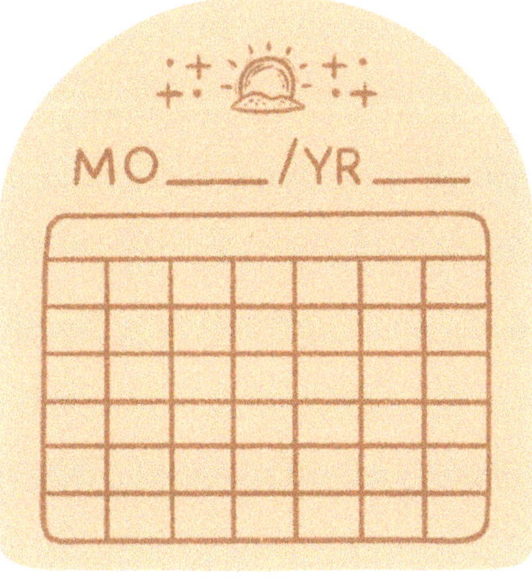

MO____/YR____

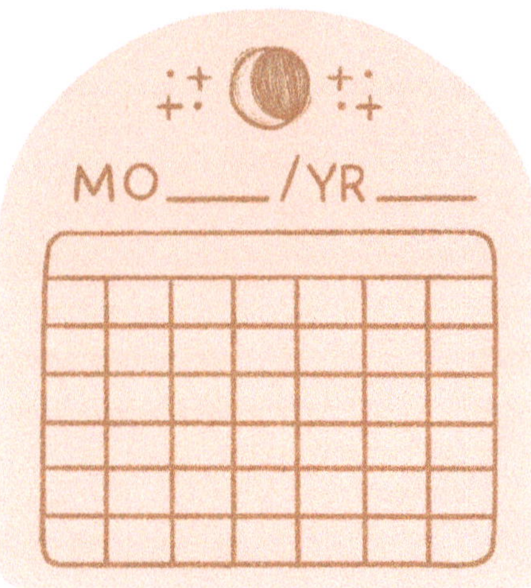

MO____/YR____

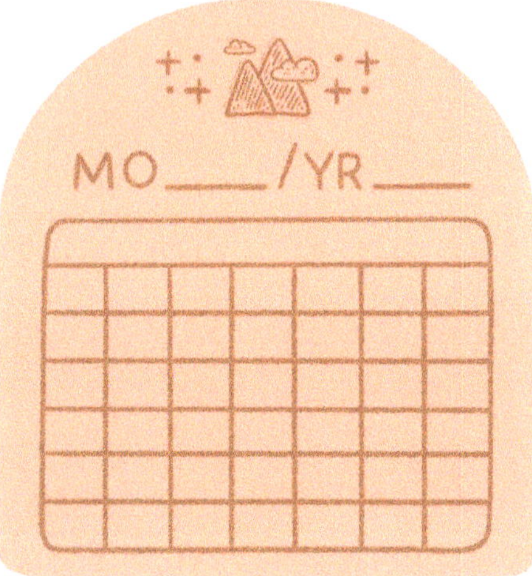

MO____/YR____

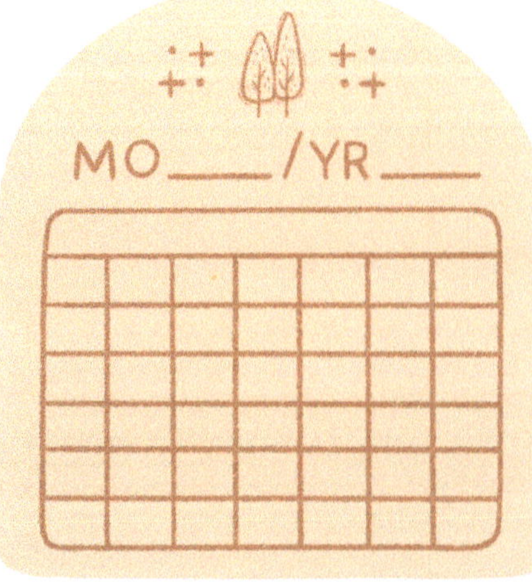

MO____/YR____

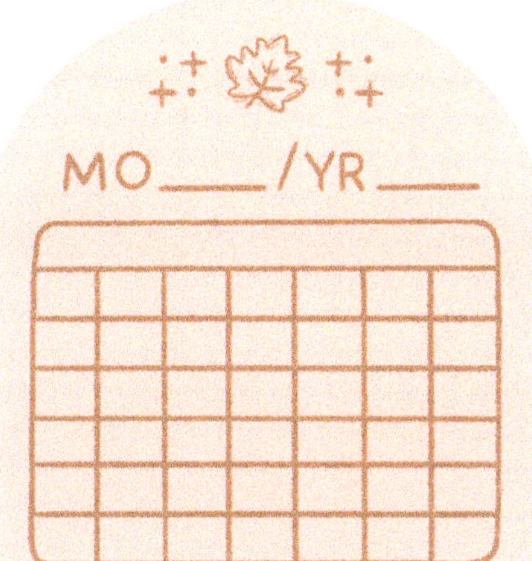

MO____/YR____

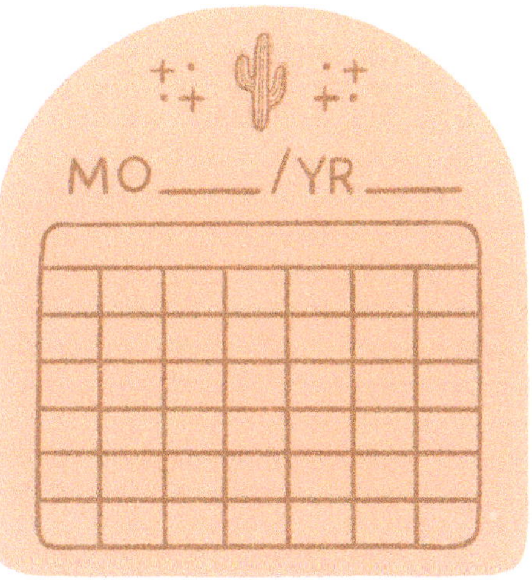

MO____/YR____

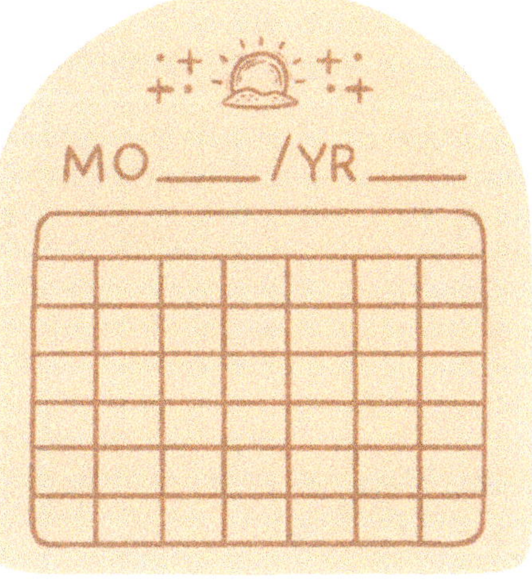

MO____/YR____

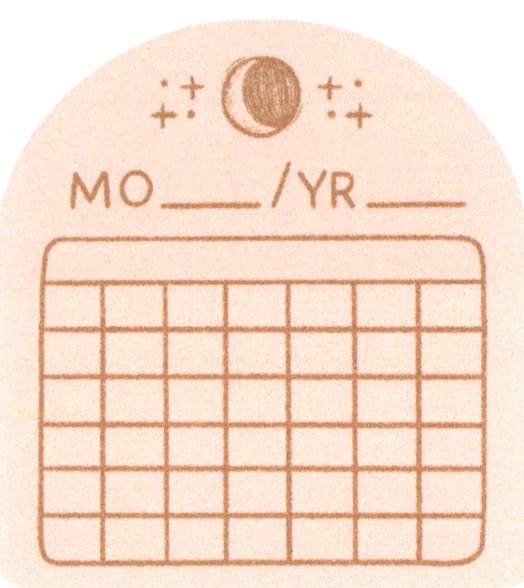
MO____/YR____

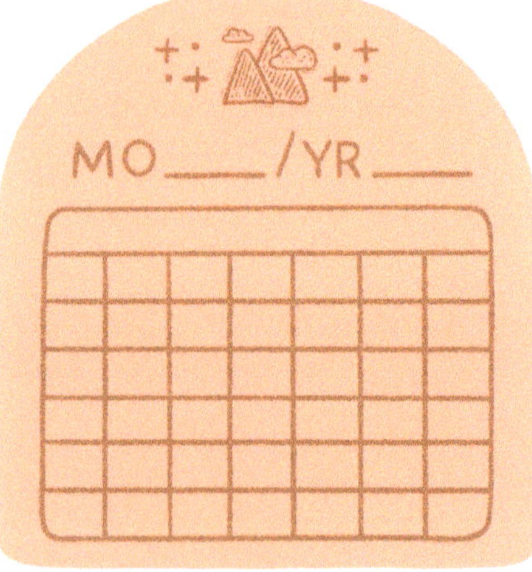
MO____/YR____

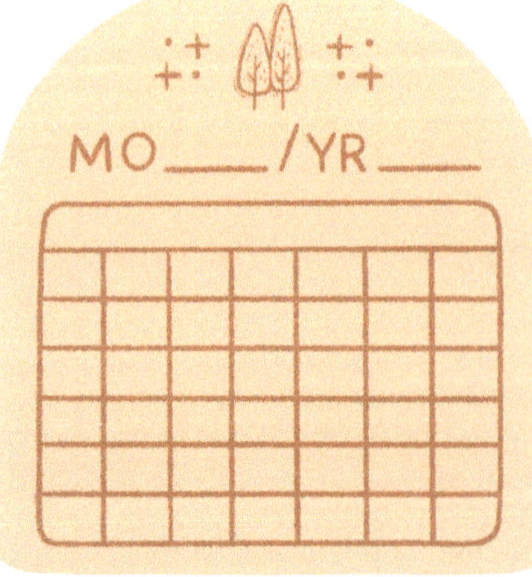
MO____/YR____

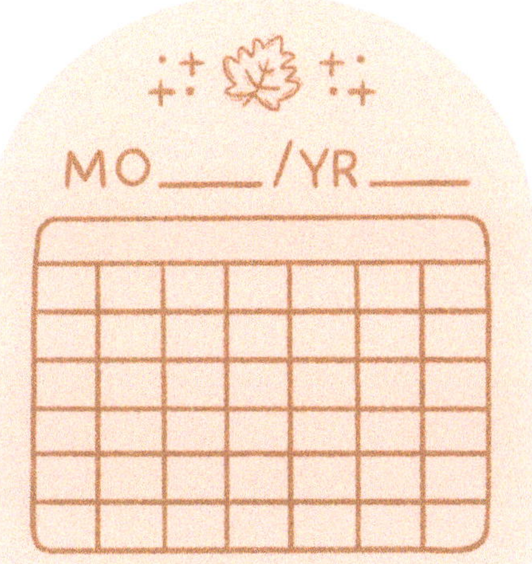
MO____/YR____

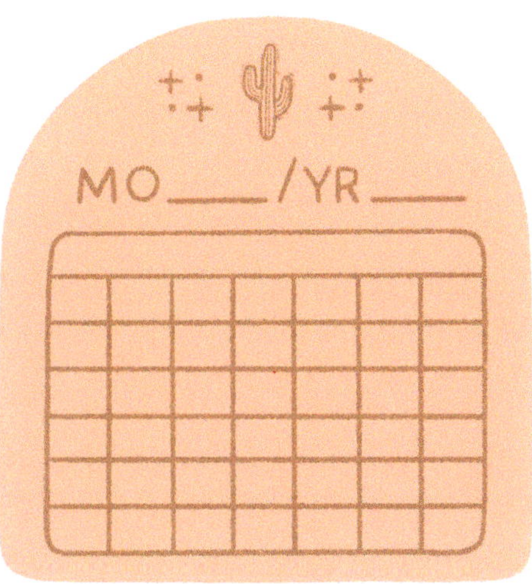
MO____/YR____

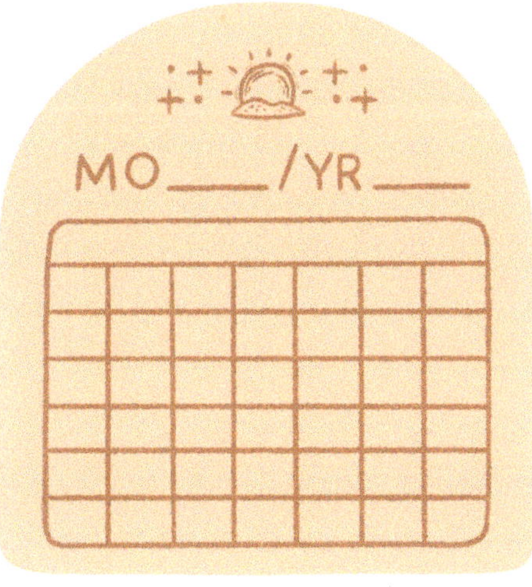
MO____/YR____

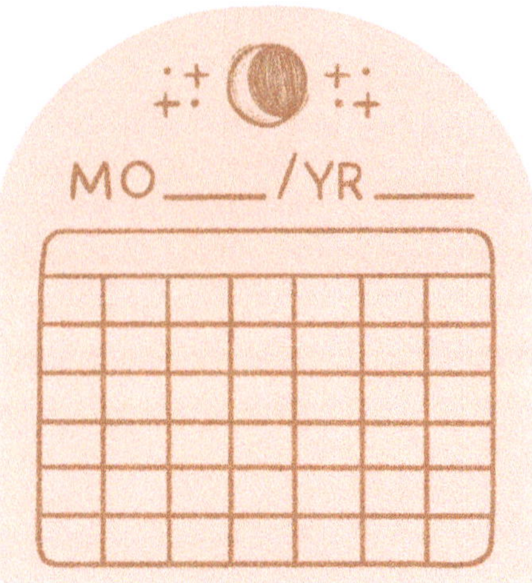

MO____/YR____

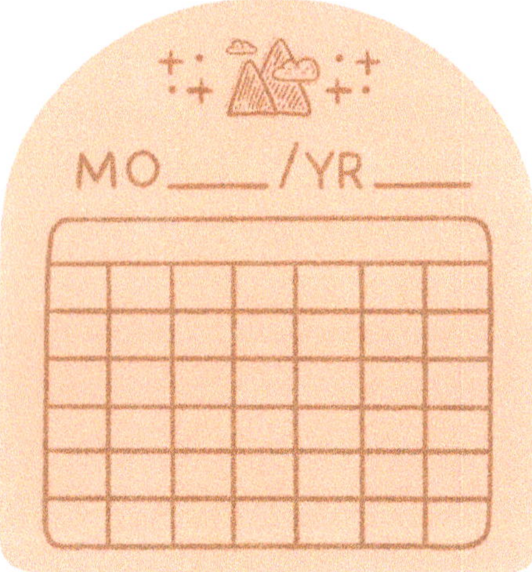

MO____/YR____

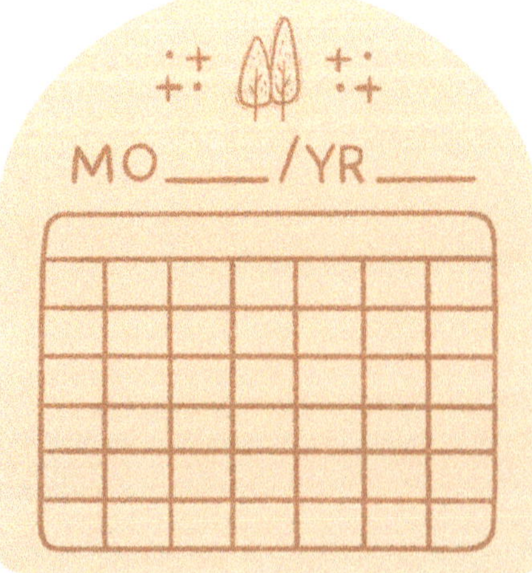

MO____/YR____

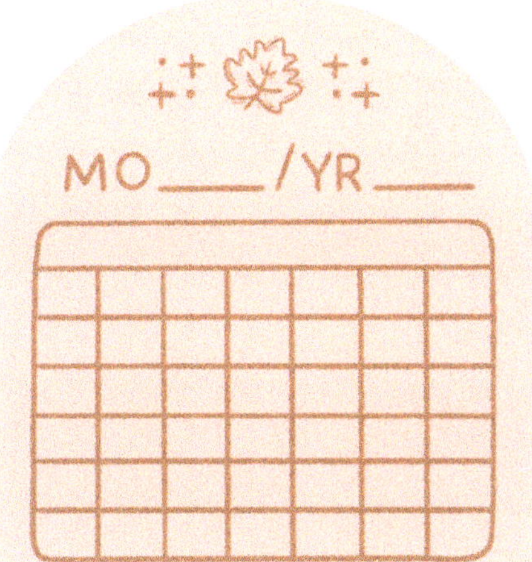

MO____/YR____

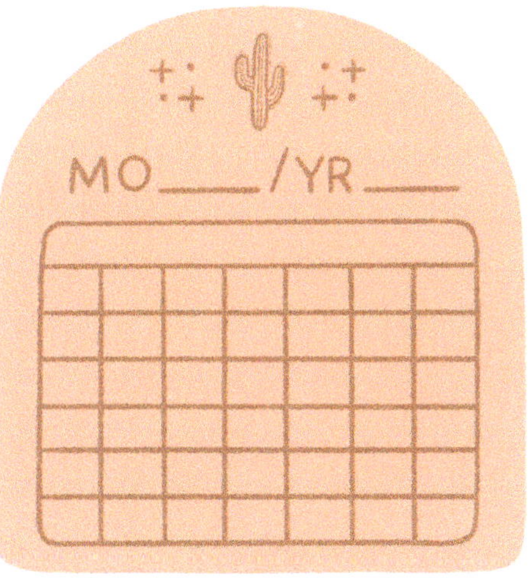

MO____/YR____

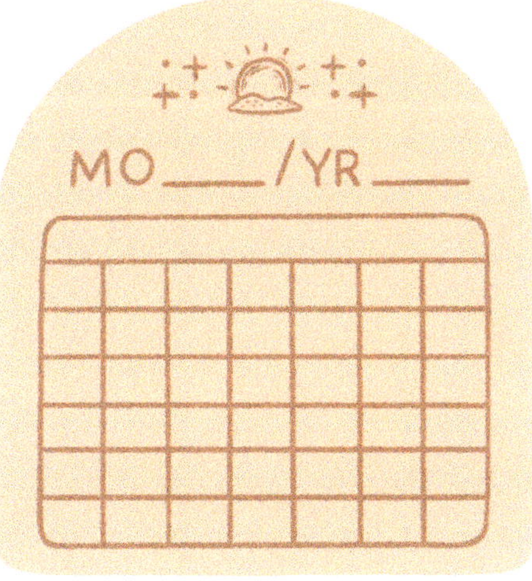

MO____/YR____

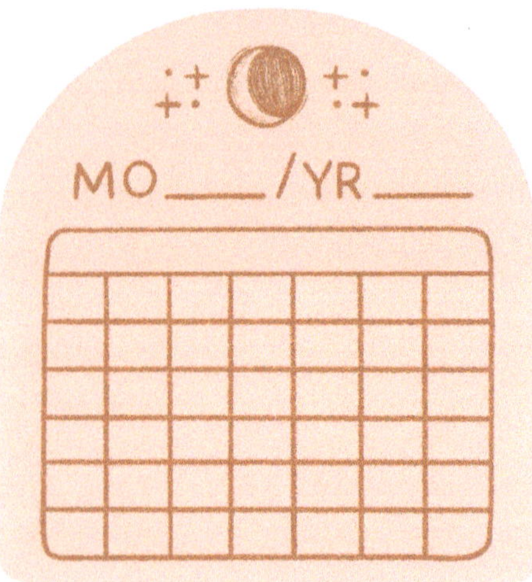
MO_____/YR_____

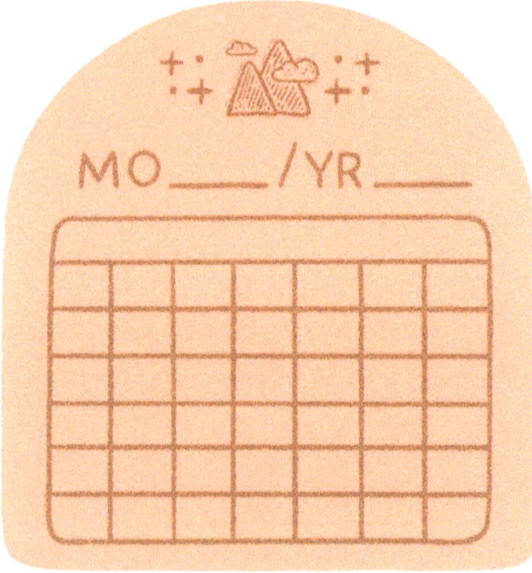
MO_____/YR_____

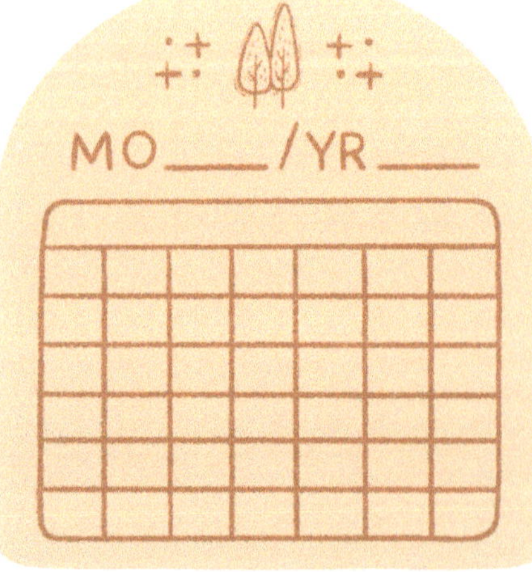
MO_____/YR_____

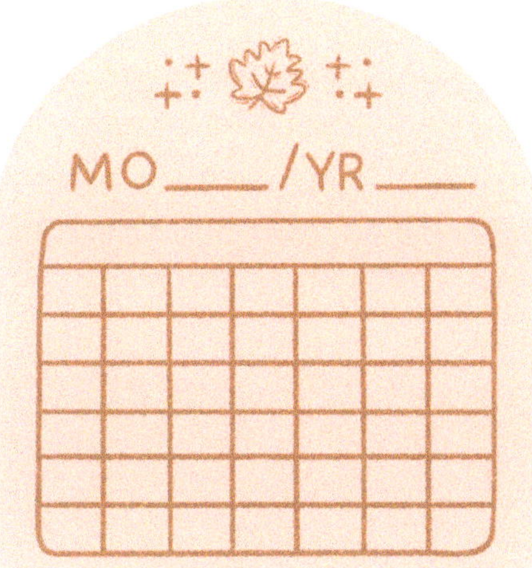

MO____/YR____

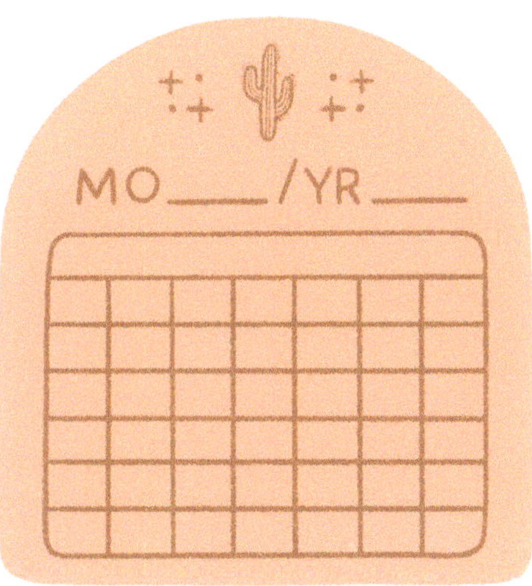

MO____/YR____

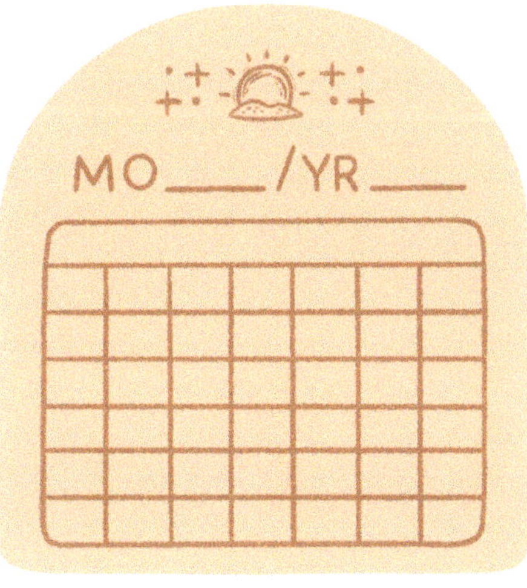

MO____/YR____

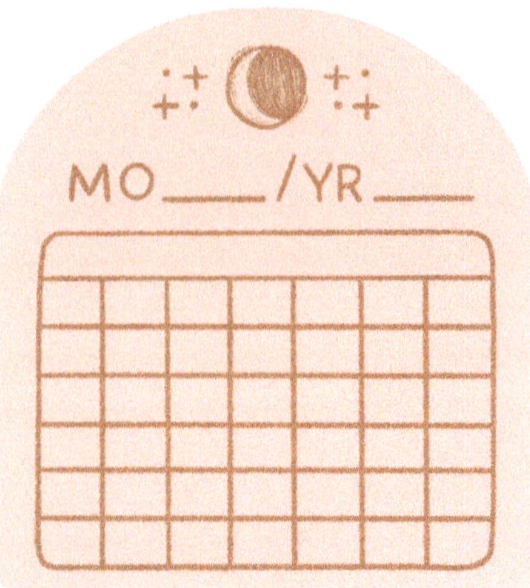
MO____ /YR____

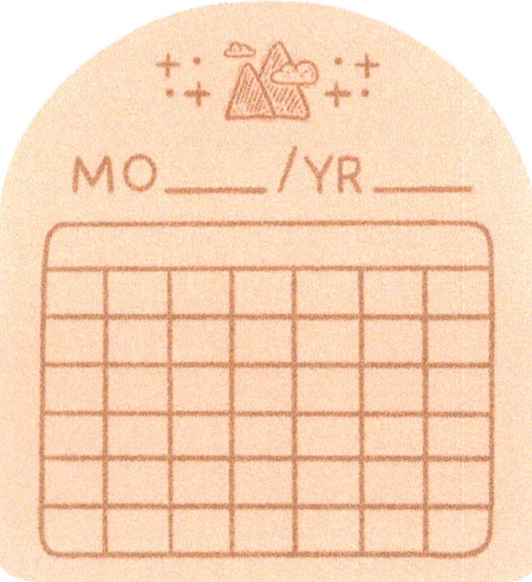
MO____ /YR____

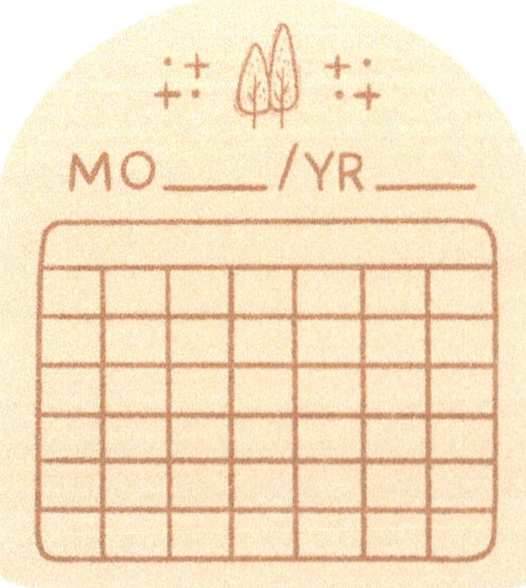
MO____ /YR____

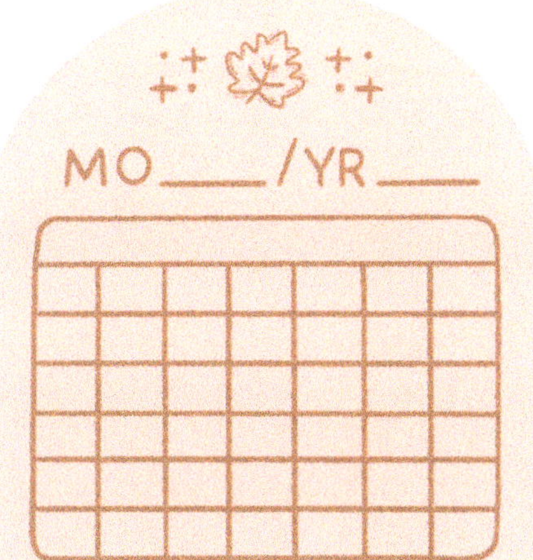

MO____/YR____

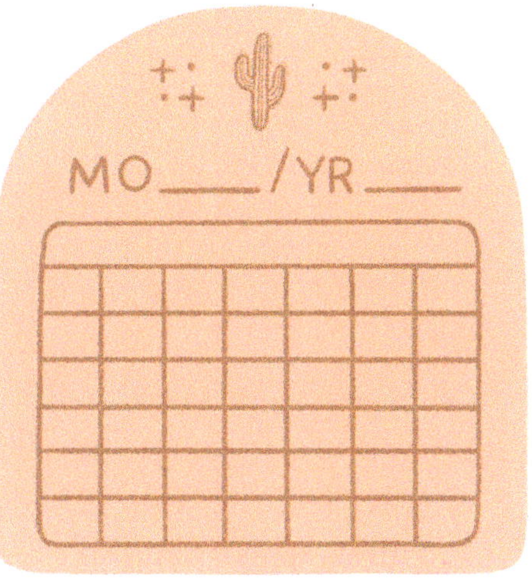

MO____/YR____

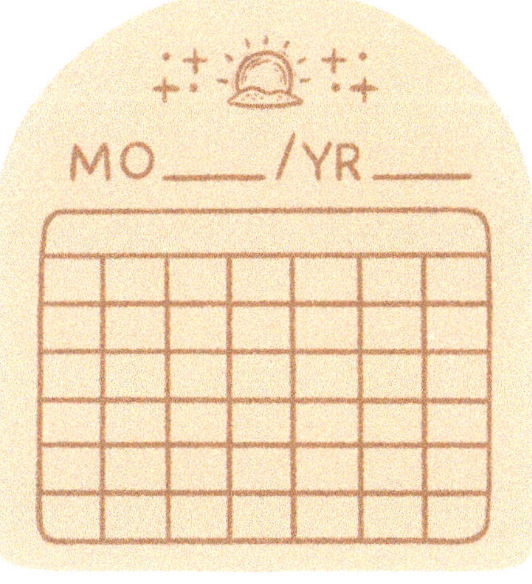

MO____/YR____

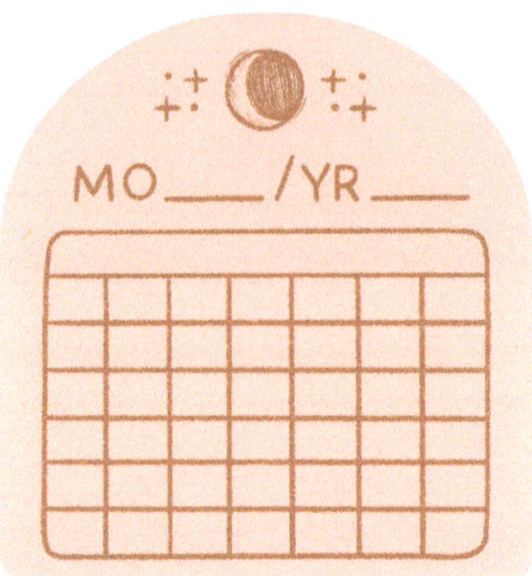
MO____/YR____
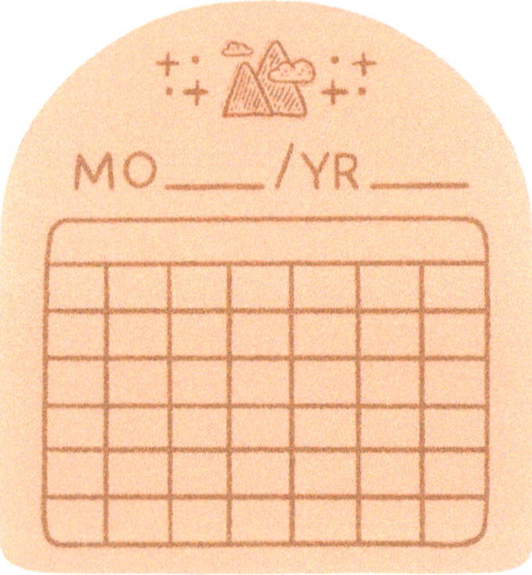
MO____/YR____
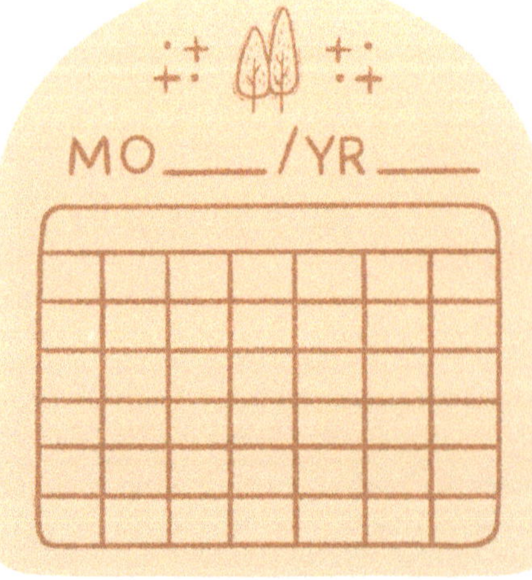
MO____/YR____

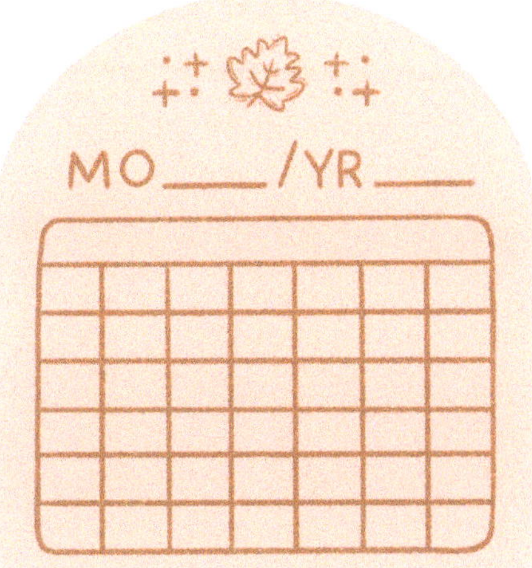

MO____/YR____

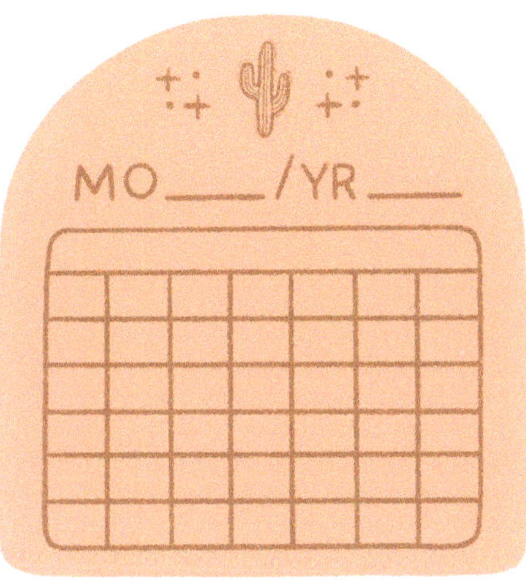

MO____/YR____

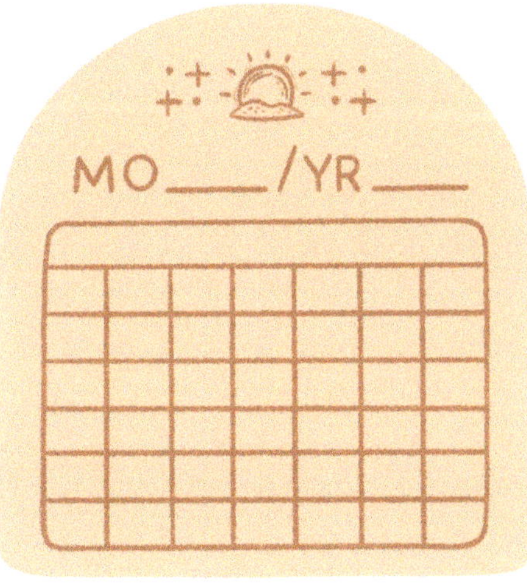

MO____/YR____

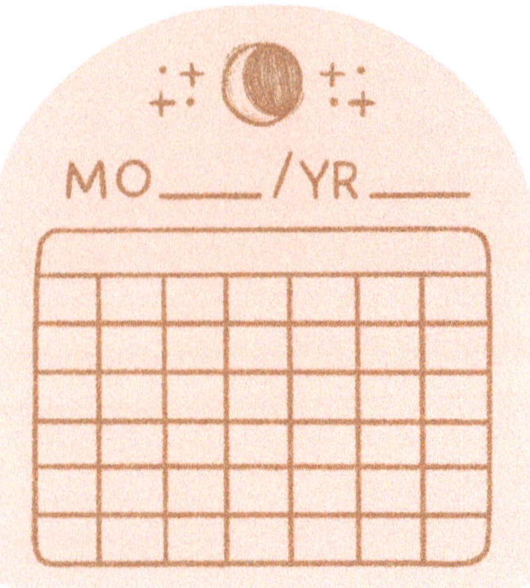
MO____/YR____

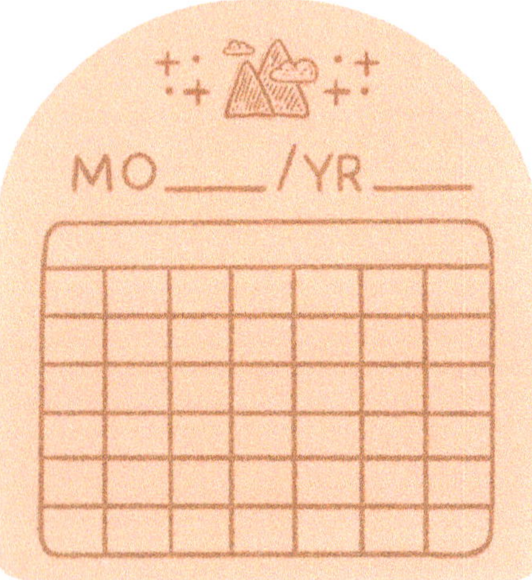
MO____/YR____

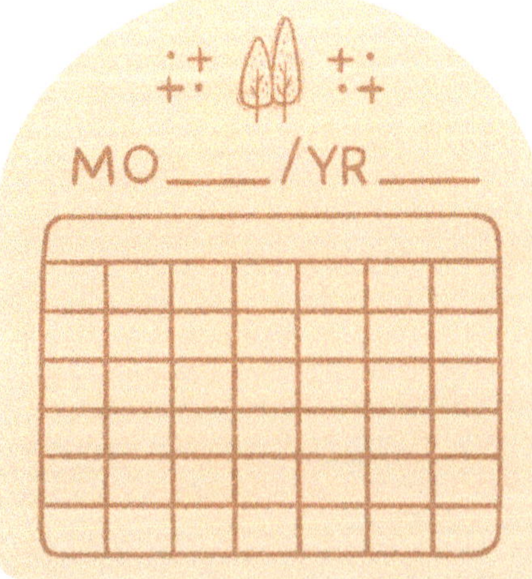
MO____/YR____

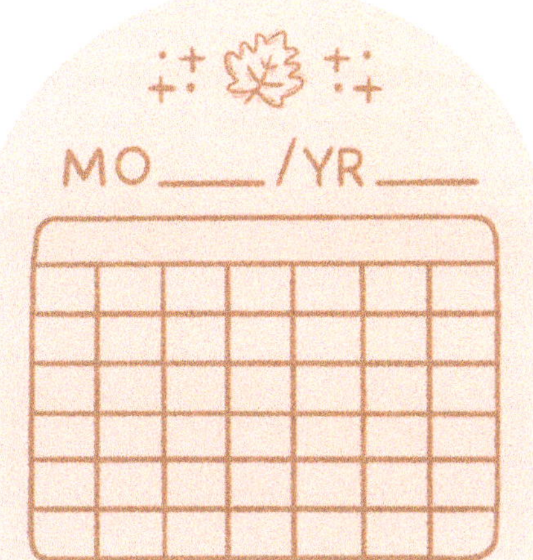
MO____/YR____

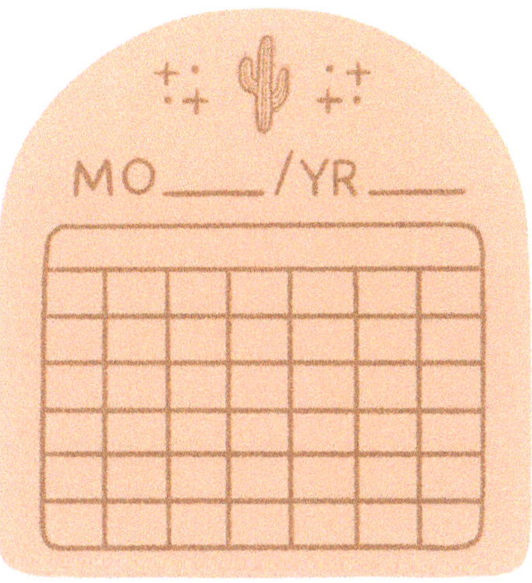
MO____/YR____

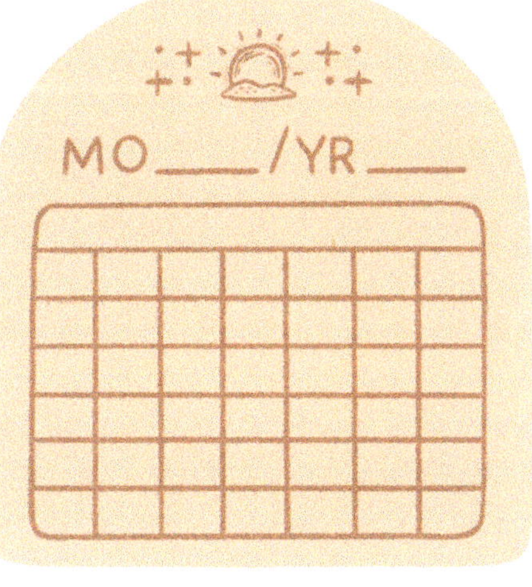
MO____/YR____

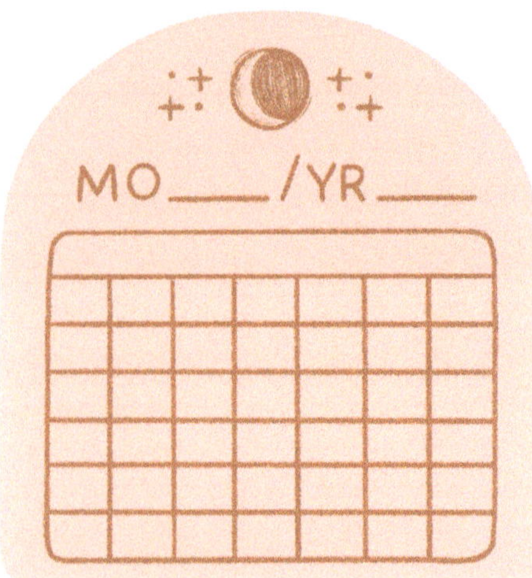

MO____/YR____

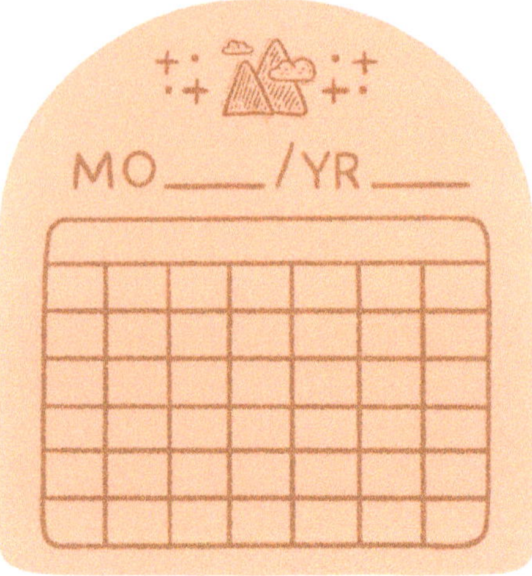

MO____/YR____

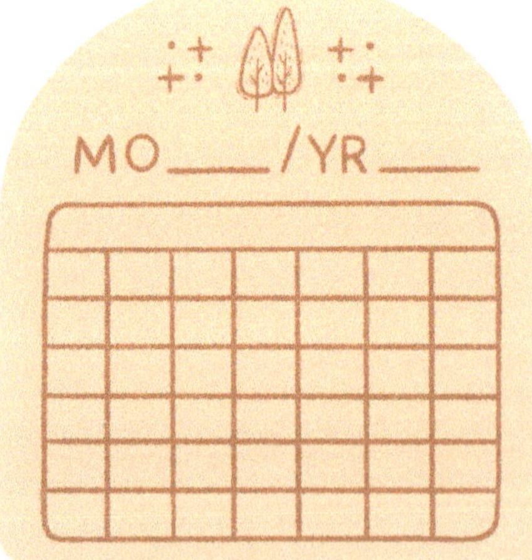

MO____/YR____

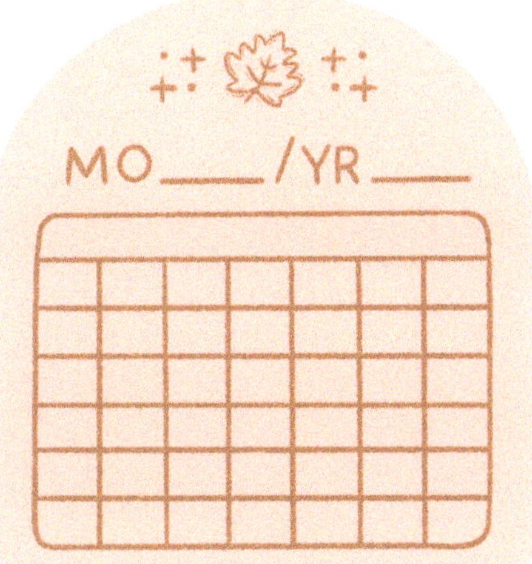
MO____/YR____

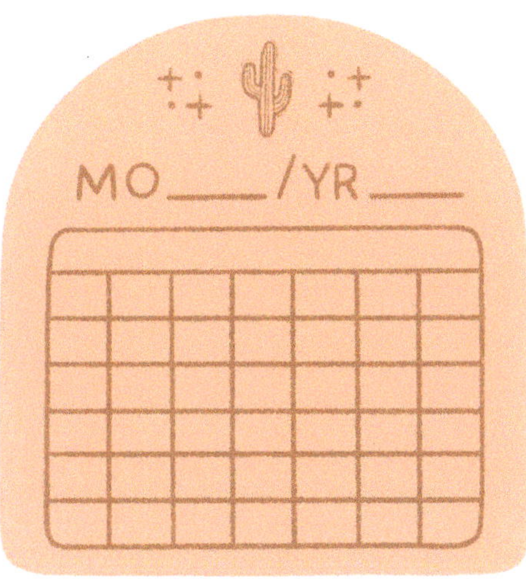
MO____/YR____

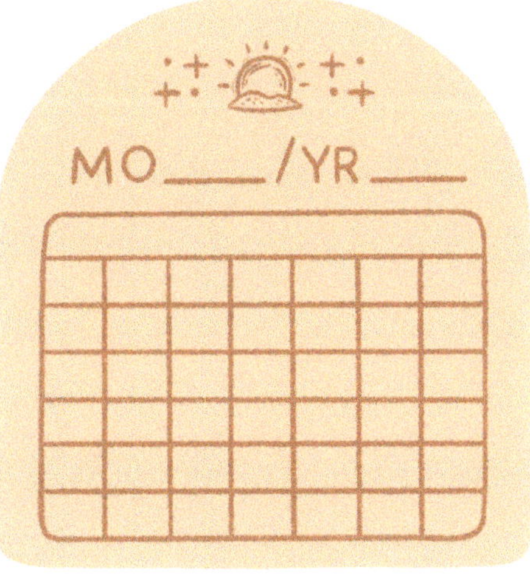
MO____/YR____

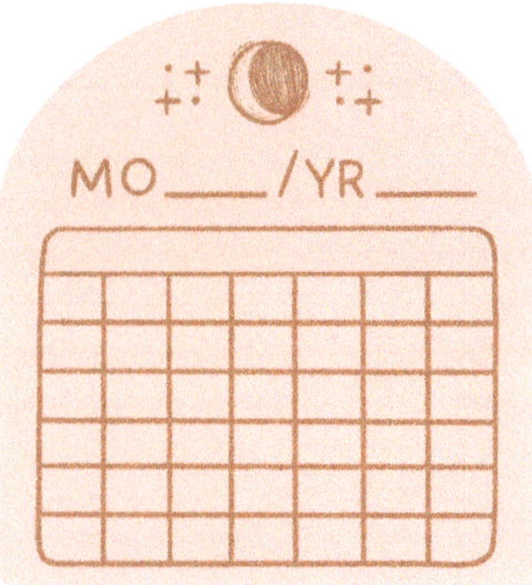
MO____/YR____

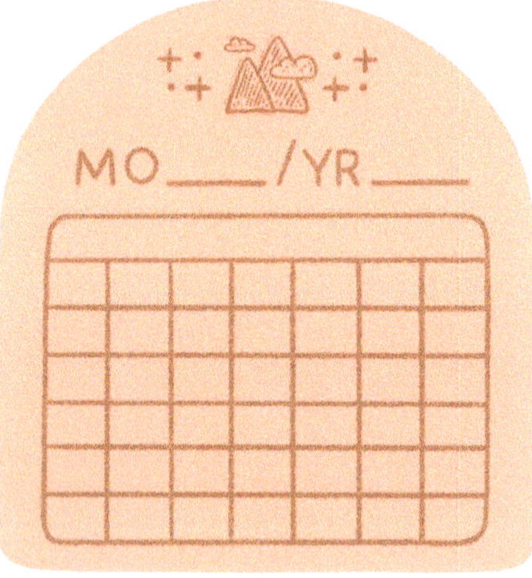
MO____/YR____

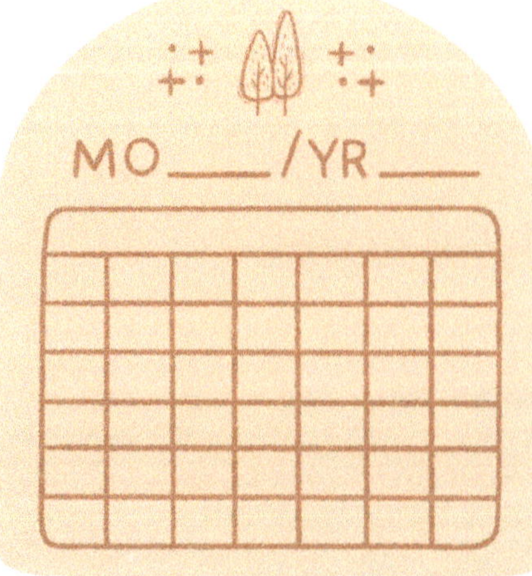
MO____/YR____

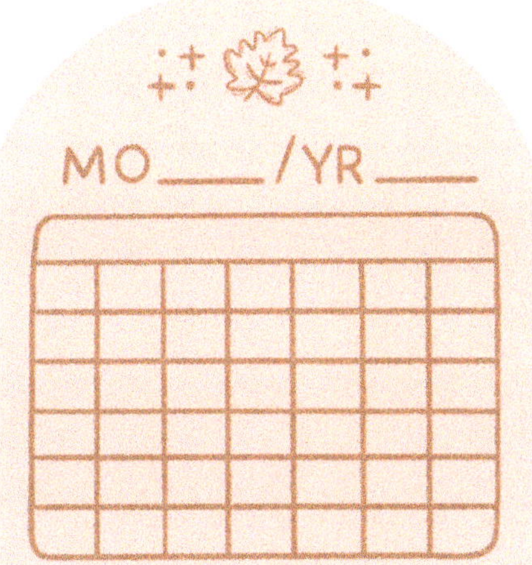

MO____/YR____

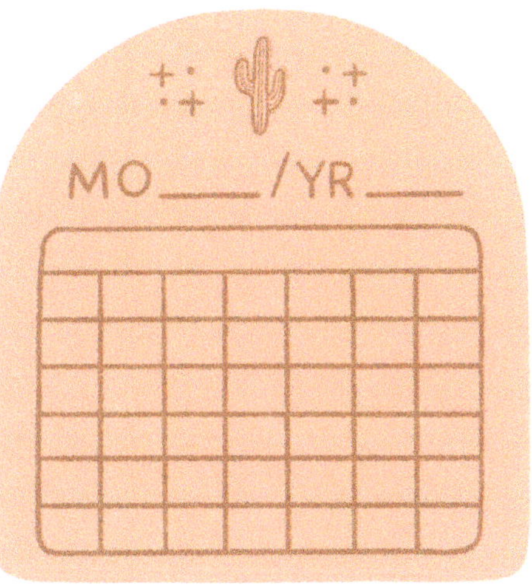

MO____/YR____

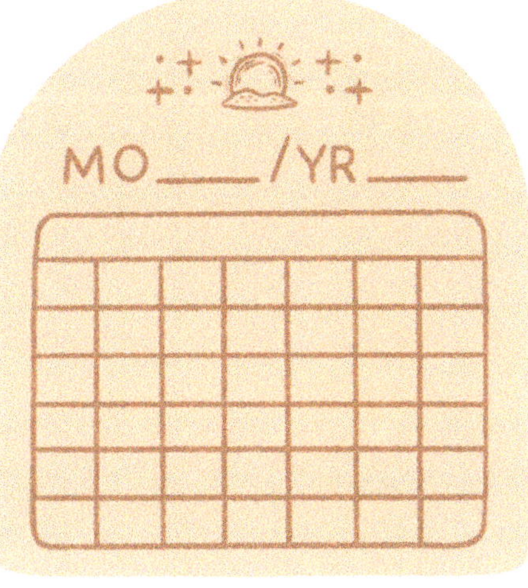

MO____/YR____

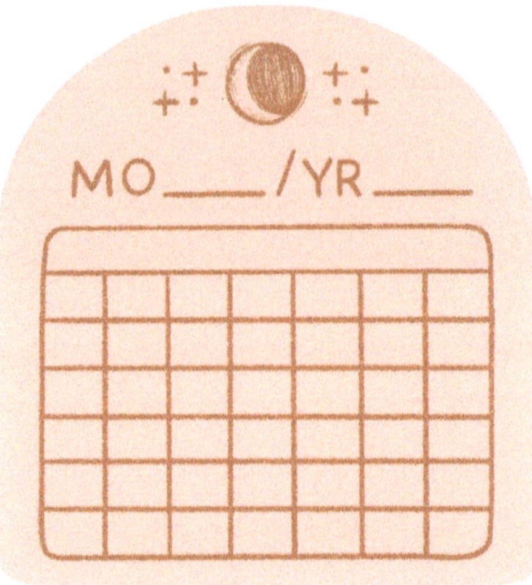

MO____/YR____

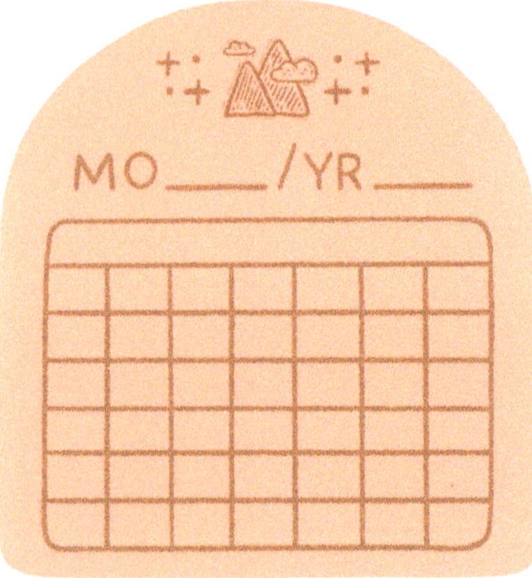

MO____/YR____

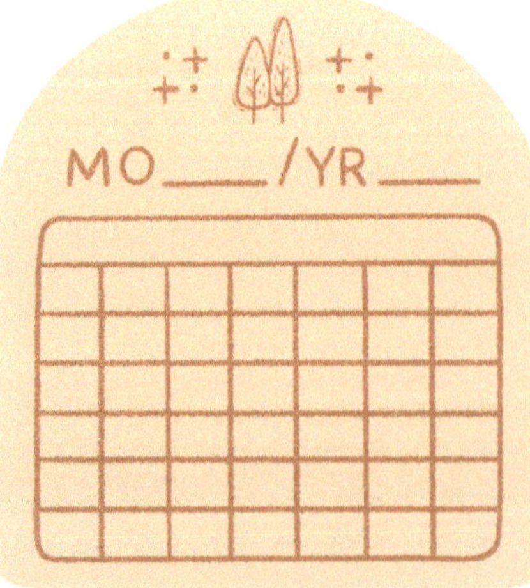

MO____/YR____

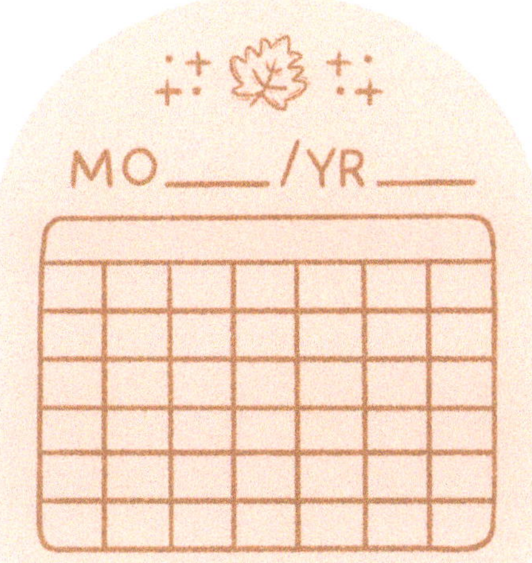

MO____/YR____

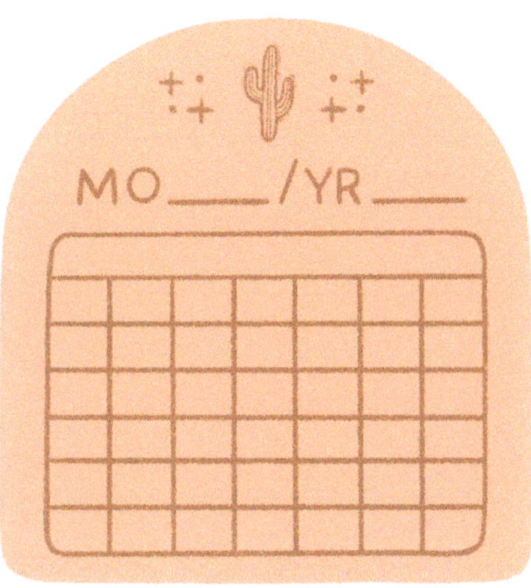

MO____/YR____

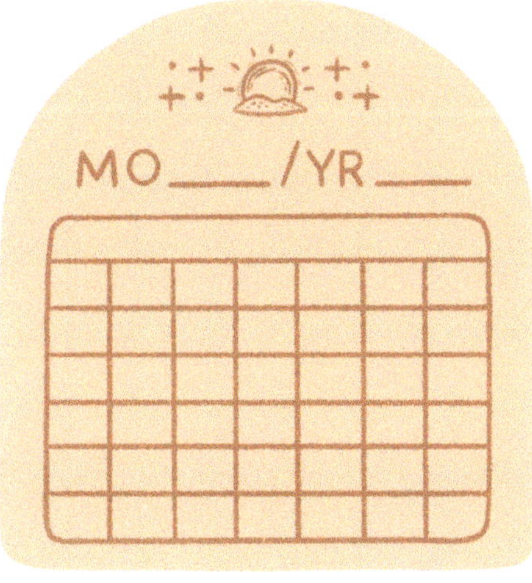

MO____/YR____

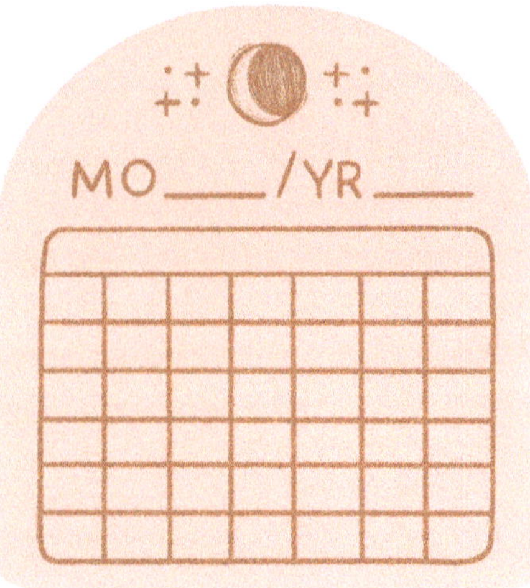

MO____/YR____

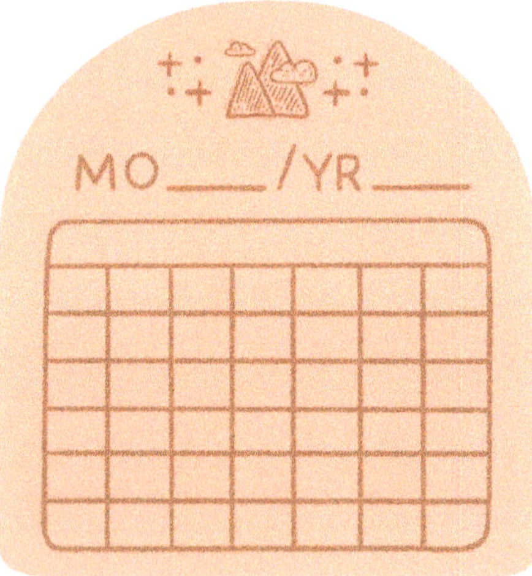

MO____/YR____

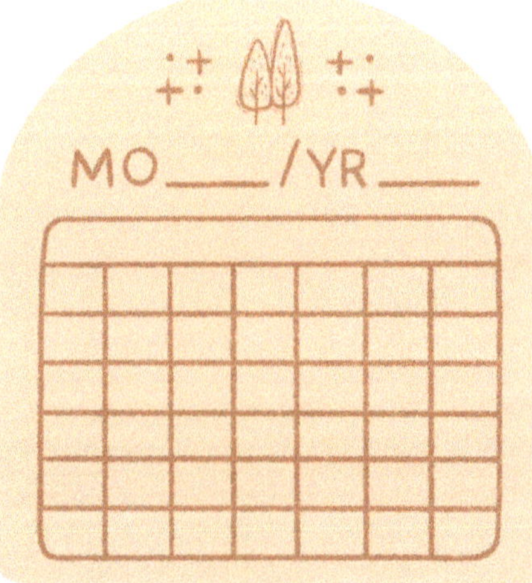

MO____/YR____

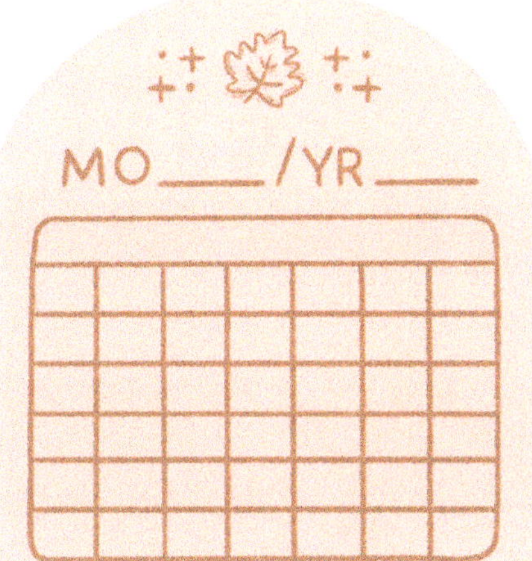

MO____/YR____

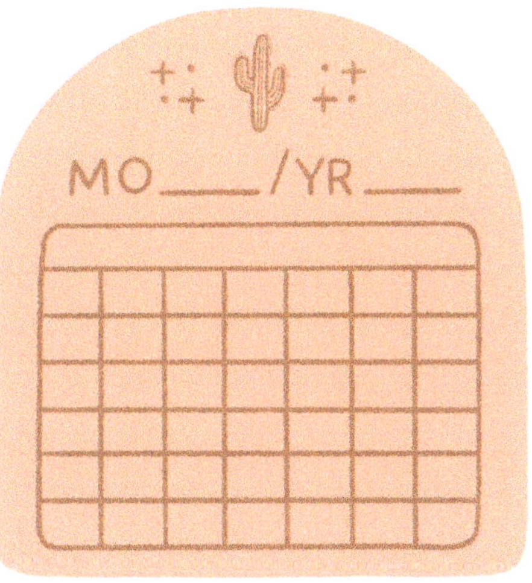

MO____/YR____

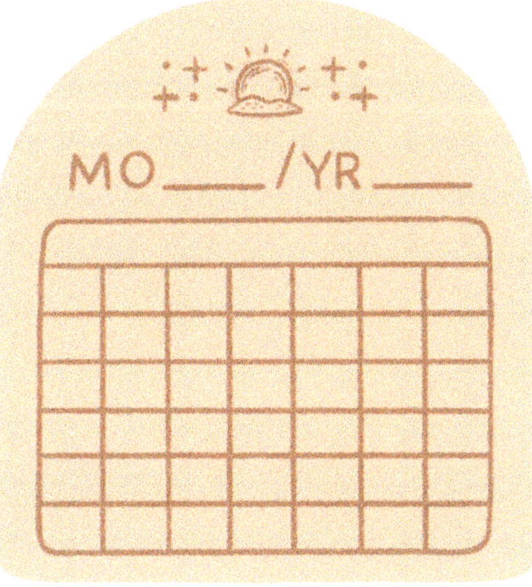

MO____/YR____

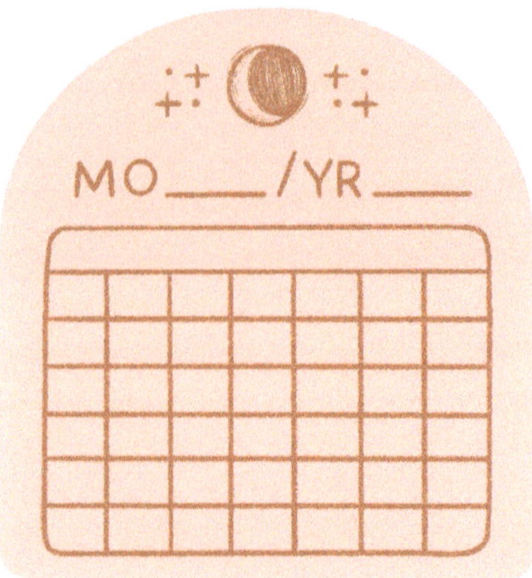
MO____ /YR____

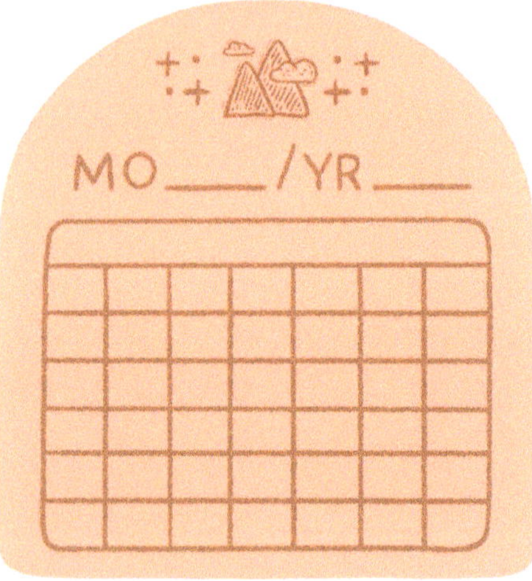
MO____ /YR____

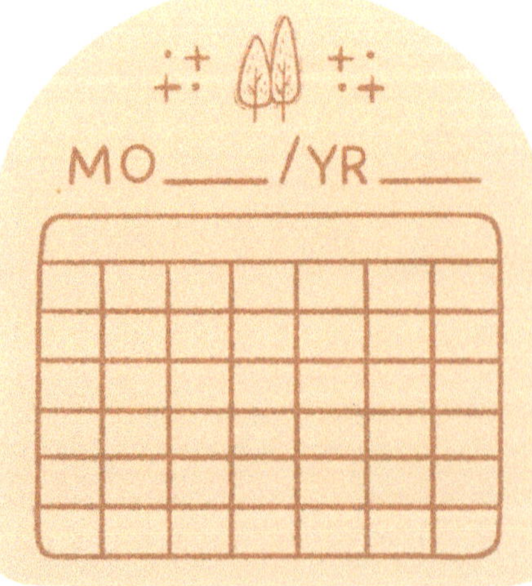
MO____ /YR____

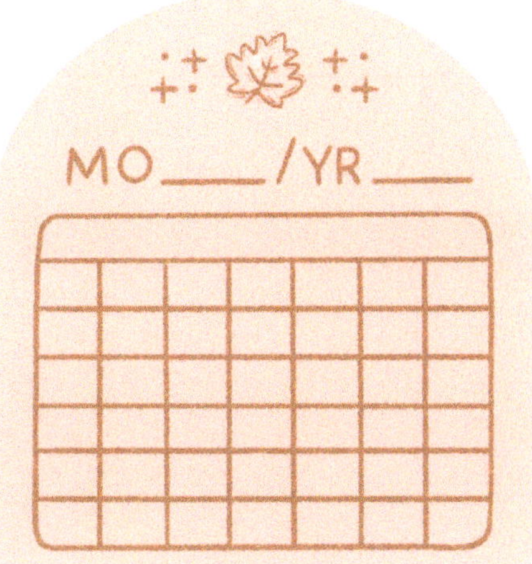

MO_____/YR_____

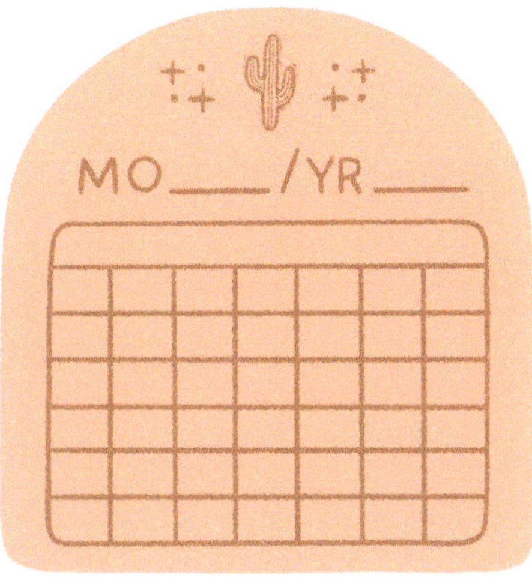

MO_____/YR_____

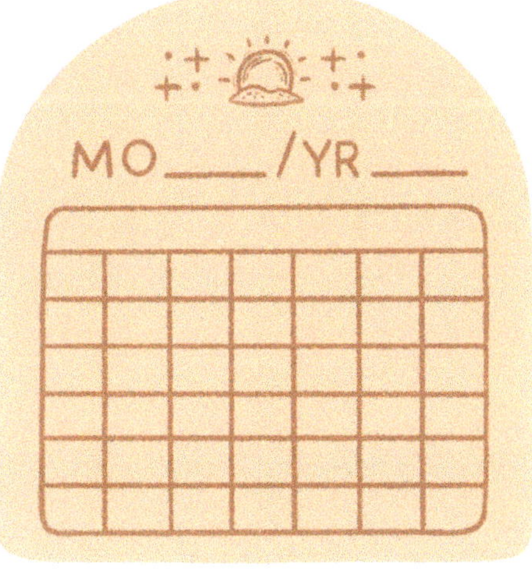

MO_____/YR_____

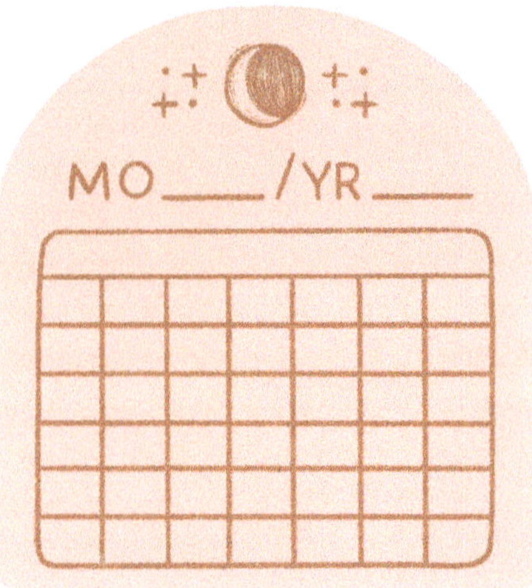
MO____/YR____

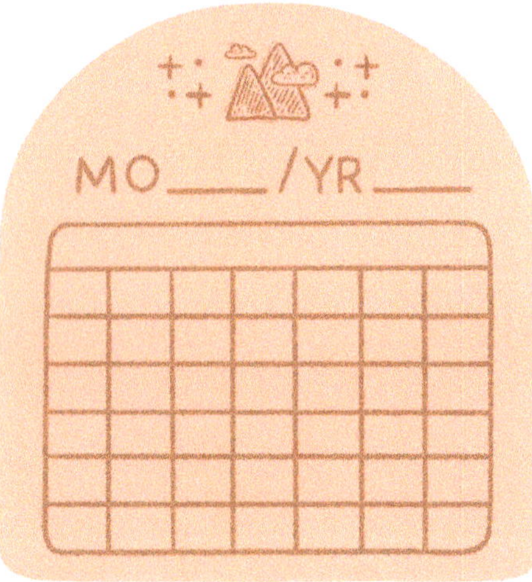
MO____/YR____

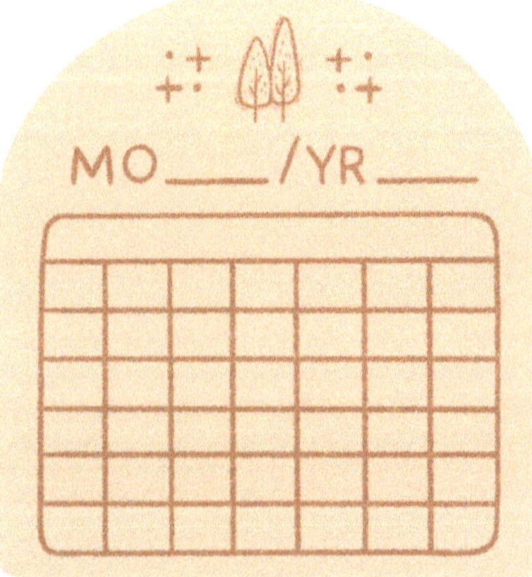
MO____/YR____

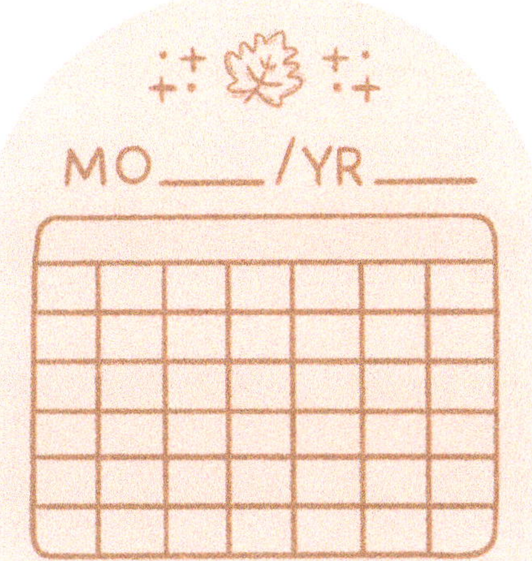

MO____/YR____

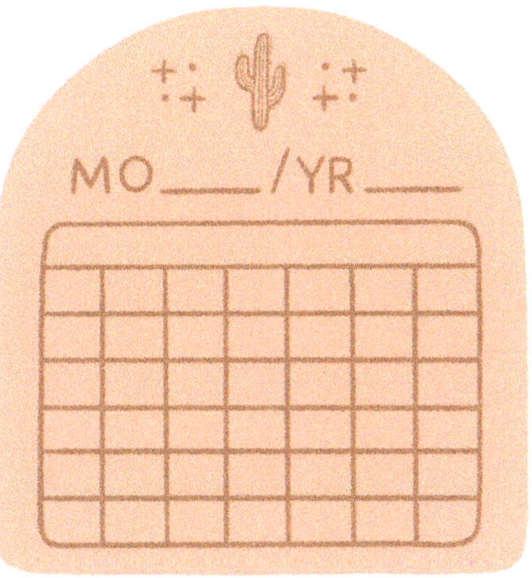

MO____/YR____

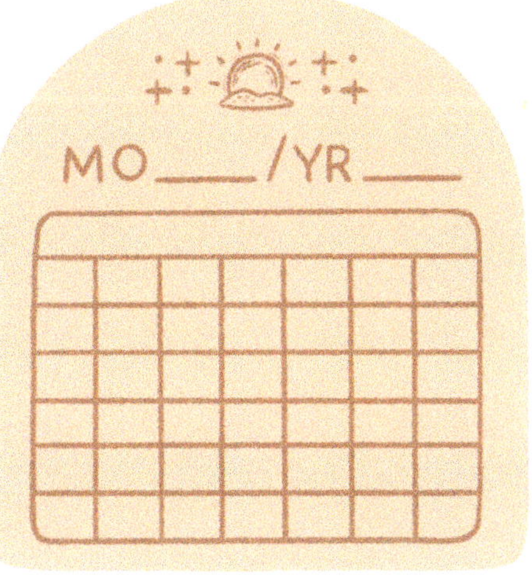

MO____/YR____

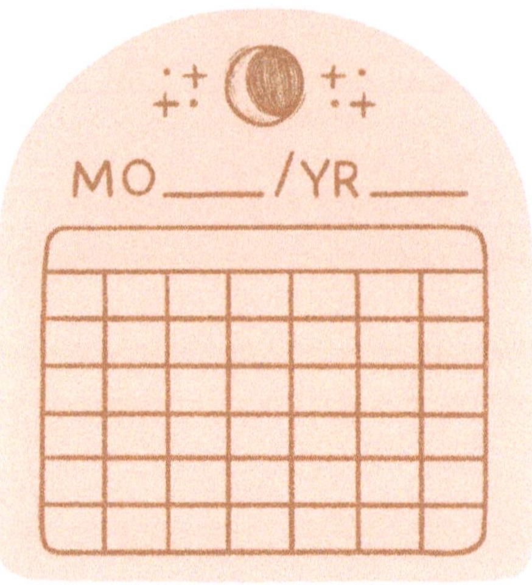
MO____/YR____

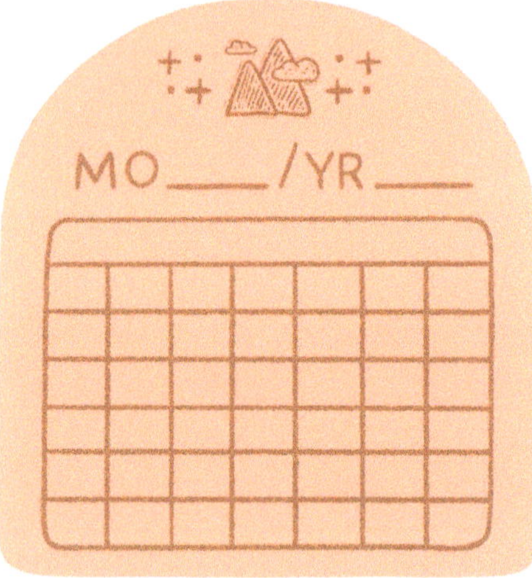
MO____/YR____

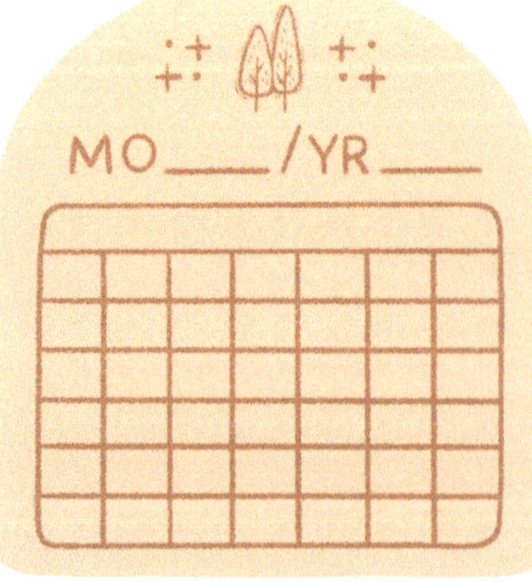
MO____/YR____

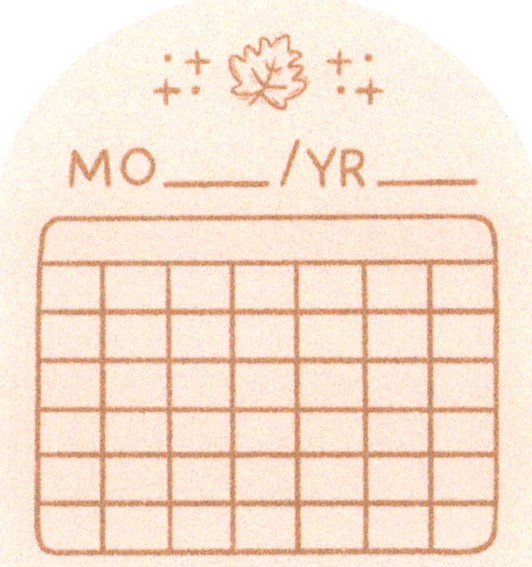

MO____/YR____

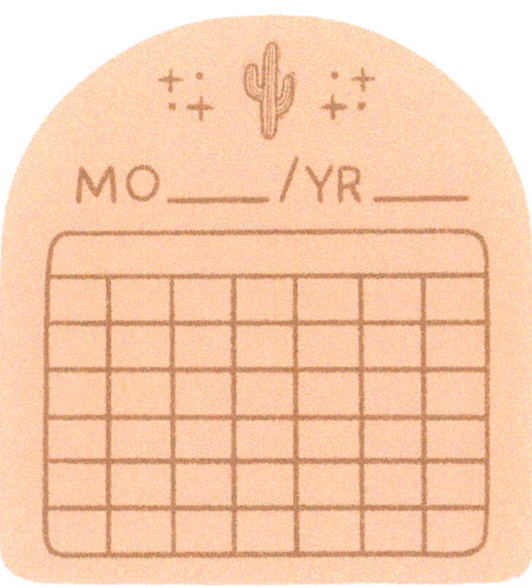

MO____/YR____

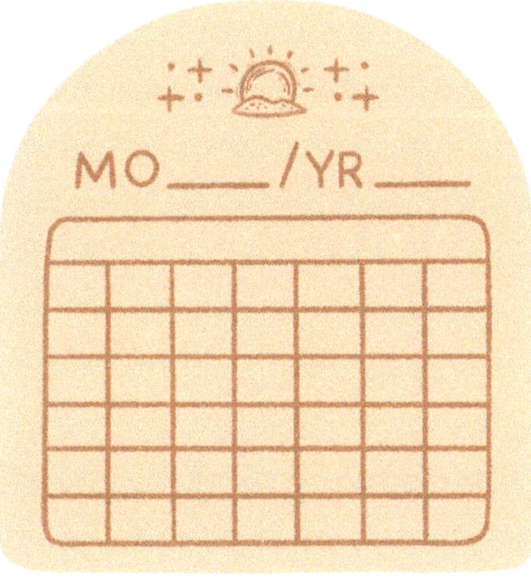

MO____/YR____

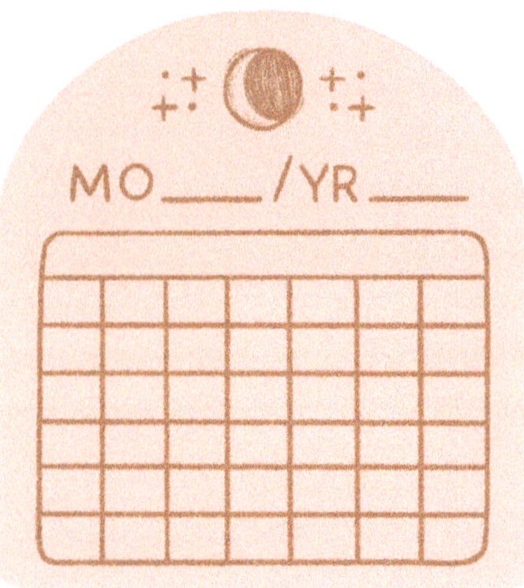

MO____/YR____

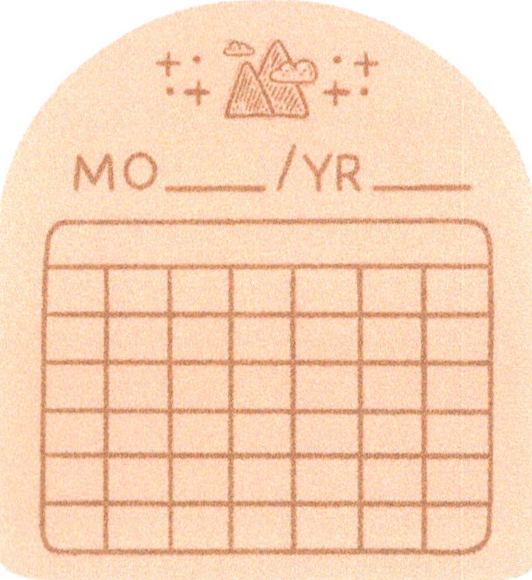

MO____/YR____

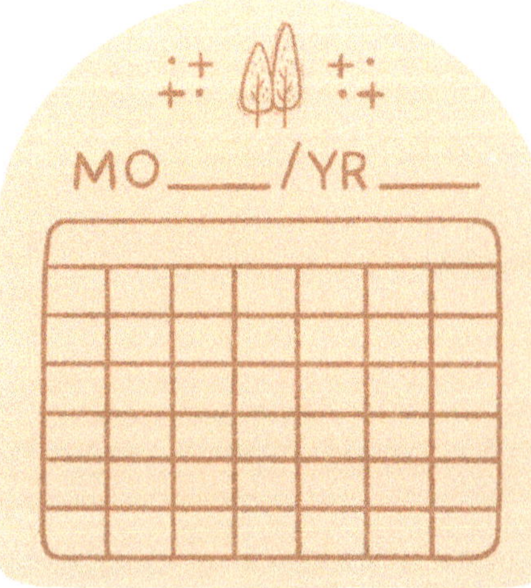

MO____/YR____

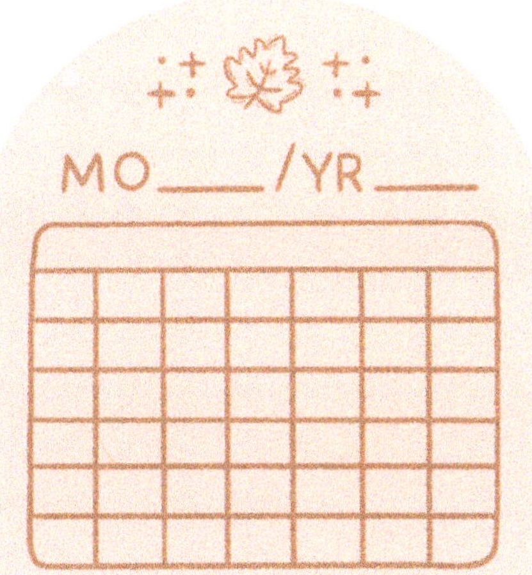
MO____/YR____

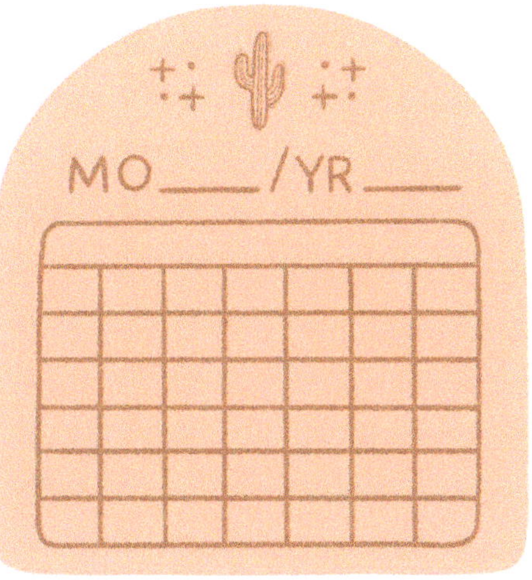
MO____/YR____

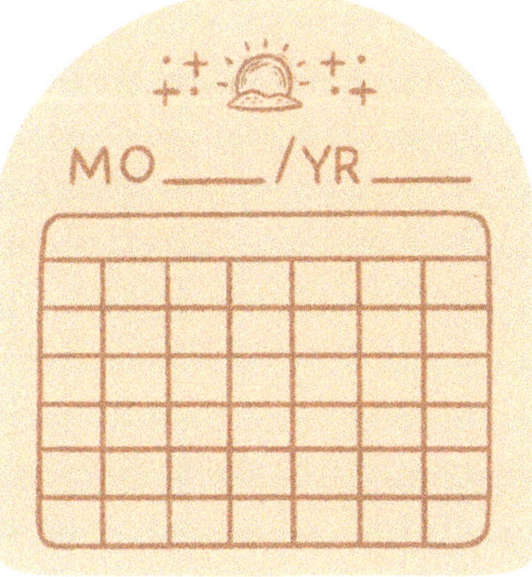
MO____/YR____

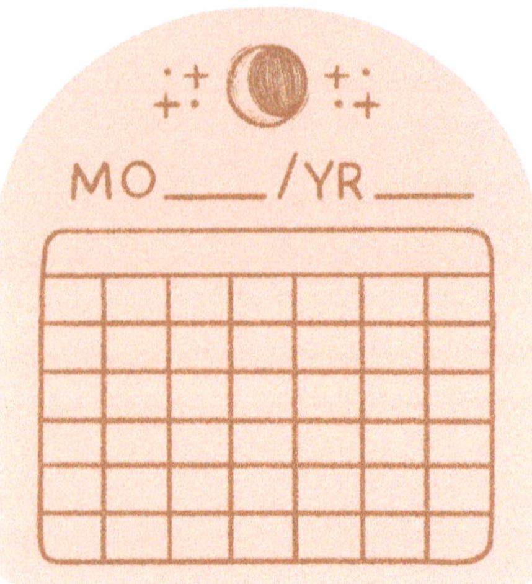
MO____/YR____

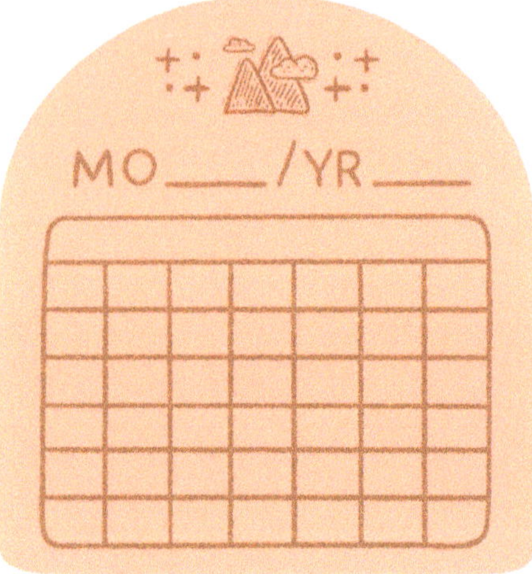
MO____/YR____

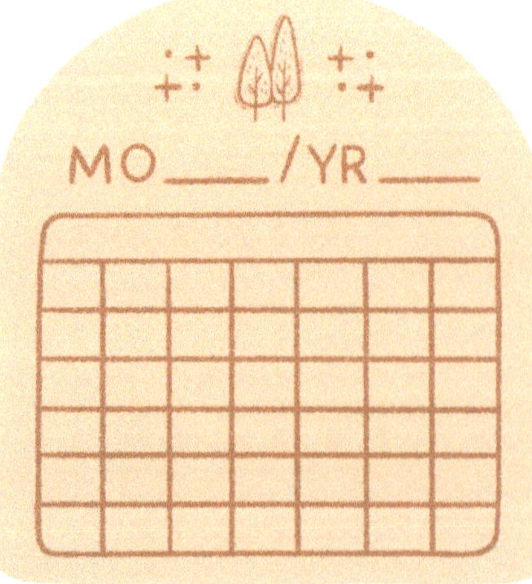
MO____/YR____

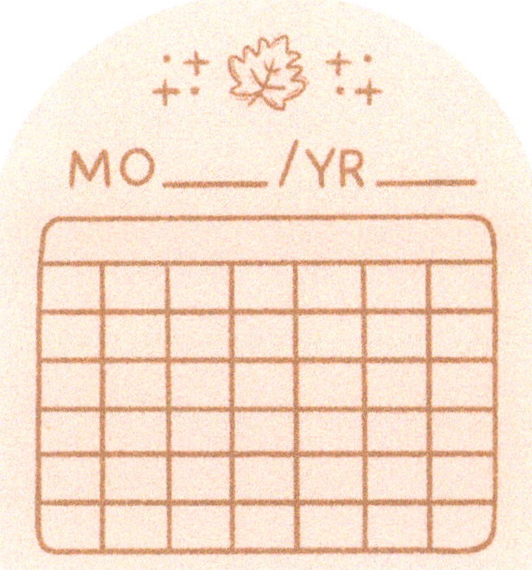
MO____/YR____

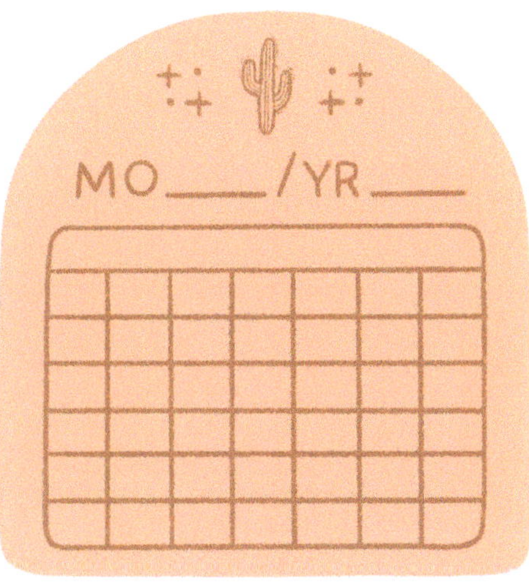
MO____/YR____

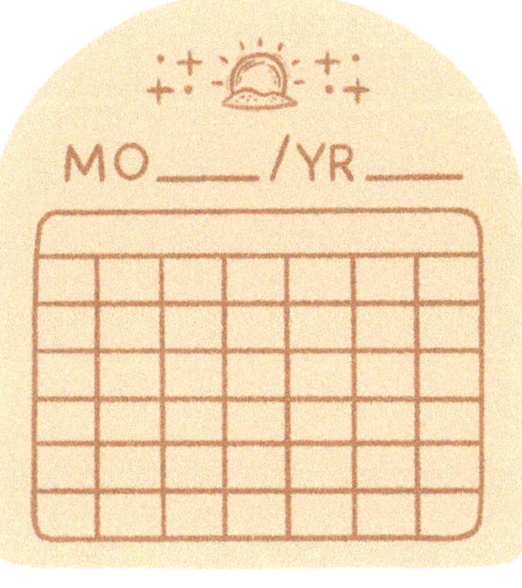
MO____/YR____

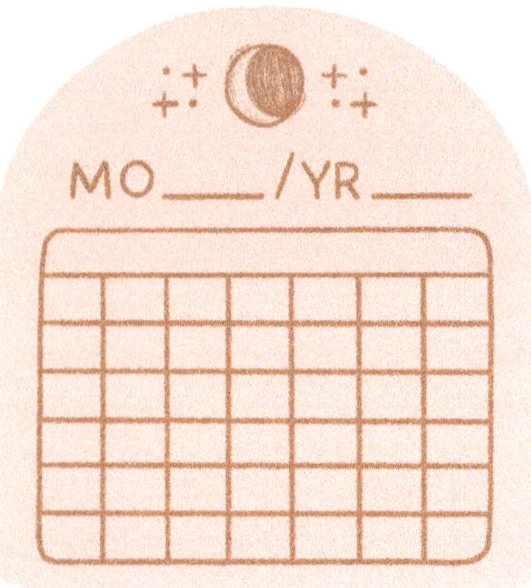
MO ____ /YR ____

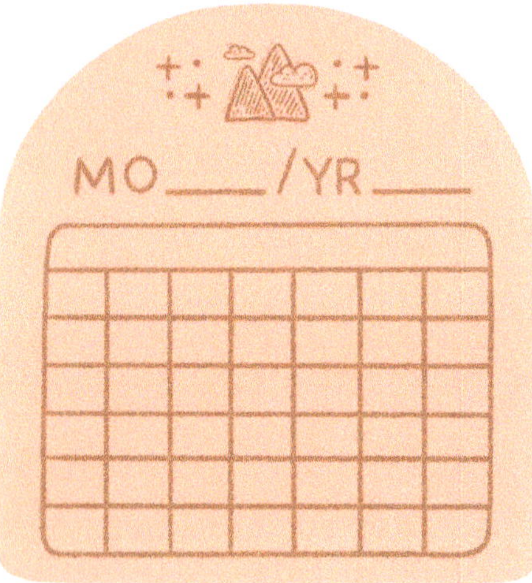
MO ____ /YR ____

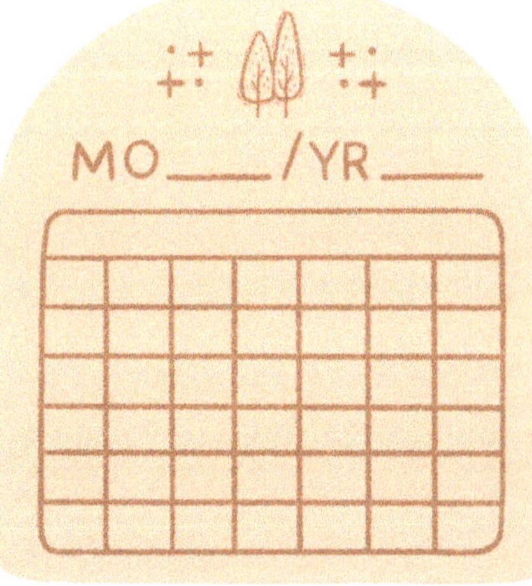
MO ____ /YR ____

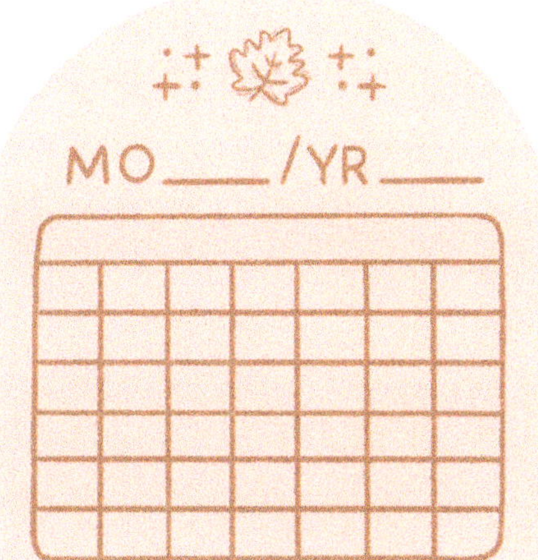

MO____/YR____

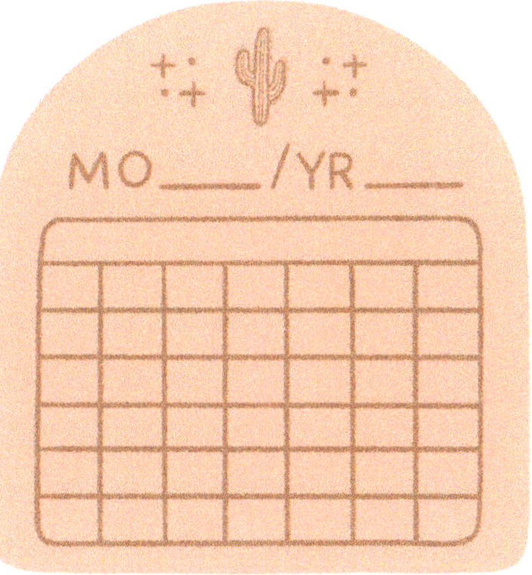

MO____/YR____

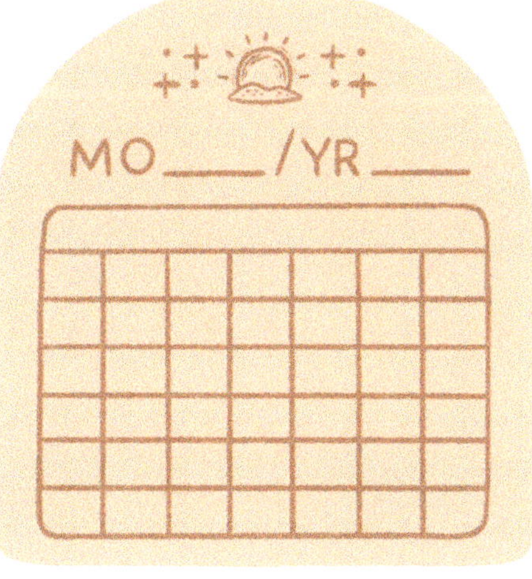

MO____/YR____

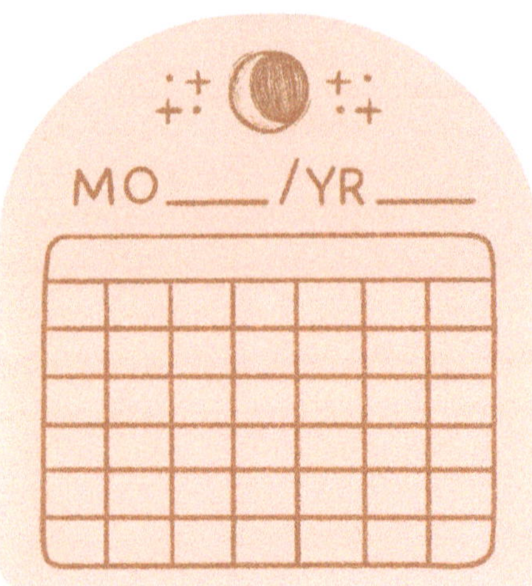

MO____/YR____

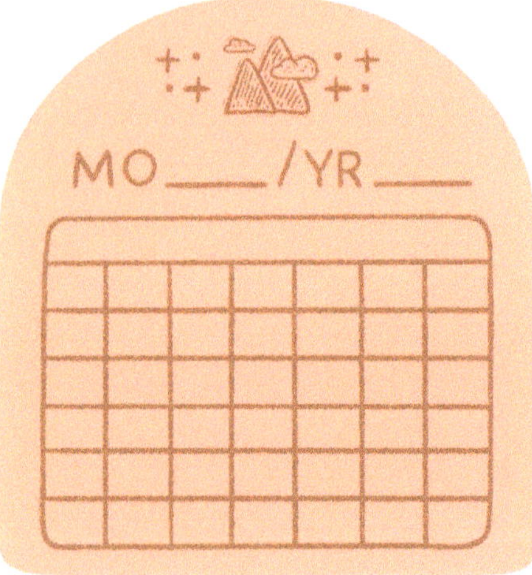

MO____/YR____

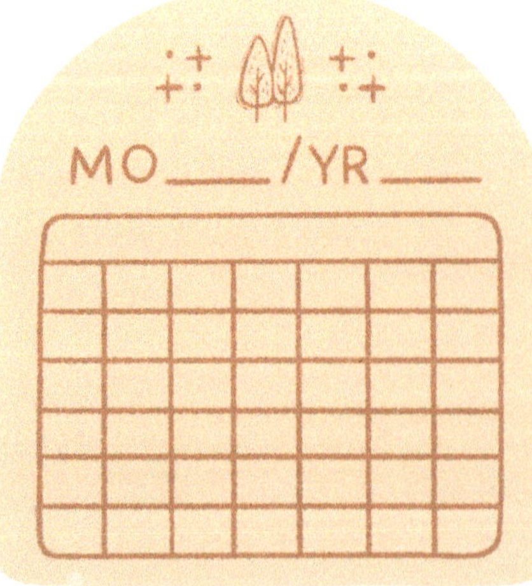

MO____/YR____

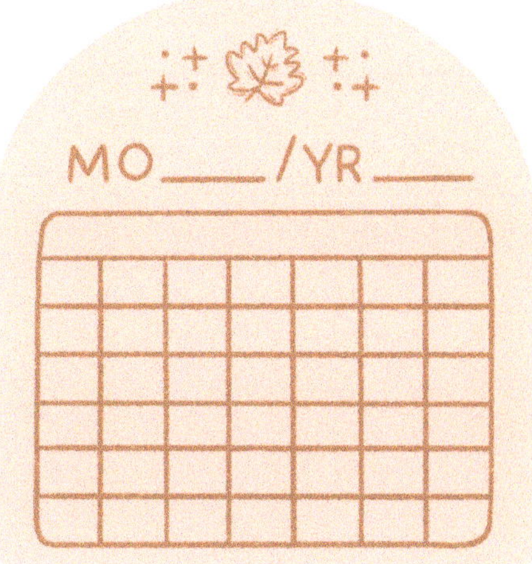

MO____/YR____

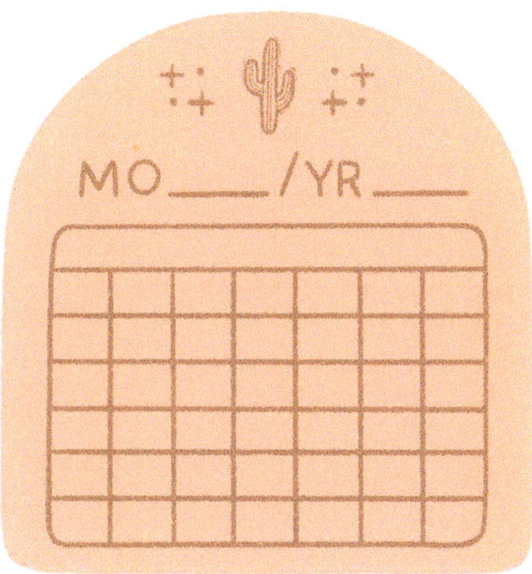

MO____/YR____

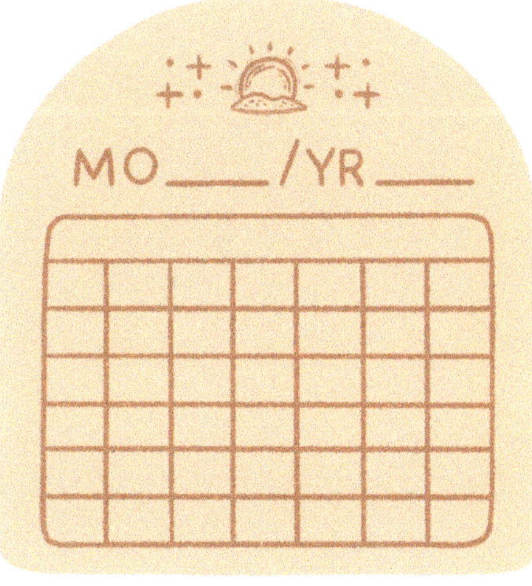

MO____/YR____

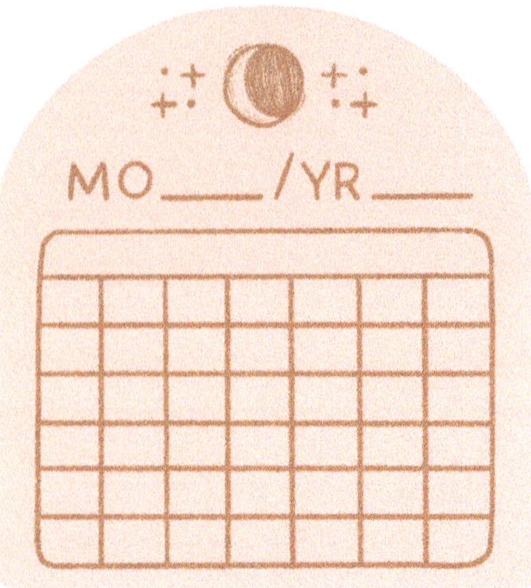
MO____/YR____

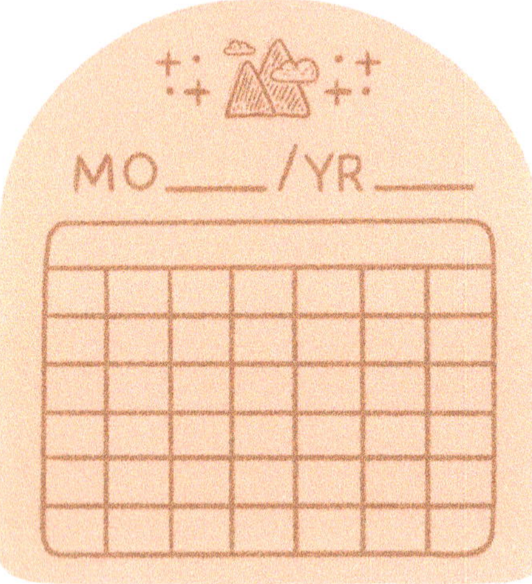
MO____/YR____

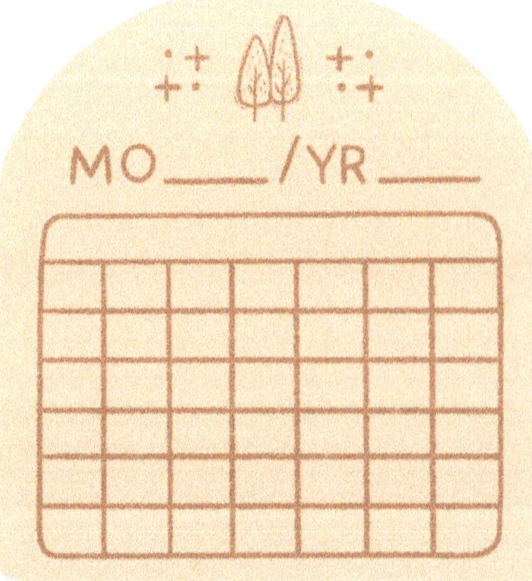
MO____/YR____

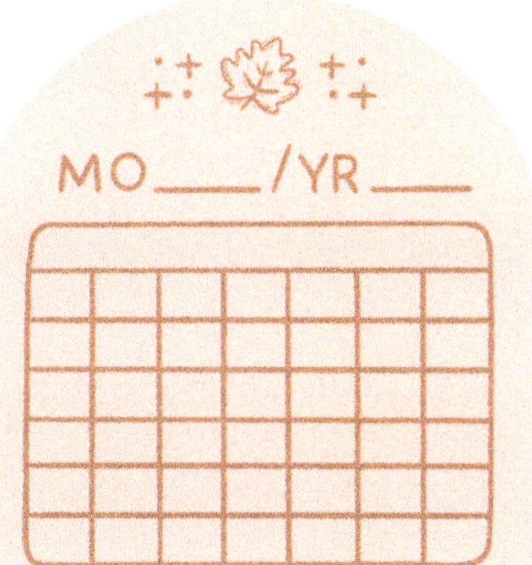
MO_____/YR_____

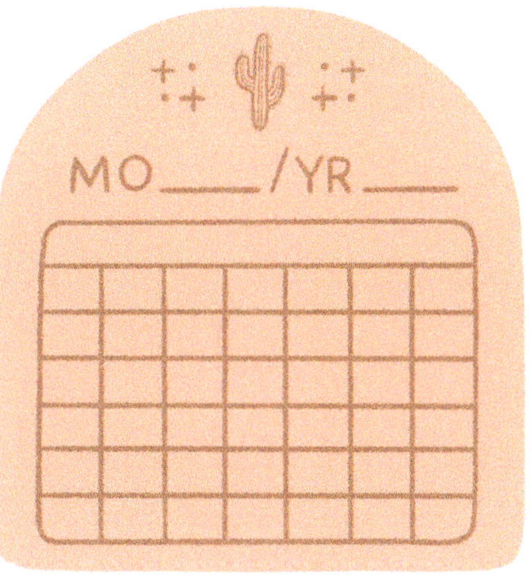
MO_____/YR_____

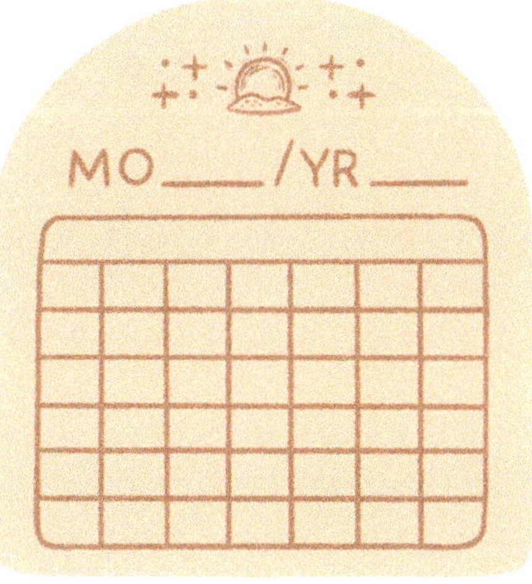
MO_____/YR_____

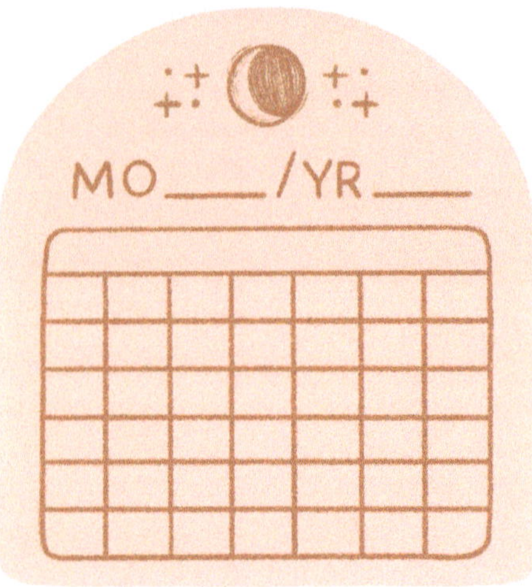
MO____/YR____

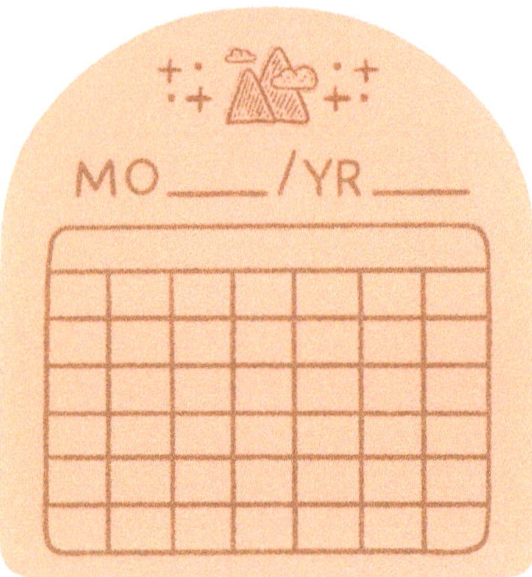
MO____/YR____

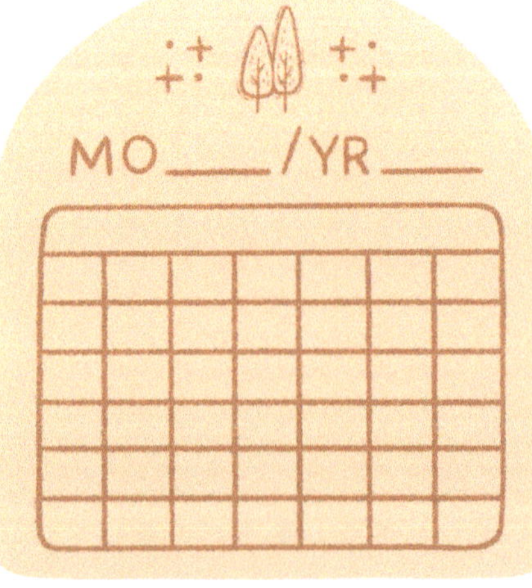
MO____/YR____

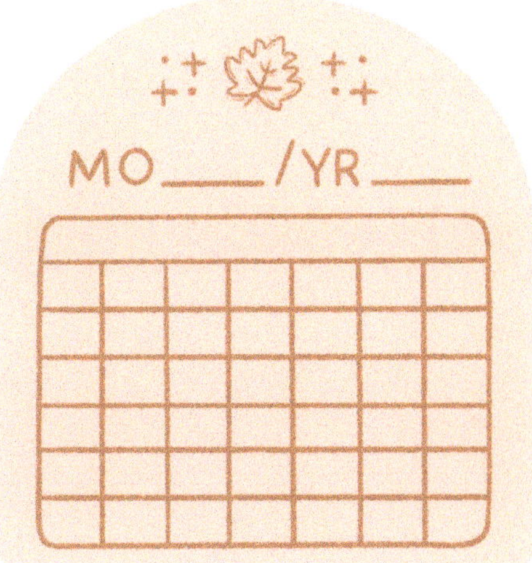
MO____/YR____

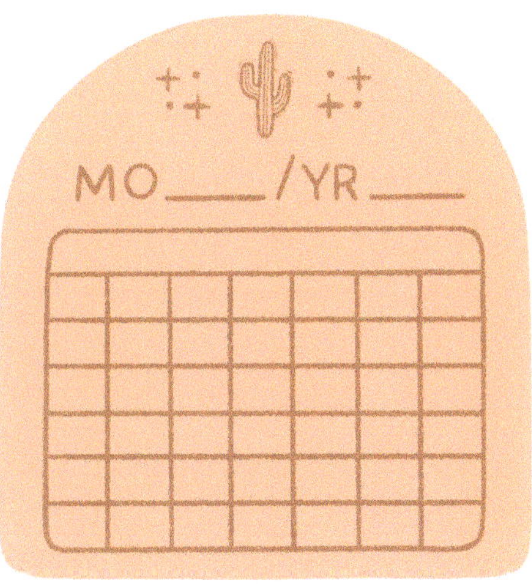
MO____/YR____

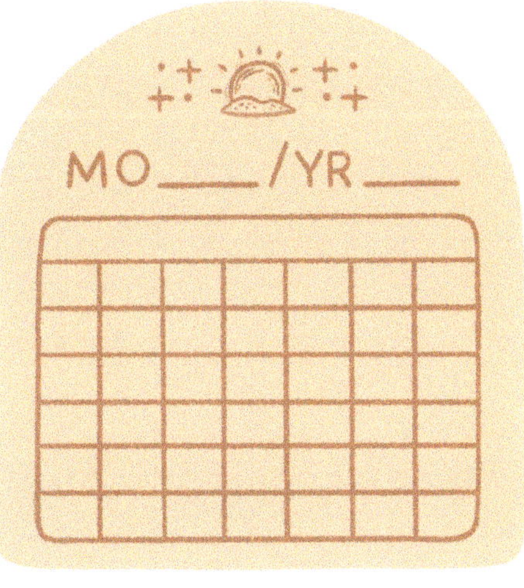
MO____/YR____

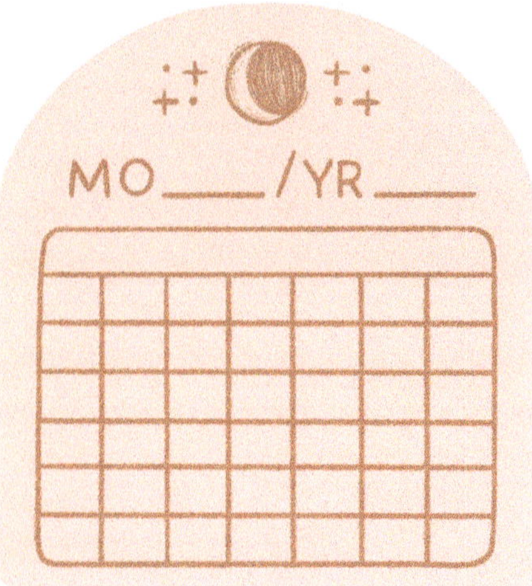

MO____/YR____

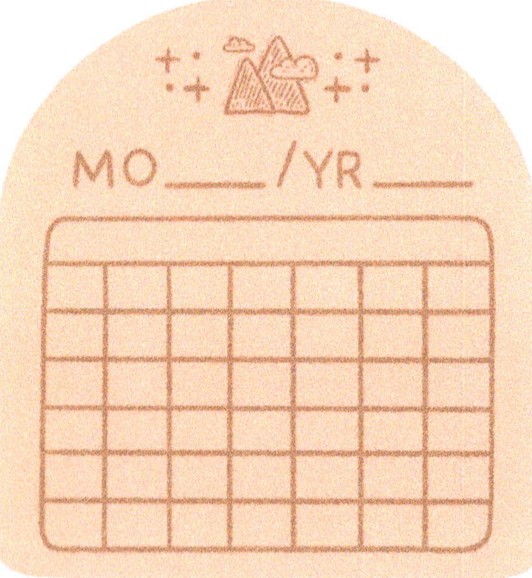

MO____/YR____

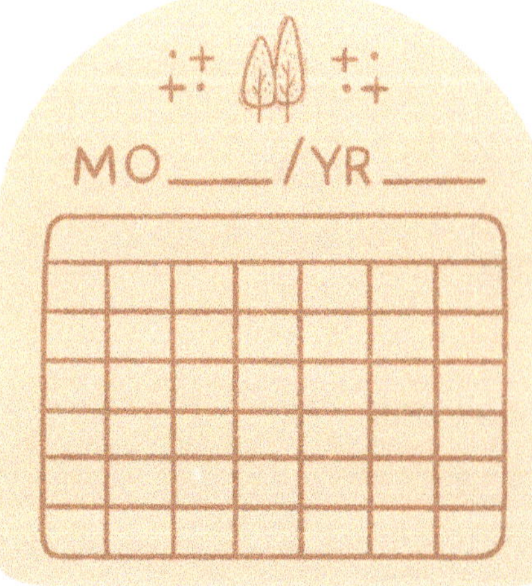

MO____/YR____

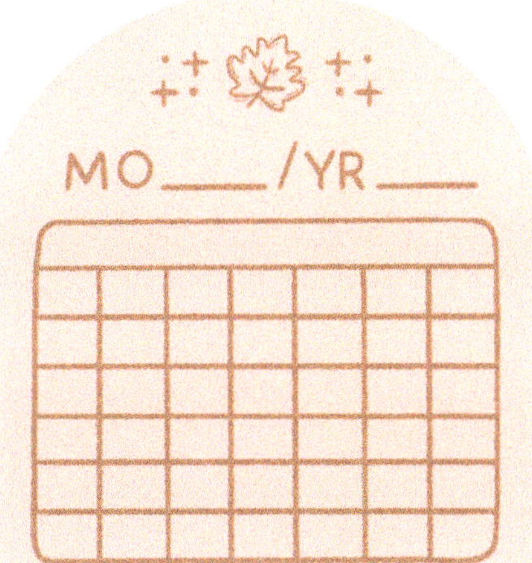
MO____ /YR____
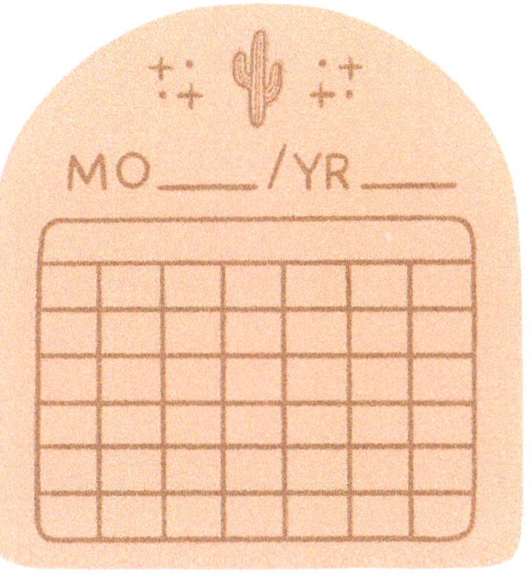
MO____ /YR____
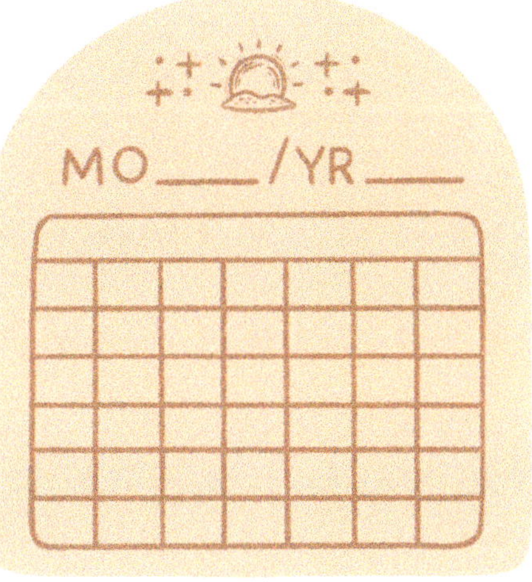
MO____ /YR____

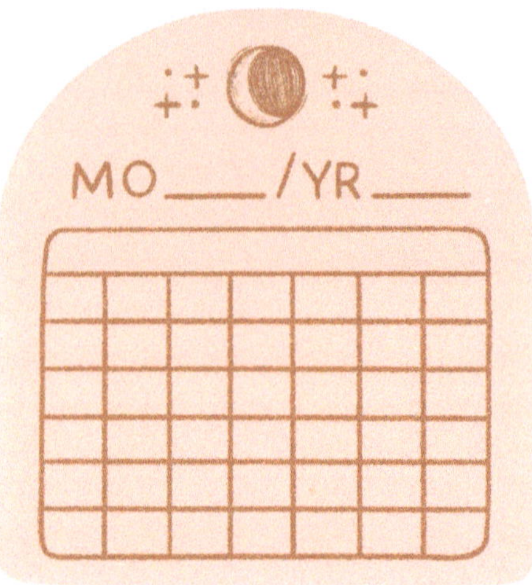

MO____/YR____

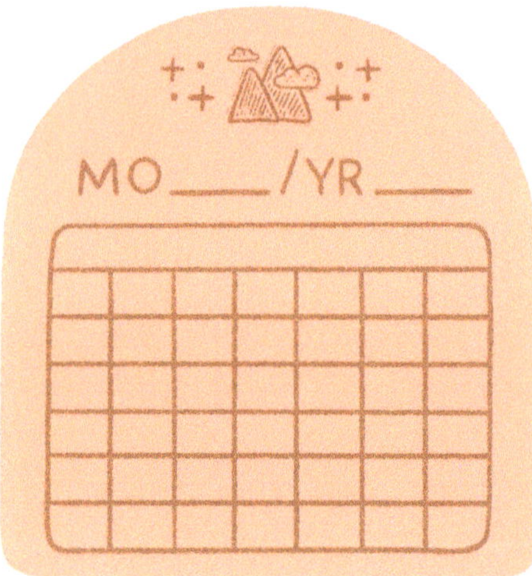

MO____/YR____

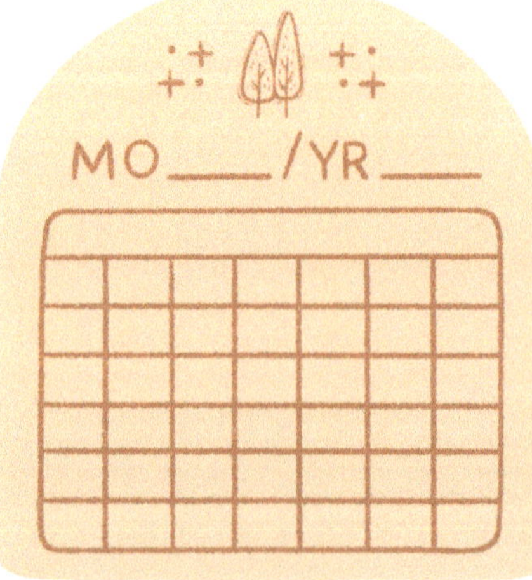

MO____/YR____

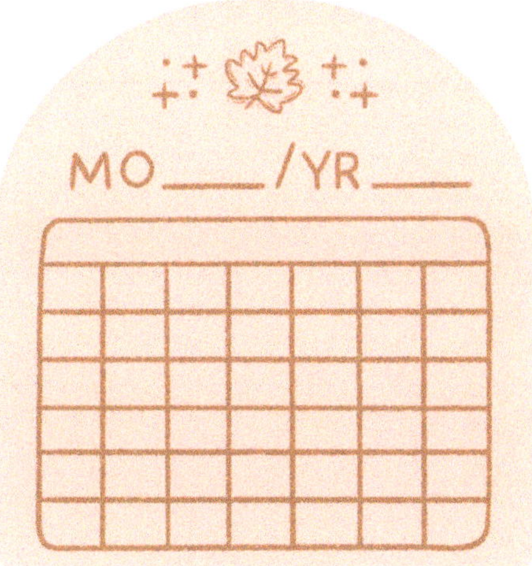
MO____/YR____

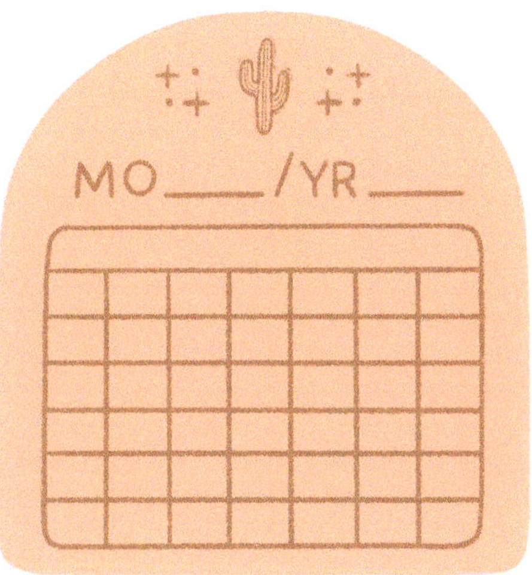
MO____/YR____

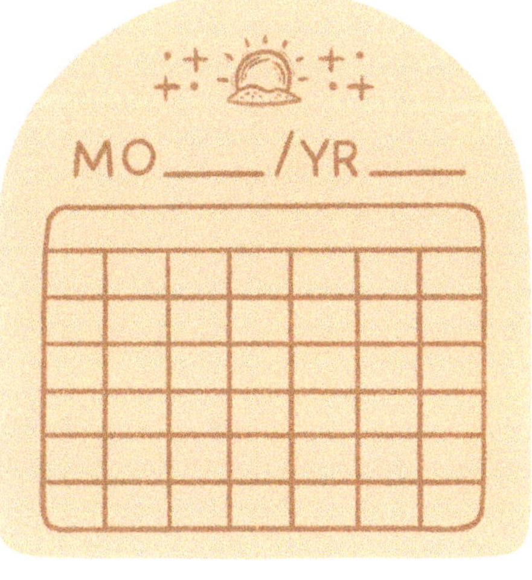
MO____/YR____

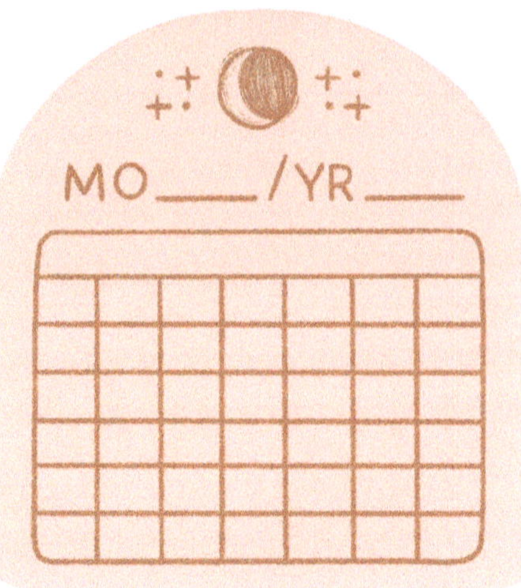
MO_____/YR_____

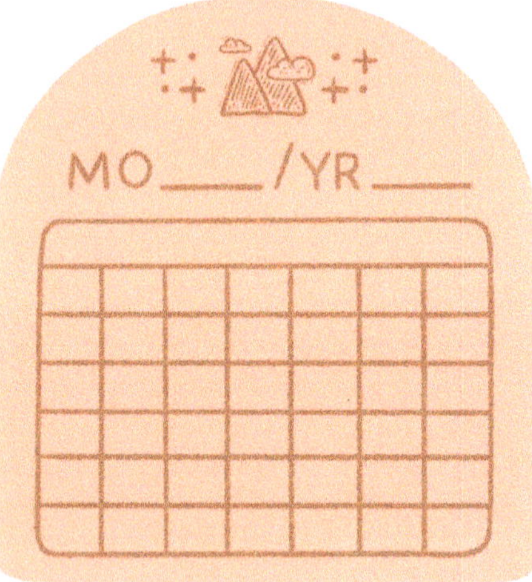
MO_____/YR_____

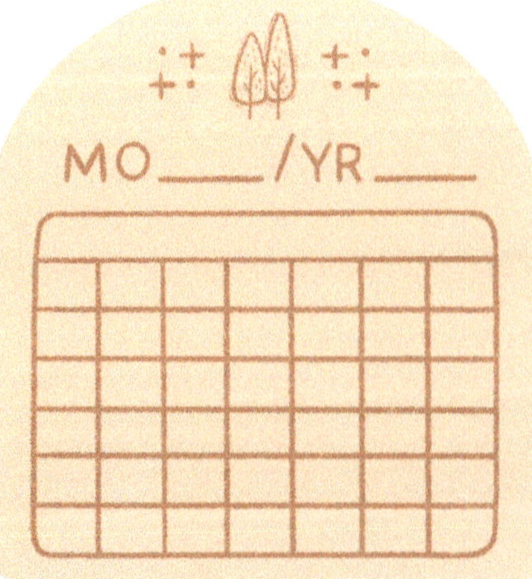
MO_____/YR_____

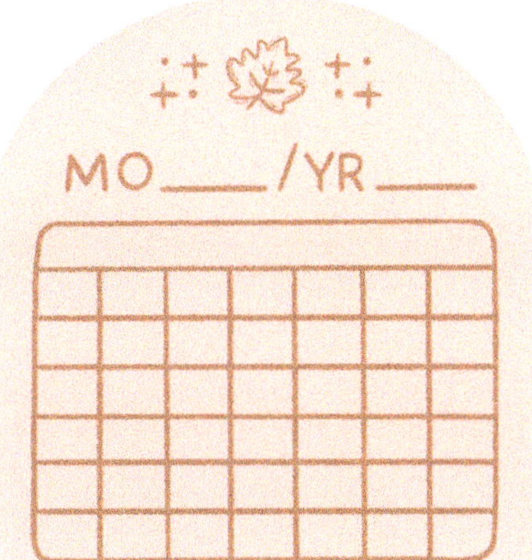

MO____/YR____

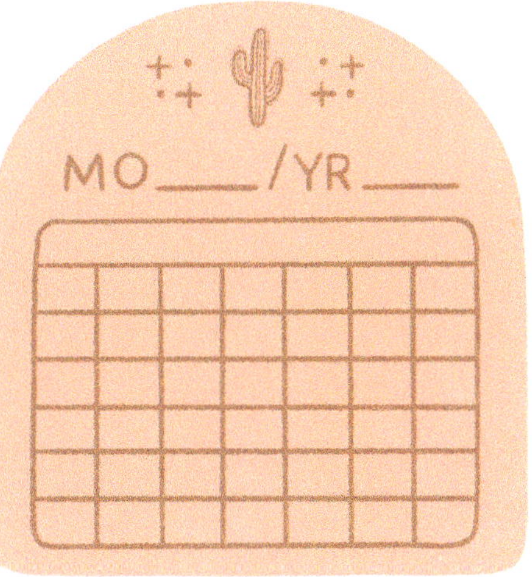

MO____/YR____

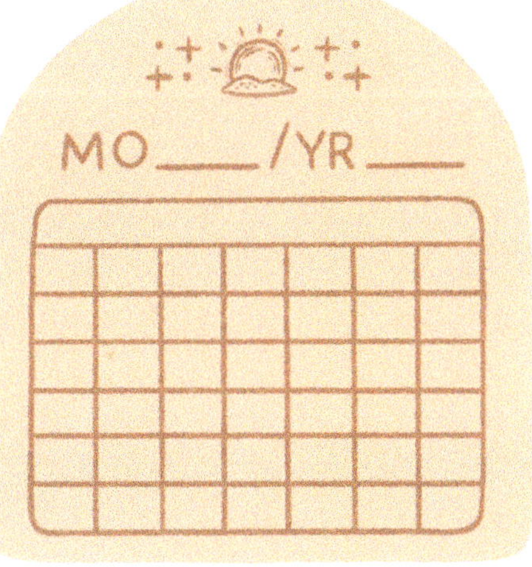

MO____/YR____

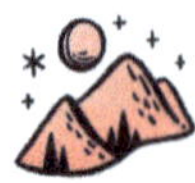

AFTERWORD: MOVING MOUNTAINS FOR DIGNITY

It is estimated that half a billion girls and women globally have no access to feminine care products or support, often resulting in their being excluded from basic education or work opportunities. These consequences starve their extraordinary potential and ultimately have devastating systemic socioeconomic effects on their families and communities. Period poverty is found not only in developing countries, but also among low-income women and girls in industrialized nations, and predominantly affects women of color, and low-income and immigrant communities. Additionally, older women living in poverty or on fixed incomes often cannot address their own needs for feminine hygiene products.

There are countless extraordinary large, small, and grassroots efforts globally — organizations, advocacy groups, legislative bills, and policy changes, primarily led by women, adolescent girls, and other menstruators — for menstrual equity and to make feminine care products affordable and accessible so that no one has to choose between purchasing food or other essentials and feminine care products. Women and girls cannot continue to bear this weight. We must have our fundamental needs met so that we can focus on the business of living our lives, learning, strengthening our communities, supporting our families, and living up to our unique potential in this world. Our human dignity must be a priority.

Twelve Moons is rooted in my heartfelt wishes for the health and nurturing of all humans. I am deeply committed to the higher purpose of meaningfully supporting communities experiencing tremendous need. A portion of the proceeds of this book will go to the Women's Refugee Commission, and the United Nations Population Fund, for dignity kits for girls and women in humanitarian crises.

RESOURCES

There is an extraordinary amount of information available written by medical doctors and other professionals and advocates to support our understanding of menstruation and menopause, and women's health in general. I have gathered supportive resources for girls and women, as well as helpful information for boys, men, and LGBTQIA+ communities. This is not an exhaustive list and there are many wonderful resources out there, but the resources provided are reputable and have been well-researched.

Because the literature and resources are growing each year, I have chosen to include and update them on the Twelve Moons website instead of in this book. Please visit twelve-moons.com for recommended reading and resources, including online tools and articles. The resource categories on the Twelve Moons website cover the following topics:

- General Health and Wellness
- Women's Health
- Menstruation
- Menopause
- Breast Health
- Aging
- Well-Being and Self-Care
- Women of Color
- LGBTQIA+ Menstruation and Menopause
- Neurodiversity
- Disability
- Reclaiming the Narrative about Menstruation and Menopause
- Growing and Adolescent Girls
- Fiction Addressing Menstruation for Growing and Adolescent Girls
- Growing and Adolescent Boys
- Parents and Caregivers of Adolescents
- Fathers and Fatherhood
- Childfree Adulthood
- Period Poverty and Menstrual Equity
- Sustainability

ACKNOWLEDGMENTS

I am so grateful to the lovely artist and kindred spirit Rhianna Wurman, with whom it has been an utter joy to spend months conceptualizing the beautiful cover art and illustrations for this book. Rhi, thank you for bringing to life my visions and love for *Twelve Moons*. My thanks also go to editor Marly Cornell, for her excellent and insightful support. I have immense gratitude for Irene Hellwig Lange, for her design expertise in the formatting of this book.

Tremendous thanks go to my dear family members and friends, who provided advice to me since I began the journey of writing and publishing *Twelve Moons*; your time and wisdom have been invaluable and so appreciated. A great many of you read through and edited several drafts of this book, and your caring and discerning contributions were like gold dust for me along the way.

Finally, I want to thank my beloved mother for her wisdom, untiring encouragement, and the beautiful conversations we shared over the course of this creative journey. Your loving heart in turn gave me mine. And to my truly wonderful husband and my endlessly adored children, thank you for your steadfast belief in me and my creation of this book, for your patience as my laptop became my constant companion, and most of all, thank you for the cocoon of love that I take shelter in. You are my everything.

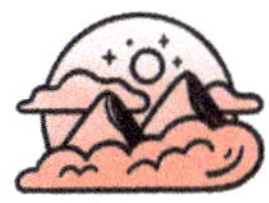

ABOUT THE AUTHOR

Jenny R. Austin is a writer, editor, and longtime advocate of children and families affected by armed conflict and displacement, family reunification, and child and maternal health and well-being. She has worked for nonprofits, philanthropies, humanitarian NGOs, United Nations agencies, as well as a couple of special independent bookshops. Jenny has written and edited many publications for nonprofit and humanitarian organizations such as UNICEF, including global field manuals for livelihoods and economic recovery in crisis and humanitarian settings for the United Nations Development Programme and the Women's Refugee Commission.

Her family and friends are her whole world, and she loves hiking, reading, baking, eating tacos, traveling, and being in nature. A graduate of the University of California, Santa Cruz, Jenny holds master's degrees from New York University and the University of Oxford on the topics of refugee studies, and family reunification and cultural memory in the context of diaspora. Born and raised in the United States, Jenny lives with her husband and children in Switzerland.

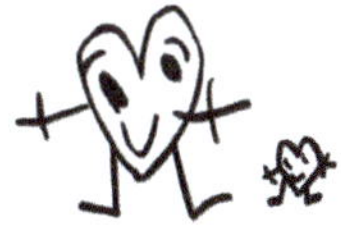

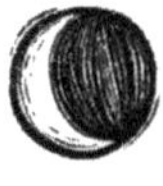